Gluten Related Disorders: People Shall not Live on Bread Alone

Special Issue Editors

Carlo Catassi
Alessio Fasano

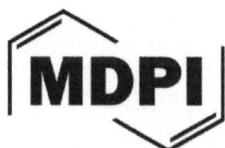

MDPI

Special Issue Editors

Carlo Catassi
Head, Department of Pediatrics
Università Politecnica delle Marche
Ancona, Italy

Alessio Fasano
Chief, Division of Pediatric
Gastroenterology and Nutrition
MassGeneral Hospital for Children
Boston, USA

Editorial Office
MDPI AG
St. Alban-Anlage 66
Basel, Switzerland

This edition is a reprint of the Special Issue published online in the open access journal *Nutrients* (ISSN 2072-6643) from 2015–2016 (available at: http://www.mdpi.com/journal/nutrients/special_issues/gluten-related-disorders).

For citation purposes, cite each article independently as indicated on the article page online and as indicated below:

Author 1; Author 2; Author 3 etc. Article title. *Journal Name*. **Year**. Article number/page range.

ISBN 978-3-03842-356-0 (Pbk)
ISBN 978-3-03842-357-7 (PDF)

Table of Contents

Section 1: Epidemiology and Pathophysiology

Section 2: Clinical Aspects

Section 3: Treatment and Follow-Up

Section 4: Experts' Guidelines

About the Guest Editors

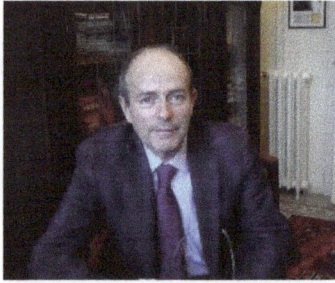

Carlo Catassi is the Head of the Department of Pediatrics at the Marche Politechnic University, Ancona Italy and Visiting Scientist at the Massachusetts General Hospital, Boston USA. During the last 20 years, he has collaborated academically and scientifically with the Center for Celiac Research originally in Baltimore and now in Boston. He is one of the world experts on celiac disease and other gluten-related disorders. His major areas of scientific interest are the epidemiology and clinical spectrum of celiac disease and non-celiac gluten sensitivity. With his research group, he performed the first population screening for celiac disease, introducing the concept of the celiac iceberg, a finding that has been replicated by hundreds of studies around the world. He is the author of more than 160 publications on peer reviewed journals cited in PubMed.

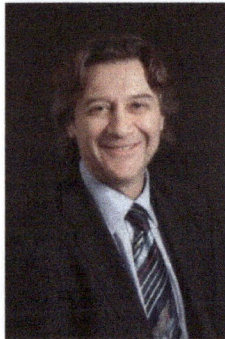

Alessio Fasano, MD, is the W. Allan Walker Chair of Pediatric Gastroenterology and Nutrition and Chief of the Division of Pediatric Gastroenterology and Nutrition at MassGeneral Hospital *for* Children (MGH*f*C). His visionary research, which established the rate of celiac disease at one in 133 people, led to the awareness of celiac disease as a growing public health problem in the United States. Dr. Fasano is also Director of the Mucosal Immunology and Biology Research Center (MIBRC) at MGH*f*C. In 2000, he and his team discovered the protein zonulin, opening up the door to a new way of looking at the function of intestinal permeability, not only as it affects the gut, but also what role it plays in both inflammation and autoimmunity throughout the body. Current research directed by Dr. Fasano encompasses both basic science focused on bacterial pathogenesis, the gut microbiome and intestinal mucosal biology, as well as translational science focused on interventional clinical trials in autoimmune and inflammatory diseases. He has published more than 270 peer-reviewed papers and has been funded from the NIH since 1995.

Preface to "Gluten Related Disorders: People Shall not Live on Bread Alone"

To the tempter that came to Him and said, "If You are the Son of God, tell these stones to become bread". Jesus replied "It is written: man shall not live on bread alone ..." (Matthew 4:4). Nowadays, many people, particularly in the Western world, have gone well beyond that holy recommendation. In a 2014 US Consumer Reports survey, 63% of participants said they felt that avoiding bread and other gluten-containing food would improve their physical or mental health. Moreover, in a 2015 Gallup Poll, 21% of Americans reported that they tried to include gluten-free foods in their diet. The "fall" of gluten might be related to the increased awareness of gluten-related disorders and the recent surge of prevalence of celiac disease (CD) and non-celiac gluten sensitivity (NCGS). This trend could still be on the rise, particularly in areas of the world undergoing a progressive "Westernization" of the diet, as suggested here by Peña and coworkers who note that the diet of people living in Central America is shifting from a maize- to a wheat based diet. Not surprisingly, in Mexico, Ontiveros et al. report that 3.7% of people purposely adhere to a gluten-free diet (GFD). Many of these individuals could be affected by NCGS; however, the frequency of this condition is difficult to ascertain due to the lack of a biomarker. This is the reason why a group of experts of gluten-related disorders recently met in Salerno to standardize the NCGS diagnostic criteria.

Despite the previously mentioned diagnostic uncertainties, well-designed studies suggest that NCGS is not only common but also more clinically variable than originally reported. In this book, three original articles add important pieces of information: (a) many patients diagnosed as having irritable bowel syndrome are clearly gluten-sensitive, and their symptoms could be adequately controlled with a gluten-free diet only; (b) "skin NCGS" is described for the first time by Bonciolini and coworkers, in non-CD subjects with skin lesions similar both to eczema and psoriasis showing itching, the presence of C3 at the dermoepidermal junction, and a rapid resolution of lesions when adopting the GFD; (c) the description of "gluten psychosis" in a pre-pubertal child presenting with a severe hallucinatory manifestation that was clearly related to the ingestion of gluten-containing food, and showing complete resolution of symptoms after starting treatment with the GFD.

Why and how gluten proteins can trigger an abnormal response ending up with clinical symptoms, particularly at the brain level, is still poorly understood, but it is likely that mechanism/s other than the adaptive, HLA-related immune response observed in CD patients, may be involved. There is currently a special interest in the effect of gluten on the so-called gut–brain axis with two not mutually exclusive theories, both starting with an increased absorption of undigested gluten peptides. Once these peptides reach the lamina propria, they may get into circulation, cross the blood–brain barrier, and ultimately interact with the opioid brain receptor, thus affecting the individual's behavior, attention and social interaction. Alternatively, these gluten peptides may cause the activation of immune cells that leave the gut mucosa, and migrate to the brain where they cause neuroinflammation leading to behavioral changes. Although these sequences of events remain to be proven, new pieces of the puzzle are becoming available. In this book, Hollon and coworkers show that gliadin exposure induces an increase in intestinal permeability in all individuals, regardless of whether or not they have CD. The results of this study suggest that gluten exposure leads to altered barrier function in both CD and NCGS, resulting in an exaggerated increase in intestinal permeability.

The quoted works are just a sample of the high-quality papers published here. As Editors of now three Special Issues on Gluten-Related Disorders, in the years 2013, 2015 and 2016 respectively, we are grateful to the *Nutrients* Editors in Chief for giving so much visibility to our scientific community and to the *Nutrients* Editorial Staff for their professionalism in handling the manuscripts. Now, the question is: would the "modern tempter" ask Jesus to transform some of the stones into gluten-free instead of regular bread? This is just a matter of speculation. From our modest point of view, we can only applaud this increasing interest in gluten-related disorders, i.e., an array of conditions affecting a growing proportion of the general population.

Carlo Catassi and Alessio Fasano
Guest Editors

Section 1:
Epidemiology and Pathophysiology

nutrients

MDPI

Review

Central America in Transition: From Maize to Wheat Challenges and Opportunities

Amado Salvador Peña * and Jakob Bart Arie Crusius

Laboratory of Immunogenetics, VU University Medical Center, Department of Medical Microbiology and Infection Control, P.O. Box 7057, 1007 MB Amsterdam, The Netherlands
* Correspondence: pena.as@gmail.com; Tel.: +31-7133-16060

Received: 15 June 2015; Accepted: 11 August 2015; Published: 26 August 2015

Abstract: The Central American countries: Guatemala, El Salvador, Honduras, Nicaragua, Costa Rica, and Panama are in transition from a dietary culture based mainly on maize to a wheat-containing diet. Several other changes are occurring, such as a decrease of parasitic and infectious diseases. The environmental changes permit a prediction of an increase of celiac disease and other autoimmune diseases such as type I diabetes and thyroid disease in these genetically heterogeneous countries. At present, celiac disease and gluten-related disorders are considered to be of no relevance at the level of public health in these nations. This review documents the presence of celiac disease in Central America. It draws attention to some of the challenges in planning systematic studies in the region since up until recently celiac disease was unknown. The aim of this review is to disseminate knowledge obtained with preliminary data, to stimulate clinical and basic scientists to study these diseases in Central America and to alert authorities responsible for the planning of education and health, to find possibilities to avoid a rise in these disorders before the epidemics start, as has occurred in the Mediterranean countries.

Keywords: celiac disease; prevalence; HLA-DQ; serological tests; anti-Endomysium antibodies; tissue transglutaminase antibodies; hygiene hypothesis; old-friend hypothesis; Central America

1. Introduction

Central America is the geographic region in the Americas between the subcontinents North and South America, to the north bordered by Mexico, to the southeast by Colombia, to the east by the Caribbean Sea and the Pacific Ocean to the west. It consists of seven countries: Belize, Guatemala, El Salvador, Honduras, Nicaragua, Costa Rica, and Panama. In this review, Belize has not been taken into consideration.

In Central America celiac disease and gluten-related disorders are not well known. Until recently only few confirmed celiac disease cases have been described. The majority of patients are adults diagnosed in national public health institutions. Some patients have been diagnosed in private clinics in Central America countries, Mexico or in the U.S.A. The tests used for diagnosis have been specific serological markers and intestinal biopsy through upper gastrointestinal endoscopy. According to recent available literature in only a small series of patients determination of the human leukocyte antigen (HLA)-based genetic susceptibility to celiac disease took place in El Salvador [1] and Costa Rica [2].

The staple food of Central American countries, since the pre-Columbian era consisted of maize, "plátanos maduros" (plantain) and cassava (called "yuca" in this region) together with beans and rice. Therefore, this diet was intrinsically gluten-free without possible gluten cross-contamination. Probably the commercial influence on consumer patterns in these countries, gluten-containing food is increasingly used. Environmental changes in the consumption culture are bound to have an effect on the composition of the intestinal flora. This tendency has been developing for decades, particularly after 1980. Gluten-containing products provided by welfare services or humanitarian organizations are now reaching rural areas.

At present tentative generalizations about the prevalence of celiac disease in these countries are risky, taking into account the high number of variables acting in Central America. Properly designed epidemiologic and genetic studies are necessary. The prevalence of celiac disease and gluten-related disorders may vary among these countries, even within one country the prevalence may vary by region.

2. Genetic and Culture Heterogeneity Are Present in the Six Central American Countries

According to a study published in Nature [3] of 52 Native American and 17 Siberian groups genotyped at 364,470 single nucleotide polymorphisms, the Native Americans descend from at least three streams of Asian gene flow. The majority descends from a single ancestral population, the "First Americans". This initial population was followed by a southward expansion along the west coast, with subsequent divisions but with little change in the gene flow after the divergence. The Chibchas known as Muisca people are according to these authors an important exception on both sides of the Panama isthmus, since they possess ancestors from both North and South America. Much later, in the 15th and 16th century the European colonizers introduce a very diverse genetic inheritance, product of the complex history of their continent of origin. Large groups of slaves imported from Africa came primarily to the Atlantic coast of Central America, although there is evidence that some also migrated to the pacific side such as El Salvador. This history emphasizes the genetic diversity without considering the migration of the post-colonial period For example, in the highlands of Guatemala the ethnic composition of the population is markedly different from that of the larger cities. This is due to the fact that colonial cities tended to act as administrative centers, so that European-descended people would gather there, relegating the original inhabitants to rural areas [4].

3. Difficulties in Diagnosis and Challenges for the Future

No epidemiological studies on celiac disease have been performed in any of the Central American countries. Some series of patients with celiac disease have been described. Their diagnosis was based on the determination in blood of specific serological tests, like the detection of IgA anti-gliadin (AGA), IgA anti-tissue transglutaminase (tTG) and/or IgA anti-Endomysium antibodies (EmA). In general the most important genetic markers of susceptibility, the HLA class-II antigens: HLA-DQ2.5 and/or HLA-DQ8 have not been taken into account. The histological findings of the duodenal biopsy specimens, based on the presence of villous atrophy and more recent on increased intraepithelial lymphocytes without villous atrophy and the response to a gluten-free diet have been taken into account to confirm the diagnosis. From the clinical point of view the inability to detect Marsh I celiac patients by specific serological tests among populations with low gluten consumption such as the rural populations of these countries is difficult. Although tropical sprue is often referred to as endemic in Central America there are no publications that suggest that it may be present. In the literature most of the patients with tropical sprue have been reported in Porto Rico, the Dominican Republic and other islands in the Caribbean [5].

In spite of the need of upper gastrointestinal endoscopy, limited availability, technical failures, lack of orientation and/or the sampling of insufficient biopsies, the "gold standard" for the diagnosis of celiac disease continues to be the small intestinal biopsy [3] in these countries. Also few pathologists appear to be interested in the proper assessment of the specimens. During endoscopy, multiple biopsies in the duodenal bulb and at least 4 in the distal duodenum should be taken. In a multicenter study carried out in children, it was confirmed that in 2.4% of 665 patients, the lesions were virtually limited to the duodenal bulb. The majority of the studies published so far do not comply with the protocol suggested by Bonamico *et al.* [6]. No data is available in Central America.

4. Results

Preliminary studies of celiac disease in Central America:

4.1. Guatemala

In Guatemala, a master thesis written by a nutritionist [7] determined the number of patients suffering from celiac disease in private clinics in gastroenterology of the capital city of Guatemala in order to develop a manual of nutritional guidance to the Guatemalan celiac patient. The results showed one case of celiac disease for every 1000 adult patients. The most frequent age of patients diagnosed was from 31 to 50 years of age, 59% were female. The "Asociación de Celíacos de Guatemala ("Celiac Patients' Association of Guatemala") was founded in Guatemala city in 2013 by Dr. E. Ligorría, who is deeply involved in the study of celiac disease and the treatment of local celiac patients. No data has been published yet. It is to be hoped that he will be able to organize systematic studies not only among the mestizos (people of mixed Native and European heritage) population but also among the indigenous Mayan descent population of Petén, the northernmost department of Guatemala. This population would be important to study the distribution of HLA antigens and the effects of the ongoing dietary transition from maize to gluten-containing products.

4.2. El Salvador

The first study using the modified Marsh classification and the full HLA-DQ typing in El Salvador has been recently published [1]. Based on serological tests, histological features of duodenal biopsy specimens and the response to a gluten-free diet, 32 individuals (23 females and 9 males) were diagnosed with celiac disease. The age at diagnosis ranges from 19 to 77 years. All patients are urban residents. Upon revision of the biopsy specimens and classification of the histological features, 28 showed the histological features that are compatible with celiac disease [6]. Twenty-three have celiac disease risk genotype: 14 HLA-DQ8 (DQA1*03/DQB1*0302; 12F and 2M), 7 HLA-DQ2.5 (DQA1*05/DQB1*02; 3F and 4M), 2 HLA-DQ2.5 and DQ8 (1F, 1M), and 9 cases (7F, 2M) who had neither DQ2.5 nor DQ8. All nine non-DQ2.5/non-DQ8 cases reported an improvement of symptoms with a gluten-free diet; two had been diagnosed abroad. Seven out of nine non-DQ2.5/non-DQ8 celiac disease patients were heterozygous carriers of allele DQA1*05 only and one had HLA-DQ2.2 (DQA1*0201/DQB1*02). One patient did not possess an HLA-DQ genotype associated with celiac disease. Another patient had also dermatitis herpetiformis.

Ethnic admixture is characteristic of El Salvador. In the ethnic categories identified in colonial times, the predominance of mestizos is important in El Salvador. Several factors influenced this outcome: (a) in El Salvador's current territory there was no place where indigenous peoples could find refuge, so that they and the Spaniards had to coexist in the same space; (b) the decrease in the indigenous population due to diseases and massacres; (c) population break up due to its exploitation for the cultivation of indigo in the 18th and 19th centuries. In El Salvador the "Asociación de Celíacos y Sensibles al Gluten de El Salvador" (ACELYSES) ("Celiac and Gluten Sensitive Association in El Salvador") is playing a predominant role in dissemination of knowledge. The primary mission is the dissemination of information on gluten-related disorders as well as promoting education and awareness among celiac disease and gluten-sensitive people, their families, public and private health institutions and other organizations which have an impact on the quality of life of celiac and gluten-sensitive people in El Salvador.

4.3. Honduras

Only isolated cases of celiac disease have been reported in Honduras. There is no celiac or gluten sensitive patient association in this country yet but the few celiacs are stimulating knowledge among the general practitioners, specialists in gastroenterology and internal medicine. They collaborate with other Celiac Associations in bordering countries.

4.4. Nicaragua

In Nicaragua, few cases are known. Possibly, this is due to the lack of knowledge of the disease. In the department of Managua (the capital of the country), the Faculty of Medical Sciences of the National Autonomous University of Nicaragua (UNAN-Managua) has conducted a study among students and faculty members. The knowledge that the respondents had about celiac disease was minimal. The teaching faculty had a higher percentage of those who knew about the disease and its clinical presentation. More surprisingly, 55.2% of faculty members involved in this study did not know about celiac disease [8].

4.5. Costa Rica

Preliminary results of 258 patients (108 male and 150 female) with celiac disease in Costa Rica with lymphocytic duodenitis and villous atrophy have been published. Mean age was 48.3 years, ranging between 16 and 90 years. Thirty-six patients were typed for the HLA-DQ2.5 and HLA-DQ8 alleles; 11 cases were positive for HLA-DQ2.5, 7 for HLA-DQ8, and 3 for both HLA-DQ2.5 and HLA-DQ8. Interestingly 15 of the 36 patients turned out to be negative, and had lymphocytic duodenitis. Further follow-up of these patients is needed since the differential diagnosis for lymphocytic duodenitis is extensive and several known causes have not yet been excluded [2].

Allele group and haplotype frequencies of HLA genes in the Costa Rica Central Valley Population, the major population of Costa Rica, have recently been determined by means of molecular typing in a sample of 130 unrelated blood donors [9]. According to these investigators the frequencies observed are consistent with a profile of a dynamic and diverse population, with a hybrid ethnic origin, predominantly Caucasian-Amerindian. The results show that the people from Costa Rica genetically are close to the Mestizo urban population from Venezuela and from Guadalajara in Mexico [9].

In Costa Rica, the "Asociación Pro-Personas Celíacas" (APPCEL) ("Pro Celiac Persons' Association") founded in 2004, is actively engaged offering psychological support as well as useful information by means of an e-newsletter and has been involved in changing the country's laws so that celiac patients may have access to safe food and properly labeled products. The "Centro de Información sobre la Enfermedad Celíaca" (CIEC), "Celiac Disease Information Center" has its headquarters in San José, Costa Rica is promoting studies and provides guidance to patients with celiac disease. They coordinate with APPCEL.

4.6. Panamá

The "Fundación Celíacos de Panamá" (FUCEPA) ("Panama Celiac Patients' Foundation") is helping celiac patients and their families by means of the dissemination of information. A good coordination exists between pediatricians and gastroenterologists interested in celiac disease. No epidemiological studies or data on the number of patients have yet been published.

5. Discussion

In Central America, celiac disease is not considered to be relevant at the level of public health. However, understanding the epidemiology of this disease and gluten related disorders is crucial for hypothesizing about causes and quantifying the burden of disease [10]. It is well known that patients with celiac disease have a greater burden of disease than the general population because of the increase risk of osteoporosis, autoimmune diseases and malignancies. As far as we know there is only one study of epidemiology ongoing in Central America. This is in El Salvador, it covers the adult population.

The statement made 10 years ago by Green *et al.* is still valid today: "There is a need for screening studies of patients with conditions associated with celiac disease to determine whether the large numbers of people with undiagnosed celiac disease currently are seeking health care" [11]. Currently, there is a need to quantify the increase in wheat allergy, as part of the increase in allergic conditions. Also it is necessary to quantify the relevance of other gluten related disorders for the awakening of the officers of national health systems to assess the total burden of these diseases and to be prepared for the application of adequate funds.

In a recent review on the prevalence of celiac disease in Latin America [12], 72 studies were included. No publication included Central American countries. According to this review, the estimated prevalence of celiac disease in Latin Americans excluding Central America ranged between 0.46% and 0.64%. The prevalence in first-degree relatives of probands with celiac disease was 5.5%. The coexistence of celiac disease and type 1 diabetes mellitus varied from 4.6% to 8.7%, depending on the methods used for diagnosis (*i.e.*, autoantibodies and/or small intestinal biopsies). In the northern border of Central America the information published from Mexico is scarce. It seems however that in the adult Mexican Mestizo population the presence of celiac disease is relatively high [13]. A recent update [14] using the weighted prevalence for double-positive serology IgA tTG and IgA EmA the prevalence was 0.59% (95% confidence interval (CI), 0.27–1.29). A high prevalence of 5.9% biopsy-proven celiac disease was found in Mexican Mestizo patients with type 1 diabetes mellitus [15].

We wish to underscore the recommendation expressed by Gonzales Burchard *et al.*: "Precisely because of this complexity, *Latinos* present a unique opportunity to disentangle the clinical, social, environmental, and genetic underpinnings of population differences in health outcomes" [16].

Other observations made in Russia and Finland are relevant to understand the value of studying regions with different genetic and environmental heterogeneity. It has been found that two adjacent populations which are equally exposed to grain products and share the same ancestry but live in different socioeconomic environment such as, Russian Karelia and Finland, exhibit a different prevalence of celiac disease. The prevalence of transglutaminase antibodies and celiac disease is lower in Russian Karelia than in Finland. To explain the differences in prevalence, the authors of the study have suggested that there exists a protective environment characterized by inferior prosperity and standard of hygiene in Karelia [17]. They emphasized that: "*The lower prevalence of celiac disease in Russian Karelia seems not to be due to differences in genetic predisposition or to the consumption of grain products, but may be associated with a protective environment characterized by poorer living conditions and standard of hygiene*".

Central America is another region in the world where the "hygiene hypothesis" [18] may apply. The improvement in the infection rates and the deworming will be responsible for an increase in celiac disease, allergy and other autoimmune diseases similar to the differences observed in Russian Karelia and in Finland. In Central America one can imagine that one of the mechanisms to explain the raise of celiac disease and other autoimmune diseases is the "old friend hypothesis" whereby the eradication of the helminthes, common in these populations, alter the numbers of T regulatory cells complementing the shift from T helper 1 (Th1) to T helper 2 (Th2) response [19,20]. In order to strengthen the awareness of celiac disease in Central America it is necessary to raise funds following the initiative of the World Gastroenterology Organization and the Asian Pacific Association of Gastroenterology in 2014 to address key issues in emergence of celiac disease in Asia [21]. Antibiotic control and more attention to the original rich staple food of Central America are two important points that may be addressed.

6. Conclusions

This review has shown the preliminary data that exist in Central America. It has made clear the heterogeneity of the populations involved and the lack of knowledge that still exists in this region. It is important to know in the planning of genetic studies that methods for genotyping HLA-DQ may not be suitable to detect the genetic variants of people with different ancestry. Therefore, the results should be validated with local populations before drawing conclusions. The collaboration of clinicians, immunologists, geneticists, pathologists, nutritionists and epidemiologists is essential to integrate the necessary knowledge on the diagnoses of these diseases in Central America and in helping to implement measures to avoid the emergence of new cases. As Greco *et al.* have estimated: "*In the near future, the burden of celiac disease will increase tremendously. Few Mediterranean countries are able to face this expanding epidemic"* [22]. Only a multidisciplinary approach may prevent a similar situation in Central America.

Acknowledgments: We like to thank Mauricio Cromeyer (Hospital de Diagnóstico Escalón, Villavicencio Plaza, Paseo General Escalón, Colonia Escalón, San Salvador, El Salvador C.A.), Karla María Zaldívar, MBA, PMP, (San Salvador, El Salvador, C.A.), Carlos Beirute Lucke, Translator and Interpreter, Ministry of Foreign Relations and Amavilia Pérez Villavicencio Celiac Disease Expert, University of Sevilla, Spain. M. Sci, Marketing and Communication Science. Celiac Disease Information Center. San José, Costa Rica for the enthusiasm with which they dedicate themselves to the study of celiac disease and provided interesting data.

Author Contributions: A.S.P and J.B.A.C. wrote the manuscript to disseminate knowledge of this emerging disease in this part of the world.

Conflicts of Interest: The authors declare no conflict of interest.

References

1. Cromeyer, M.; Gutierrez, R.A.; Zaldivar, K.; Crusius, J.B.A.; Peña, A.S. Celiac disease in El Salvador. In *Celiac Disease and Non-Celiac Gluten Sensitivity*; Rodrigo, L., Peña, A.S., Eds.; Omnia Science: Barcelona, Spain, 2014; pp. 75–88.
2. Brenes-Pino, F.; Herrera, A. Small Intestine Biopsy and its Interpretation: Preliminary Results in Costa Rica. In *Celiac Disease and Non-Celiac Gluten Sensitivity*; Rodrigo, L., Peña, A.S., Eds.; Omnia Science: Barcelona, Spain, 2014; Volume 229, pp. 203–218.
3. Reich, D.; Patterson, N.; Campbell, D.; Tandon, A.; Mazieres, S.; Ray, N.; Parra, M.V.; Rojas, W.; Duque, C.; Mesa, N.; *et al.* Reconstructing Native American population history. *Nature* **2012**, *488*, 370–374. [CrossRef] [PubMed]
4. Perez Villavicencio, A.; Beirute Lucke, C.; Peña, A.S. Perspectives to take into account when studying celiac disease in China and Central America. In *Celiac Disease and Non-Celiac Gluten Sensitivity*; Rodrigo, L., Peña, A.S., Eds.; Omnia Science: Barcelona, Spain, 2014; pp. 61–64.
5. Batheja, M.J.; Leighton, J.; Azueta, A.; Heigh, R. The face of tropical sprue. *Case. Rep. Gastroenterol.* **2010**, *4*, 168–172. [CrossRef] [PubMed]
6. Bonamico, M.; Mariani, P.; Thanasi, E.; Ferri, M.; Nenna, R.; Tiberti, C.; Mora, B.; Mazzilli, M.C.; Magliocca, F.M. Patchy villous atrophy of the duodenum in childhood celiac disease. *J. Pediatr. Gastroenterol. Nutr.* **2004**, *38*, 204–207. [CrossRef] [PubMed]
7. Portillo Vargas, J.E. Elaboración de un Manual de Orientación Nutricional Para el Paciente con Enfermedad Celiaca en Guatemala. Master's Thesis, Universidad de San Carlos de Guatemala, Guatemala City, Guatemala, 2006.
8. González Moncada, C.I.; Arguello Portobancl, R.; Herrera Vallecillo, M. Conocimiento de la Comunidad Universitaria (UNAN-Managua) Sobre la Enfermedad Celiaca. 2013. Available online: https://prezi.com/ nrtc6wd2qjpw/linea-de-base-enfermedad-celiaca-2013/ (accessed on 24 October 2013).
9. Arrieta-Bolanos, E.; Maldonado-Torres, H.; Dimitriu, O.; Hoddinottc, M.A.; Fowlesc, F.; Shahc, A.; Órlich-Pérezd, P.; McWhinnieb, A.J.; Alfaro-Bourrouete, W.; Buján-Bozaf, W.; *et al.* HLA-A, -B, -C, -DQB1, and -DRB1,3,4,5 allele and haplotype frequencies in the Costa Rica Central Valley population and its relationship to worldwide populations. *Hum. Immunol.* **2011**, *72*, 80–86. [CrossRef] [PubMed]
10. West, J.; Fleming, K.M.; Tata, L.J.; Card, T.R.; Crooks, C.J. Incidence and prevalence of celiac disease and dermatitis herpetiformis in the UK over two decades: Population-based study. *Am. J. Gastroenterol.* **2014**, *109*, 757–768. [CrossRef] [PubMed]
11. Green, P.H. The many faces of celiac disease: Clinical presentation of celiac disease in the adult population. *Gastroenterology* **2005**, *128*, S74–S78. [CrossRef] [PubMed]
12. Parra-Medina, R.; Molano-Gonzalez, N.; Rojas-Villarraga, A.; Agmon-Levin, N.; Arango, M.T.; Shoenfeld, Y.; Anaya, J.M. Prevalence of celiac disease in Latin America: A systematic review and meta-regression. *PLoS ONE* **2015**, *10*, e0124040. [CrossRef] [PubMed]
13. Remes-Troche, J.M.; Ramirez-Iglesias, M.T.; Rubio-Tapia, A.; Alonso-Ramos, A.; Velazquez, A.; Uscanga, L.F. Celiac disease could be a frequent disease in Mexico: Prevalence of tissue transglutaminase antibody in healthy blood donors. *J. Clin. Gastroenterol.* **2006**, *40*, 697–700. [CrossRef] [PubMed]

14. Remes-Troche, J.M.; Nunez-Alvares, C.; Uscanga-Dominguez, L.F. Celiac disease in Mexican population: An update. *Am. J. Gastroenterol.* **2013**, *108*, 283–284. [CrossRef] [PubMed]

15. Remes-Troche, J.M.; Rios-Vaca, A.; Ramirez-Iglesias, M.T.; Rubio-Tapia, A.; Andrade-Zarate, V.; Rodríguez-Vallejo, F.; López-Maldonado, F.; Gomez-Perez, F.J.; Uscanga, L.F. High prevalence of celiac disease in Mexican Mestizo adults with type 1 diabetes mellitus. *J. Clin. Gastroenterol.* **2008**, *42*, 460–465. [CrossRef] [PubMed]

16. Gonzalez Burchard, E.; Borrell, L.N.; Choudhry, S.; Naqvi, M.; Tsai, H.-J.; Rodriguez-Santana, J.R.; Chapela, R.; Rogers, S.D.; Mei, R.; Rodriguez-Cintron, W.; *et al.* Latino populations: A unique opportunity for the study of race, genetics, and social environment in epidemiological research. *Am. J. Public Health* **2005**, *95*, 2161–2168. [CrossRef] [PubMed]

17. Kondrashova, A.; Mustalahti, K.; Kaukinen, K.; Viskari, H.; Volodicheva, V.; Haapala, A.-M.; Ilonen, J.; Knip, M.; Mäki, M.; Hyöty, H.; *et al.* Lower economic status and inferior hygienic environment may protect against celiac disease. *Ann. Med.* **2008**, *40*, 223–231. [CrossRef] [PubMed]

18. Kondrashova, A.; Seiskari, T.; Ilonen, J.; Knip, M. Hyoty, H. The "Hygiene hypothesis" and the sharp gradient in the incidence of autoimmune and allergic diseases between Russian Karelia and Finland. *APMIS* **2013**, *121*, 478–493. [CrossRef] [PubMed]

19. Rook, G.A.; Brunet, L.R. Old friends for breakfast. *Clin. Exp. Allergy* **2005**, *35*, 841–842. [CrossRef] [PubMed]

20. Rook, G.A.; Brunet, L.R. Microbes, immunoregulation, and the gut. *Gut* **2005**, *54*, 317–320. [CrossRef] [PubMed]

21. Makharia, G.K.; Mulder, C.J.; Goh, K.L.; Ahuja, V.; Bai, J.C; Catassi, C.; Green, P.H.R.; Gupta, S.D.; Lundin, K.E.A.; Ramakrishna, B.S.; *et al.* Issues associated with the emergence of coeliac disease in the Asia–Pacific region: A working party report of the World Gastroenterology Organization and the Asian Pacific Association of Gastroenterology. *J. Gastroenterol. Hepatol.* **2014**, *29*, 666–677. [CrossRef] [PubMed]

22. Greco, L.; Timpone, L.; Abkari, A.; Abu-Zekry, M.; Attard, T.; Bouguerrà, F.; Cullufi, P.; Kansu, A.; Micetic-Turk, D.; Mišak, Z.; *et al.* Burden of celiac disease in the Mediterranean area. *World J. Gastroenterol.* **2011**, *17*, 4971–4978. [CrossRef] [PubMed]

nutrients

MDPI

Review

Intestinal Microbiota and Celiac Disease: Cause, Consequence or Co-Evolution?

María Carmen Cenit [1,2,*], **Marta Olivares** [1], **Pilar Codoñer-Franch** [2,3] and **Yolanda Sanz** [1,*]

[1] Microbial Ecology, Nutrition & Health Research Group, Institute of Agrochemistry and Food Technology, National Research Council (IATA-CSIC), Avda. Agustín Escardino, 7, 46980 Paterna, Valencia, Spain; m.olivares@iata.csic.es

[2] Department of Pediatrics, Dr. Peset University Hospital, Avda. Gaspar Aguilar, 80, 46017 Valencia, Spain; pilar.codoner@uv.es

[3] Department of Pediatrics, Obstetrics and Gynecology, University of Valencia, Av Blasco Ibáñez, 13, 46010 Valencia, Spain

*   Correspondence: mccenit81@gmail.com (M.C.C.); yolsanz@iata.csic.es (Y.S.); Tel.: +34-963-90-0022 (M.C.C. & Y.S.); Fax: +34-963-63-6301 (M.C.C. & Y.S.)

Received: 28 May 2015; Accepted: 6 August 2015; Published: 17 August 2015

Abstract: It is widely recognized that the intestinal microbiota plays a role in the initiation and perpetuation of intestinal inflammation in numerous chronic conditions. Most studies report intestinal dysbiosis in celiac disease (CD) patients, untreated and treated with a gluten-free diet (GFD), compared to healthy controls. CD patients with gastrointestinal symptoms are also known to have a different microbiota compared to patients with dermatitis herpetiformis and controls, suggesting that the microbiota is involved in disease manifestation. Furthermore, a dysbiotic microbiota seems to be associated with persistent gastrointestinal symptoms in treated CD patients, suggesting its pathogenic implication in these particular cases. GFD *per se* influences gut microbiota composition, and thus constitutes an inevitable confounding factor in studies conducted in CD patients. To improve our understanding of whether intestinal dysbiosis is the cause or consequence of disease, prospective studies in healthy infants at family risk of CD are underway. These studies have revealed that the CD host genotype selects for the early colonizers of the infant's gut, which together with environmental factors (e.g., breast-feeding, antibiotics, *etc.*) could influence the development of oral tolerance to gluten. Indeed, some CD genes and/or their altered expression play a role in bacterial colonization and sensing. In turn, intestinal dysbiosis could promote an abnormal response to gluten or other environmental CD-promoting factors (e.g., infections) in predisposed individuals. Here, we review the current knowledge of host-microbe interactions and how host genetics/epigenetics and environmental factors shape gut microbiota and may influence disease risk. We also summarize the current knowledge about the potential mechanisms of action of the intestinal microbiota and specific components that affect CD pathogenesis.

Keywords: microbiota; celiac disease; gluten-free diet; dysbiosis

---

1. Introduction

Celiac disease (CD) is a chronic immune-mediated inflammatory disease affecting the small bowel, triggered by gluten ingestion in genetically susceptible individuals. Even though CD is an infra-diagnosed disorder, it is currently considered the most common food intolerance, affecting approximately 1% of European ancestry individuals.

CD is a complex multifactorial disorder involving both genetic and environmental factors. For a long time, the only securely established genetic factors contributing to CD risk were various genetic variants located within the HLA region (those encoding the HLA-DQ2/DQ8 heterodimers) [1]. Gluten peptides presented by HLA-DQ2/DQ8 heterodimers stimulate HLA-DQ2 and HLA-DQ8 restricted T cells, triggering a complex immune response involving both the innate and adaptive immune system. With the introduction of GWAS (*genome wide association studies*) and the Immunochip study, an additional 39 non-HLA regions of susceptibility have been associated with CD development, some of which are shared with other autoimmune diseases [2–7]. CD is a complex immune-related disorder with the best characterized genetic component; however, only an approximate 31% of its heritability has been explained so far, suggesting that other genetic factors besides gene–gene and gene–environment interactions might be involved in disease development [1]. Interestingly, most of those chromosome regions associated with CD predisposition contain genes with immune related functions and some CD susceptibility genes and/or their altered expression play a role in bacterial colonization and sensing. Studies have also revealed an altered expression of non-specific CD risk-genes involved in host–microbiota interactions in the intestinal mucosa of CD patients, such as those of Toll-like receptors (TLRs) and their regulators [8]. Furthermore, 81% of CD associated genetic variants are located in noncoding regions of the genome [9], suggesting that one of the main mechanisms by which genetic variation could have an impact on CD is by affecting the gene expression levels. Thus, the altered expression of CD-risk genes, as well as other non-specific CD genes triggered by genetic and epigenetic factors, may contribute to disturbing the host–microbiota interaction, and shift immune balance in CD subjects. Similar findings have been reported for inflammatory bowel disease (IBD) [10], a disorder characterized by a deregulated immune response against the microbiota, triggered by specific genetic determinants [11].

CD commonly appears in early childhood after the first exposures to dietary gluten, which is its main environmental trigger. However, there are increasing numbers of subjects experiencing CD onset in early and late adulthood [12], which suggests that additional environmental factors must play a role in CD development. In fact, other environmental factors that influence the early gut microbiota composition such as birth delivery mode and milk-feeding type, intestinal infections and antibiotic intake, have also been associated with the risk of developing CD [13–18]. Thus, a number of epidemiological studies indicate that several perinatal factors participate in conjunction to modulate CD risk.

Many complex immune-mediated diseases have been linked to changes in the composition of the gut microbiota and its genome (microbiome), including CD [19–23]. It has also recently been observed that the microbiota differs among the different subgroups of CD patients stratified according to specific clinical manifestations [24]. Moreover, although the vast majority of patients diagnosed with CD respond to a GFD there is a subgroup of CD patients that do not show clinical improvement after adherence to a GFD [24]. In particular, patients suffering persistent symptoms on a long-term GFD also show an altered microbiota composition [25]. CD14 is, together with TLR-4, involved in the recognition and signal transduction of bacterial endotoxin or lipopolysaccharide, a major component of the bacterial cell wall of Gram-negative bacteria. The CD14/TLR-4 complex, upon binding, triggers innate host defense mechanisms, such as the release of pro-inflammatory cytokines. Soluble CD14 (sCD14) is commonly used as an indicator of innate immunity cell activation in response to mucosal translocation of Gram-negative bacteria or their components [26]. Interestingly, it has recently been reported that sCD14 protein seropositivity is increased in untreated CD patients [27]. These increased sCD14 serum levels in CD could be the consequence of translocation of commensal intestinal bacteria, which could aggravate CD pathogenesis. Taken together, all this evidence suggests a role for the microbiota in disease manifestation, pathogenesis and risk. It also opens up the possibility of finding new strategies for alleviating the symptoms of specific patient subgroups or reducing the risk of the disease by intentional modulation of the intestinal microbiota.

Here, we review the current knowledge about host–microbe interactions and how host genetics/epigenetics and environmental factors shape the gut microbiota and may influence disease risk. We also summarize the current understanding of the potential mechanisms of action of the intestinal microbiota and its specific components in CD pathogenesis.

2. Host Immune–Microbiota Interactions

Initially, microbes were viewed solely as pathogens that cause and propagate infectious diseases. Nowadays, it is well established that human beings harbor microbial communities with key beneficial health functions. Indeed, most of these microbes are commensal and play an important role in our metabolism, mediating food digestion, and in the development and polarization of immune responses, preventing pathogens from invading our body [25]. The microbiota, namely the microbial communities harbored by the host, outnumber human cells by a factor of 10 and encode hundreds of genes that are absent in the human genome [28].

The human immune system and gut microbiota clearly interact with each other in such a way that one shapes the other to a large extent. The immune system plays a crucial role in protecting humans from invading pathogens and in maintaining the self-tolerance. However, in the case of autoimmunity, the breakdown of physiological mechanisms responsible for maintaining tolerance to self-antigens leads the immune system to attack the body's own tissues. It has been suggested that dysbiosis may affect autoimmunity by altering the balance between tolerogenic and inflammatory members of the microbiota and, therefore, the host immune response.

The human immune system has developed different mechanisms to tolerate commensal microbes and prevent pathogens invading the host [29]. In this respect, the microbiota increases the epithelial barrier function through the production of different metabolites, such as short-chain fatty acids (SCFAs) and mucus. The microbiota also promotes the production of antimicrobial molecules such as regenerating islet-derived protein III (REGIII)-γ and REGIII-β by epithelial cells in the intestine [29]. Researchers report that germ-free mice and mice treated with broad-spectrum antimicrobials showed a reduced proliferation of intestinal epithelial cells (IECs) and also a lower production of antimicrobial peptides [30,31]. Furthermore, this host–microbiota relationship also ensures the establishment of immune homeostasis so that the host's immune system does not attack the commensal microbes. Pattern-recognition receptors (PRRs), including TLRs, located on IECs and also on antigen presenting cells (APCs) at the interface between the host and microbiota, recognize and integrate signals from microbial associated motifs and regulate intestinal barrier function and immune responses [23]. The inflammatory response triggered by TLR signaling can be further controlled either by intracellular regulators, which can inhibit TLR signaling pathways, or by the production of anti-inflammatory cytokines that are also modulated by the microbiota [29]. In addition, several studies have found that different functions of macrophages, dendritic cells and neutrophils, which are an essential part of the innate immune system, are modulated by the microbiota [32,33]. Furthermore, the gut microbiota seem to play a critical role in differentiating a second type of Natural Killer (NK) cells (IL-22$^+$NKp46$^+$) which belongs to the group of innate lymphoid cells (ILCs) with an important role in regulating homeostasis and inflammation [34].

Other studies also support a role of the gut microbiota in the development and function of the adaptive immune system. Specific microbial groups are associated with the initiation of specific T cell responses; for instance, *Bacteroides fragilis* induces the differentiation of Treg cells, promoting an anti-inflammatory immune response [35]. Furthermore, *Clostridium* spp., belonging to clusters IV and XIVa, have also been associated with the differentiation of CD4$^+$ T cells into IL-10 producing-Treg cells in the germ-free mice intestinal mucosa, colonized with a specific bacterial mixture of clostridia [36]. Segmented filamentous bacteria (SFB) comprise a group of Gram-positive clostridia-related bacteria that strongly stimulate immune responses. Indeed, SFB have been associated with a pro-inflammatory response, inducing the differentiation of naïve CD4$^+$ T cells into Th17 cells [37]. SFB mediate a state of controlled inflammation, which primes the gastrointestinal tract to be ready for pathogen invasion, thus protecting the host against acute infections (e.g., *Citrobacter rodentium*, a bacterial pathogen affecting animals that causes acute intestinal inflammation similar to enteropathogenic *Escherichia coli* (EPEC) in humans) [37]. However, SFB colonization could also lead to adverse host effects. SFB can therefore be considered as examples of pathobionts, which are potentially pathogenic microorganism comprising the indigenous microbiota but that may contribute to disease under certain circumstances (triggered by environmental or genetic factors), possibly involving increased numbers or adaptive mutations [38–41]. Therefore, the specific host genetic makeup and environmental factors could contribute to promoting or preventing the colonization of particular microorganisms, influencing their numbers and virulence features, thereby shaping a pro-inflammatory or anti-inflammatory intestinal milieu. CD is well characterized by an upregulated Th1 immune response (increased IFN-γ) and consequently a Th1 polarized inflammation even observed in patients following a GFD. Recent studies have suggested that the increased expression of Th1 cytokines observed in CD may have partly resulted from the microbiota imbalance and/or the altered expression of PPRs which could play a role in shifting responsiveness towards Th1-type immunity [8,42,43]. Human genetics and host-associated microbial communities have been related independently to a wide range of chronic diseases, including CD. We now know that environmental factors and host genetics interact to regulate microbiota acquisition and to maintain healthy gut microbiota stability [44,45]. In turn, these three components seem to interact strongly, maintaining gut integrity and immune gut homeostasis. The disruption of gut integrity and disturbance of immune gut homeostasis caused by modifying one or more of the three interacting components may trigger the development of diseases such as CD (Figure 1) [46].

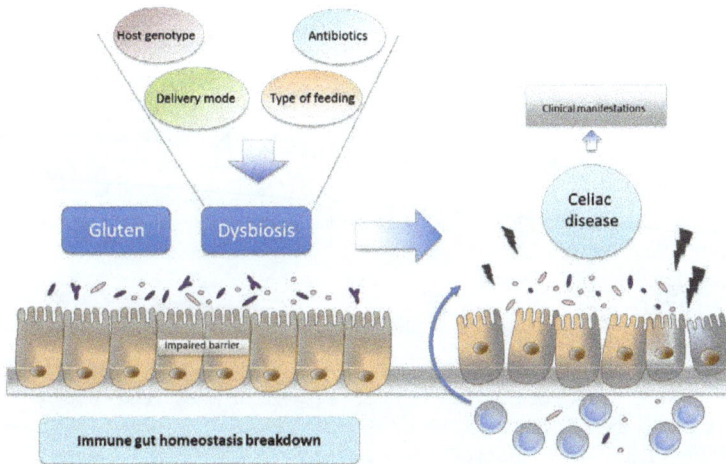

Figure 1. Proposed model for celiac disease (CD) pathogenesis. Specific host genetic makeup and environmental factors could promote the colonization of pathobionts and reduce symbionts, thus leading to dysbiosis. Dysbiosis may contribute to disrupting the immune homeostasis and gut integrity, thereby favoring CD onset and aggravating the pathogenesis.

3. Host Genetics and Intestinal Microbiota

Although gut microbiota composition shows large inter-individual variability, family members have more similar microbiota than unrelated individuals and, indeed, the same bacterial strains are shared among family members [47–49]. These similarities between the microbiota of related members most likely reflect the influence of the host genetic makeup although the shared environmental factors have also been shown to have an effect. Over 30 years ago, a study reported that the fecal microbiota of monozygotic human twins was much more similar than that of dizygotic twins [47].

Some years ago, researchers tested whether specific taxa co-segregated as quantitative traits linked to genetic markers using quantitative trait loci (QTL) analysis in mice [50]. The QTL detection approach revealed 18 host-associated QTLs having a linkage with the abundance of 26 specific microbial taxa. In addition, they established that one QTL is often associated with more than one taxon, indicating that human genetics may strongly influence the microbiota community structure. Interestingly, a QTL associated with abundance of specific bacterial taxa (the genus *Lactococcus* and the family Coriobacteriaceae) was found to contain important genes for mucosal immunity: Irak3 (encoding IL-1 receptor-associated kinase 3, which modulates the Myeloid differentiation primary response gene 88 (*Myd*88)-dependent TLR-2 pathway), *Lyz*1 and *Lyz*2 (two primary mouse lysozyme genes), *Ifng* (the interferon-γ gene) and *Il22* (the interleukin-22 gene) [50].

In addition, candidate gene approaches showed that a single host gene can have a remarkable effect on the microbiota composition [51]. Not surprisingly, most of the genes that have been identified as genes associated with microbiota changes encode factors involved in bacterial sensing and immune reactions, while some others are involved in metabolism [52]. The first human gene for which variation was shown to influence the gut microbiota was Mediterranean fever (*MEFV*) [51]. Specifically, this study revealed that changes in the human gut microbiota are associated with a single mutation in *MEFV*, which leads to a hereditary autoinflammatory disorder affecting people with Mediterranean ancestors, the so-called familial Mediterranean fever.

PRRs as well as antimicrobial peptides are key factors controlling the intestinal microbiota composition. Indeed, deficiencies in these genes lead to changes in the composition of the gut microbiota [52]. Animal studies have indicated that genes coding for inflammasome-related proteins, which are also involved in the recognition of microbial or other damage signals, influence intestinal microbiota composition and colitis development. Actually, deficient mice in the pyrin 6 member of the nucleotide-binding oligomerization domain-like receptor (Nlrp6) showed different fecal microbiota characterized by increased representation of Bacteroidetes (Prevotellaceae) and TM7, reduced IL-18 production by epithelial cells and exacerbation of colitis induced by exposure to dextran sodium sulfate [53]. Very recently, a study has reported that NLRP6 inflammasome regulates goblet cell mucus secretion, showing that NLRP6 inflammasome-deficient mice are highly susceptible to persistent infection since they are unable to clear enteric pathogens from the mucosal surface [54]. Some years ago, the capacity of interferon (IFN) signaling pathways to modulate the microbiota composition was demonstrated in mice [55]. Thompson *et al.* revealed that the microbiota was less stable in IFN regulatory factor 9 (*Irf9*) knock out mice, which is primarily involved in type I IFN signaling than in control mice [55].

GWAS have revealed that genes involved in innate and adaptative immunity are associated with inflammatory diseases [5,56,57]. Interestingly, several of these genes have been shown to have a role in shaping the microbiota. Particularly, many of the IBD-susceptibility genes regulate host–microbial interactions [57]. Some of these loci are involved in bacterial sensing and immune reactions and might contribute to explaining the relationship between IBD and intestinal dysbiosis. For instance, nucleotide-binding oligomerization domain containing 2 (NOD2) is an intracellular sensor of bacterial peptidoglycan strongly expressed in Paneth cells, regulating their function, which is to release granules containing antimicrobial peptides in response to bacteria [58]. *NOD2* has been identified as a susceptibility gene for Crohn's disease and different NOD2 polymorphisms have been associated with loss-of-function of the protein. Recently, a study focusing on IBD revealed a significant association between NOD2 risk allele counts and increased relative abundance of Enterobacteriaceae [59]. Furthermore, NOD2-deficient mice display a diminished ability to kill bacteria and increased loads of commensal bacteria, demonstrating that NOD2 is essential for regulating intestinal microbiota [60]. Subsequent studies have demonstrated that NOD2 genotypes also affect human microbial composition [61]. NOD2-deficient mice displayed increased responses to TLR stimulation, which might mirror the situation in genetically susceptible individuals [62]. Therefore, it is tempting to speculate that NOD2 polymorphisms could increase susceptibility to Crohn's disease by suppressing TLR homeostasis, which would trigger a pathogenic response to the commensal microbiota. A recent study focusing on IBD demonstrated reproducible effects of a number of host genes on the microbiome taxonomic structure across two or more cohorts; some of the studied genes have known involvement in microbial handling while others are of unknown function [59]. Interestingly, beside NOD2, tumor necrosis factor (ligand) superfamily member 15 (TNFSF15) and subunit beta of interleukin 12 (IL12B) showed significantly conserved directionality effects on bacterial taxa between at least one pair of studies. A functional enrichment analysis showed that genes regulating the innate immune response, the JAK-STAT pathway and other immunity-related pathways, seem to be related with microbiome features [59]. Most likely some of those genotype-microbiome associations may be IBD-independent and relevant to individuals with other diseases such as CD.

Another study described that the β-1, 4-n-acetyl-galactosaminyltransferase 2 (*B4galnt2*) gene, encoding a mucosal surface glycan with an important role in host–microbiota interaction, influences the abundance of specific bacterial taxa microbiota composition [63]. A recent study reported the link between Cystic fibrosis transmembrane conductance regulator (*CFTR*) gene variants and shifts in fecal microbiota [64]. Furthermore, a rare polymorphism located within the immunity-related GTPase family M (*IRGM*) gene (involved in autophagy and with a potential role in microbiota homeostasis) is reported to show a significant correlation with a *Prevotella*-predominant enterotype [65].

Another recent study has compared the microbiota of 416 twin pairs, identifying many specific members of the gut microbiota whose abundances were influenced by the host genetic makeup, while other members seem to be determined by environmental factors [44]. Specifically, the family Christensenellaceae showed the highest heritability, forming a co-occurrence network with other heritable bacteria and Archaea in lean individuals; however, Bacteroidetes seem to be mostly determined by the environment. Interestingly, the study showed that Christensenellaceae was enriched in lean individuals, and was associated with reduced weight gain in mice. Therefore, the results indicate that host genetics influence gut microbiome composition, and may do so in ways that impact host metabolism [44]. All the above evidence would indicate that host genetic factors influence both the composition of gut microbiota and disease risk.

To date, several loci have been associated with microbiota composition; however, it is worth mentioning that it is as yet unknown how the complete human genome influences the microbiome. A variety of evidence suggests that a substantial number of genetic factors in humans may contribute with a relatively weak effect on the microbiota composition. Future studies should focus on analyzing all the host alleles underlying heritability of the gut microbiome as this would shed more light on the relationship between host genotype and microbiome composition.

4. CD Genetics and Intestinal Microbiota

CD is a disorder with a complex non-Mendelian pattern of inheritance, involving major histocompatibility complex (MHC) and non-MHC genes. The main genetic risk factor for CD falls within the MHC region, a region located on 6p21 responsible for the strongest association signals observed in most immune-mediated diseases, which contains hundreds of genes with immunological functions. Specifically, the alleles encoding human leukocyte antigen (HLA)-DQ2 have been identified as playing a key role in the genetic risk conferred by the MHC region. In fact, these HLA-associated alleles are much more frequently found in patients with CD (up to 95%) than in the general population (up to 35%). The main function of the MHC II molecules is to present bacterial antigens to T cells and to activate the immune system.

Some years ago, a prospective study in a cohort of 164 infants with a family history of the disease reported association between CD genetic risk (HLA-DQ genotype) and intestinal microbiota composition. In this study, the HLA-DQ2/8 genotype and the type of feeding (maternal or formula) were shown to influence, in conjunction, the intestinal microbiota composition [66]. In addition, specific decreases in *Bifidobacterium* spp. and *B. longum* and increases *Staphylococcus* spp. were associated with higher genetic risk of developing CD, regardless of milk-feeding type [66]. A recent microbiome analysis performed using next generation sequencing on a sub-cohort of 22 infants, all breast-fed and vaginally delivered, confirmed that the HLA-DQ genotype, in itself, influences the intestinal microbiota composition [67]. The high risk (HLA-DQ2 genotype) infant group showed an increased proportion of Firmicutes and Protebacteria and a reduction in Actinobacteria (including the genus

Bifidobacterium) [67]. Furthermore, several studies based on different animal models have also indicated the presence of certain MHC polymorphisms that influence fecal microbiota composition [68,69].

To date, we have limited knowledge of the mechanisms by which the HLA-DQ genotype could selectively influence colonization and composition of the gut microbiota. The main function of MHC II molecules is to activate MHC restricted T cells. Therefore, we can speculate that different degrees of T cell activation, depending on the antigen presented to the T cells, could contribute to regulating the gut microbiota by enhancing B cell responses. These responses could involve the release of protective antibodies or promote T cell maturation into different effector cells such as Th1, Th2, Th17 or Foxp3$^+$ Treg cells, the latter with immunosuppressive activity, which could contribute to developing tolerance towards the intestinal microbiota [70]. One murine study has supported this hypothesis, indicating that the repertoire of thymus-derived Treg cells is profoundly influenced by microbiota composition [71]. In turn, gut colonization dictated by the genotype could influence the risk of developing CD. Thus, De Palma *et al.* described an increased abundance of *Staphylococcus* spp. in the group of infants with higher genetic risk (HLA-DQ2) of developing CD. Staphylococcal superantigens bind directly to HLA class II molecules and strongly activate T cells. *HLA class II* polymorphisms can determine the strength of the superantigen HLA class II binding, by governing the magnitude of the induced immune activation and therefore the outcome of super antigen-mediated diseases [72].

The fucosyltranferase 2 (*FUT2*) gene is responsible for synthesizing ABH blood group antigens in the mucus and other secretions. Homozygous individuals for *FUT2* gene loss-of-function mutation show a non-secretor phenotype, which has been associated with an increased susceptibility of developing Crohn's disease [73]; this mutation is also associated with CD [74]. In addition, FUT2 non-secretor status has been associated with increased serum lipase activity in asymptomatic subjects and an increased risk for chronic pancreatitis [75], a disorder strongly linked to CD [76]. A recent study described how *FUT2* genotype and *FUT2* gene expression could explain differences in gut microbiota composition. The non-secretor individuals were demonstrated to have an altered mucosa-associated microbiota in their intestinal tract, characterized by reduced diversity, richness and abundance of *Bifidobacterium spp.*, a bacterial genus that may play an important role in autoimmune disease risk [77–79]. To better understand CD etiology, the CD genetic component has been extensively studied by performing GWAS and the Immunochip study [7]. Currently, it is well-established that 39 non-MHC loci are also associated with the risk of developing CD. Some of these 39 non-MHC loci harbor genes related to bacterial colonization and sensing and would, therefore, be potential candidate loci to investigate the possible interactions between the gut microbiota composition and host genotype. Furthermore, other candidate loci are those harboring disease-associated single nucleotide polymorphism (SNPs) with the potential to develop regulatory roles in the expression of genes related to microbiota handling.

5. Epigenetics and Intestinal Microbiota: A New Emerging Field

Nowadays, it is well established that there are changes in gene expression or cellular phenotype triggered by epigenetic modifications, such as methylation or non-coding RNAs (ncRNAs), defined as RNA molecules transcribed from DNA but not translated into proteins. These are involved in post-transcriptional regulation of gene expression, among others, and not caused by changes in the DNA sequence. Interestingly, blood DNA methylation patterns are associated with gut microbiota profiles [80] and a recent study has also indicated the relationship between microbiota and methylation level of the free fatty acid receptor 3 gene, involved in metabolism and the inflammatory response [81]. Furthermore, methylation level at the IFNG locus is correlated with the immune response to microbial components and with the expression of IFN-γ in ulcerative colitis patients [82]. The relationship between ncRNAs and gut microbiota is a new research field. Until now, different studies have reported a link between miRNAs, a group of small ncRNAs, and microbiota [83]. Dalmasso *et al.* studied whether miRNAs are involved in microbiota-mediated regulation of host gene expression based on comparisons between germ-free mice and germ-free mice colonized with the microbiota from pathogen-free mice. They showed nine miRNAs differentially expressed in the ileum and colon of colonized mice compared to germ-free mice [84]. A similar study was performed by Singh *et al.* showing that the murine miRNA signature in the caecum is affected by the microbiota [85]. Moreover, authors found that 34 putative miRNA target genes encode for proteins involved in the regulation of the intestinal barrier function and immune response, indicating the interplay between microbiota and caecal miRNA signature [85]. Modifications of histone acetylation, related to local relaxation of the chromatin and access for transcription machinery by histone deacetylase (HDACs) are also critical in epigenomic regulation. HDACs are inhibited by commensal bacterial-derived SCFAs in innate and adaptive immune cell populations, suggesting that the metabolic activity of commensal bacterial can modify the epigenome of host cells and in turn alter their development and function [86]. In fact, SCFAs derived from commensal bacteria exert anti-inflammatory effects in the colon, partially by stimulating histone acetylation of Forkhead box P3 (FoxP3) locus in naïve CD4$^+$ T cells and, thereby increasing FoxP3 expression and promoting the differentiation of Tregs [87]. However, research into the role of epigenetics in regulating the cross talk between the host and the microbiota is in the early stages, while studies related to CD have yet to be undertaken.

6. Environmental Factors and Intestinal Microbiota

Besides host genetics, environmental factors also influence microbiota composition; indeed, diet is one of the main drivers of gut microbiota composition and function [45,88–91]. The milk-feeding type (breast-milk *versus* formula) exerts an important effect on gut microbiota composition [91]. Breast milk promotes gut colonization by *Bifidobacterium* spp., leading to the association of this bacterial genus with the beneficial properties of infants' health attributed to breast-feeding. Retrospective studies have shown that longer breast-feeding, and particularly, maintenance of breast-feeding when gluten is introduced, reduces the risk of developing CD or delays its onset [92]. However, subsequent prospective studies have not confirmed this protective effect of longer breast-feeding on CD [93,94]. These discrepancies could be related to the influence of additional confounding factors, which remain uninvestigated systematically as yet. In fact, a recent study has found that mothers with CD present a decrease in several immune markers IL-12p70, transforming growth factor (TGF)-β1 and secretory IgA (sIgA) and in numbers of *Bifidobacterium* spp. in breast-milk compared to healthy mothers [95]. Therefore, these differences in breast milk composition could be one of the additional factors influencing the protective effects of breast-feeding on infant health. Furthermore, wheat gliadins and other gluten peptides have been identified in breast milk using specific IgA-antibodies against gliadin, and the presence of gluten in breast milk may play a role in the induction of oral tolerance in breastfed infants [96]. Thus, it is tempting to speculate that the breast milk of mothers with CD following a GFD lacks this stimulus and other protective factors, which might influence the future gluten tolerance of their offspring. However, there are no robust prospective studies revealing how differences in breast milk composition and intestinal microbiota acquisition and evolution early in life might ultimately protect or contribute to CD onset.

The mode of delivery (vaginally or cesarean section) also has a strong influence on shaping the initial gut microbiota composition [97]. This is one of the perinatal and early postnatal environmental factors that clearly influences gut microbiota composition and is also associated with CD susceptibility [98]. The greater risk of developing CD in children born by elective caesarean section might be attributed to the delay in intestinal colonization by bifidobacteria, and the reduced bacterial diversity observed in caesarean-born compared to vaginally delivered infants [97].

GFD also seems to cause changes in the intestinal microbiota composition as well as in the immune response induced by the altered microbiota of immunocompetent cells *in vitro* [99]. In healthy adults, the GFD associated with a reduced intake of complex polysaccharides caused shifts in gut microbiota composition. Particularly, there were decreases in *Bifidobacterium* spp., *Clostridium lituseburense* group, *Fecalibacterium prausnitzii*, *Lactobacillus* spp. and *Bifidobacterium longum* after adherence to a GFD, whereas *Escherichia coli*, *Enterobacteriaceae* and *Bifidobacterium angulatum* numbers increased [99].

Therefore, alterations detected in CD patients under a GFD could partly be due to the dietary effect and not only to the underlying disease.

Antibiotics and other commonly used drugs are also well known environmental factors exerting a profound impact on the microbiota composition, potentially modifying its functional role in health and disease [100]. Recently, a positive association between antibiotic exposure and CD development has been reported, as it has been the case for other inflammatory disorders [18]. This association suggests that perturbation of the microbiota by antibiotics may play a role in CD onset and pathogenesis.

7. Intestinal Dysbiosis and Its Potential Pathogenic Role in CD

Most observational studies in children and adults with CD have shown alterations in the intestinal microbiota composition compared to control subjects [21,22,101,102]. In this context, we performed studies using different quantitative methods to assess microbiota composition, such as fluorescence *in situ* hybridization (FISH) and quantitative PCR. Our results found reduced numbers of *Bifidobacterium* spp. and *B. longum* and increased numbers of *Bacteroides* spp. in stools and duodenal biopsies of CD patients, untreated and treated with a GFD, compared to control subjects [21,22]. We also found higher enterobacteria and staphylococci numbers in untreated CD patients compared with controls, but the balance was almost restored in CD subjects on a long-term GFD [21]. Likewise, other studies in children have reported an increased prevalence of *Bacteroides vulgatus* and *E. coli* in CD biopsies before and after GFD compared to controls, as well as lower numbers of *Lactobacillus* and *Bifidobacterium* and higher numbers of *Bacteroides, Staphylococcus* and enterobacteria in stools of children with CD compared to healthy controls [101]. Although there are ecological differences in the upper and lower part of the intestinal tract that influence the microbiota composition, our studies also showed that the alterations associated with CD were similar in both duodenal biopsies and fecal samples [21]. A study carried out by Schippa *et al.* analyzed the dominant mucosa-associated microbiota of duodenal biopsies by using temperature gradient gel electrophoresis (TTGE), revealing that the CD patients, before and after GFD, have a particular microbiota profile [103]. The authors also reported an increase in *Bacteroides vulgatus* and *Escherichia coli* in CD patients compared to controls [103]. Another analysis of proximal small intestine biopsies from 45 children with CD and 18 controls revealed that the microbiota from CD patients collected during the Swedish CD epidemic (2004–2007) differed only slightly from the microbiota found in controls currently. However, rod-shaped bacteria were found to constitute a significant fraction of the proximal small intestine microbiota in children born during the Swedish CD epidemic (1985–1996) detected by scanning electron microscopy and further analyzed by 16S rRNA gene sequencing, suggesting that such alterations could contribute to the fourfold increase in disease incidence at that time; nevertheless, the lack of similar associations in samples taken more recently (2004–2007) contradict this theory [104]. Other studies have analyzed the metabolites derived from intestinal microbiota activity, revealing significant differences between treated CD patients and healthy controls, suggesting there is a metabolic signature for the CD microbiome [102]. A very recent study has also reported that CD patients with gastrointestinal symptoms have different microbiota composition when compared with controls and patients with dermatitis herpetiformis, suggesting that the microbiota may play a role in the manifestation of the disease [24]. Furthermore, a dysbiotic microbiota seems to be associated with persistent gastrointestinal symptoms in treated CD, clearly indicating its pathogenic implication in these particular cases [105]. Nevertheless, we should also mention that other authors report no differences in mucosa-associated duodenal microbiome composition and diversity using a 16S–23S rRNA interspacer region-based profiling method [106] and there is lack of consensus and understanding of what constitutes a CD-promoting microbiota.

From the studies described above, it is still unclear whether the changes in the microbiota are a cause or a secondary consequence of CD development. The fact that intestinal dysbiosis has been observed not only in newly diagnosed CD patients but also in those treated with a GFD supports a primary role of gut microbiota in CD. Thus, it would seem that the microbiota are predisposed to

CD, although the role of GFD in the microbiota alterations detected in treated CD patients cannot be disregarded [99].

A deeper characterization has been undertaken of the CD microbiota by isolating bacterial strains and analyzing their pathogenic features. Interestingly, *E. coli* clones belonging to virulent phylogenetic groups (B2 and D) isolated from untreated and treated CD patients present a higher number of virulence genes, encoding P fimbriae, capsule K5 and hemolysin, than those isolated from healthy controls [107]. A similar finding was reported by Schippa *et al.* in Crohn's disease [43]. The authors characterized adhesive and invasive capabilities of *E. coli* strains found in adult and pediatric Crohn's disease patients as well as in controls, and reported significant differences related to the disease. They identified particular *E. coli* variants (adherent invasive *Escherichia coli* strains) in the intestine of Crohn's disease patients, suggesting that these could be generated via evolutionary phenomena driven by a persistent inflammatory state [43]. Furthermore, the abundance of *Bacteroides fragilis* strains coding for metalloproteases is increased in both untreated and treated CD patients, and this strongly supports a pathogenic role of intestinal dysbiosis and specific pathobionts in CD [108]. In fact, *Bacteroides fragilis* and, particularly, the strains producing metalloproteases are frequently involved in opportunistic infections and they aggravate colitis in animal models [109]. The isolation and identification of clones belonging to the genus *Staphylococcus* also revealed that *S. epidermidis* carrying the *mecA* gene (methicillin resistant gene) was more abundant in the CD patients (treated and untreated) than in controls [110].

Different study models have also indicated the possible mechanisms of action of intestinal dysbiosis in CD (Figure 2). Specific alterations in the microbiota could contribute to the etiopathogenesis of CD by providing proteolytic activities that influence the generation of toxic and immunogenic peptides from gluten, and compromise the intestinal barrier function. In general, some gluten peptides (gliadin) partially resist gastrointestinal digestion and disrupt the intestinal integrity by altering the expression or localization of tight junction proteins and increasing epithelial permeability. In this respect, the microbiota may facilitate the access of gliadin peptides to the lamina propria and its interaction with infiltrated lymphocytes and APCs responsible for triggering the immune response via different mechanisms. *In vitro* studies indicate that the proteolytic activity of the intestinal microbiota may modify gliadin peptides differently, increasing or reducing their toxicity. *Bacteriodes fragilis* clones isolated from the intestinal microbiota of CD patients showed gliadin-hydrolyzing activity, and some of them generated peptides that maintain their immunogenicity, eliciting inflammatory cytokine production by Caco-2 cell cultures, and showing a greater ability to permeate the Caco-2 cell monolayer [108]. In contrast, different bifidobacteria and, particularly, *B. longum* CECT 7347 (also termed *B. longum* IATA-ES1) reduced the cytotoxic and inflammatory effects of gliadin peptides generated during gastrointestinal digestion [111]. Regarding the mechanism of action on the intestinal barrier function, CD-triggers (gliadin and IFN-γ) decreased the goblet cell numbers in intestinal loops of inbred Wistar-AVN rats, and enterobacteria isolated from CD patients, such as *Escherichia coli* CBL2 and *Shigella* CBD8, aggravated this effect [112]. Furthermore, exposure to these enterobacteria caused increased mucin secretion and greater disruption of tight junctions. By contrast, *Bifidobacterium bifidum* CECT 7365 (also named *B. bifidum* IATA-ES2) increased the number of goblet cells and the production of metalloproteinase inhibitors, and reduced gliadin translocation to the lamina propria, which could contribute to gut mucosal protection [112]. Other probiotic bacteria such as *Lactobacillus rhamnosus* GG contributed *in vitro* to the maintenance of normal intestinal permeability in Caco-2 cell cultures exposed to gliadin [113].

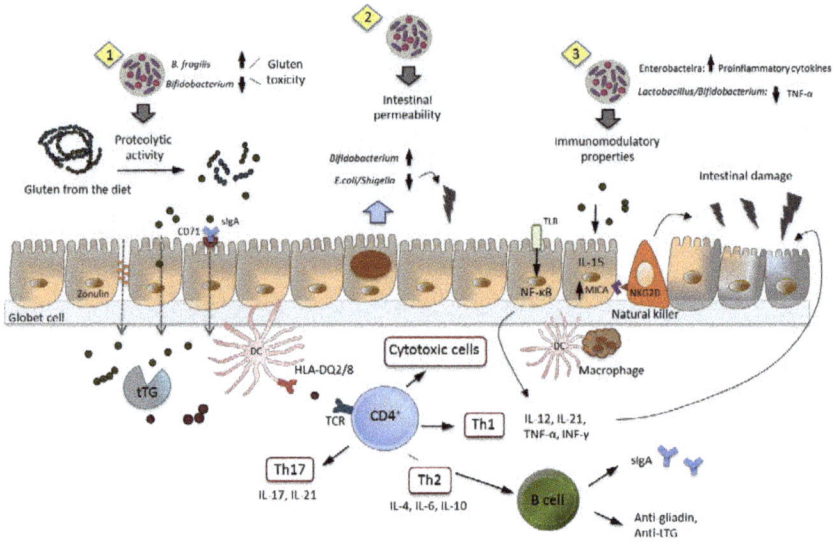

Figure 2. Potential mechanisms of action of intestinal microbiota components in CD. Schematic representation of CD pathogenesis and the potential role of intestinal dysbiosis. Some gluten peptides cross the intestinal epithelium and can be deamidated by the tissue transglutaminase (tTG), which increases their ability to bind the HLA-DQ2/8 molecules of antigen-presenting cells and to trigger an adaptive immune response, involving Th1, Th2 and Th17 cells. This leads to the release of pro-inflammatory cytokines (IFN-γ, interleukin (IL)-21, *etc.*) and the production of CD antibodies. Other gluten peptides activate the innate immune response by interacting with epithelial cells and APCs and, thus, triggering the activation of inflammatory pathways (NFκB) and the production of inflammatory cytokines such as IL-15. In particular, IL-15 increases the expression of the MICA molecule at epithelial cell surface and triggers activation of intraepithelial lymphocytes through engagement of NKG2D, leading to an innate-like cytotoxicity toward epithelial cells and enhanced CD8 T cell-mediated adaptive response, contributing to villous atrophy. The microbiota could contribute to the etiopathogenesis of CD by (2) providing proteolytic activities that influence the generation of toxic and immunogenic peptides from gluten and by mediating host-microbe interactions which could influence (1) the intestinal barrier and (3) immune function (e.g., via regulation of the cytokine network of pro-inflammatory and anti-inflammatory factors). Adapted from [114].

The composition of the gut microbiota also seems to influence the release of pro-inflammatory cytokines triggered by gluten peptides. For instance, a mixture of bacteria isolated from CD patients during the Swedish CD epidemic (*Prevotella* spp., *Lachnoanaerobaculum umeaense* and *Actinomyces graevenitzii*) induced IL-17A mRNA expression in *ex vivo* biopsies of intestinal mucosa of CD patients [115]. Thus, researchers have hypothesized that those bacteria could contribute to breakdown in gluten tolerance by increasing the IL-17 response. By contrast, in gliadin-sensitized HLA-DQ8 transgenic mice, a strain of *Lactobacillus casei* reduced the TNF-α levels in jejunal tissue sections [116]. In a model of newborn rats sensitized with IFN-γ and orally administered gliadin, *B. longum* CECT 7347 reduced TNF-α and increased IL-10 in intestinal tissue samples [117].

On the one hand, *B. longum* CECT 7347 and *B. bifidum* CECT 7365 reduced the inflammatory cytokine secretion (IFN-γ and TNF-α) induced by the fecal microbiota of CD patients while, on the other, they increased IL-10 secretion in peripheral blood mononuclear cell cultures [118]. *Escherichia coli* CBL2 and *Shigella* CBD8 isolated from CD patients, boosted the production of IL-12 and IFN-γ, and the expression of HLA-DR and CD40 in co-cultures of monocyte-derived dendritic cells (MDDCs) and Caco-2 cells compared to *B. longum* CECT 7347 or *B. bifidum* CECT 7365 [119].

20

8. Role of Probiotics in CD: Human Intervention Studies

The potential use of probiotics in CD management is supported by the intestinal dysbiosis generally associated with CD and the role attributed to these potentially beneficial bacteria (*i.e.*, "probiotics") in maintaining gut barrier function and regulating the response of the innate and adaptive immune system. Based on this hypothesis, three randomized, double-blind placebo-controlled human intervention trials have been conducted in CD patients to date [120–122]. In one of these interventions, *B. infantis* NLS was administered to untreated CD patients to evaluate the effect of the probiotic independently of the GFD. This study reported an improvement in some gastrointestinal symptoms, specifically indigestion and constipation, in untreated CD patients after the administration of *B. infantis* NLS. Furthermore, it did not improve diarrhea or abdominal pain nor modify intestinal permeability or the pro-inflammatory status measured as the serum level in some cytokines and chemokines [120]. Another intervention study evaluated the influence of *B. longum* CECT 7347 in CD children on a GFD in order to assess whether this bifidobacteria probiotic could improve the efficacy of the GFD. This trial revealed a decrease in peripheral CD3+ T lymphocytes and a trend in the reduction of TNF-α serum levels after *B. longum* CECT 7347 administration, and also a relevant reduction of *Bacteroides fragilis* numbers and sIgA in stools when compared to the placebo group [121]. A recent three-month trial has also evaluated the effect of combining the strains *B. breve* BR03 and *B. breve* B632, as compared to a placebo, in children with CD on a GFD. The study reported that *B. breve* strains decreased the production of the pro-inflammatory cytokine TNF-α in children with CD on a GFD [122].

9. Concluding Remarks and Future Perspectives

To date, different studies have demonstrated associations between intestinal dysbiosis, CD and gastrointestinal manifestations of the disease. Microbiota imbalances have been observed not only in untreated CD patients but also in patients following a GFD. In addition, specific bacterial strains isolated from patients with active and non-active CD have been shown to have increased virulence features. These findings suggest that microbiota alterations are not only a mere consequence of the inflammatory status characteristics of the active phase of the disease. These alterations could play both a secondary role by aggravating CD pathogenesis and generating a vicious-circle, and a primary role by contributing to disease onset. Prospective studies in healthy infants at family risk of CD are also underway to decipher the co-evolution of the gut microbiome and the host genome in response to environmental factors and possible causal relationships with CD onset. We expect that CD results from the combination of an altered human genome and microbiome in conjunction with as yet unknown epigenetic modifications, partly due to different environmental factors, which together influence mucosal gene expression and the mucus layer, prompting self- and gluten reactivity in the host. Future progress in this area will be crucial to provide new clues to help improve CD management and primary prevention. This will also help us progress beyond the obscure scenario of unsuccessful intervention trials focusing only on the inclusion of gluten in the infant's diet.

Acknowledgments: This work was supported by grant AGL2014-52101-P from the Spanish Ministry of Economy and Competitiveness (MINECO). The scholarships to MO from CSIC are fully acknowledged. MCC is a recipient of a Sara Borrell postdoctoral fellowship from the Instituto de Salud Carlos III at the Spanish Ministry of Health (Spain) CD14/00237.

Conflicts of Interest: The authors declare no conflict of interest

References

1. Wijmenga, C.; Gutierrez-Achury, J. Celiac disease genetics: Past, present and future challenges. *J. Pediatr. Gastroenterol. Nutr.* **2014**, *59* (Suppl. 1), S4–S7. [CrossRef] [PubMed]

2. Van Heel, D.A.; Franke, L.; Hunt, K.A.; Gwilliam, R.; Zhernakova, A.; Inouye, M.; Wapenaar, M.C.; Barnardo, M.C.N.M.; Bethel, G.; Holmes, G.K.T.; *et al.* A genome-wide association study for celiac disease identifies risk variants in the region harboring IL2 and IL21. *Nat. Genet.* **2007**, *39*, 827–829. [CrossRef] [PubMed]

3. Hunt, K.A.; Zhernakova, A.; Turner, G.; Heap, G.A.R.; Franke, L.; Bruinenberg, M.; Romanos, J.; Dinesen, L.C.; Ryan, A.W.; Panesar, D.; *et al.* Newly identified genetic risk variants for celiac disease related to the immune response. *Nat. Genet.* **2008**, *40*, 395–402. [CrossRef] [PubMed]

4. Dubois, P.C.A.; Trynka, G.; Franke, L.; Hunt, K.A.; Romanos, J.; Curtotti, A.; Zhernakova, A.; Heap, G.A.R.; Adány, R.; Aromaa, A.; *et al.* Multiple common variants for celiac disease influencing immune gene expression. *Nat. Genet.* **2010**, *42*, 295–302. [CrossRef] [PubMed]

5. Trynka, G.; Hunt, K.A.; Bockett, N.A.; Romanos, J.; Mistry, V.; Szperl, A.; Bakker, S.F.; Bardella, M.T.; Bhaw-Rosun, L.; Castillejo, G.; *et al.* Dense genotyping identifies and localizes multiple common and rare variant association signals in celiac disease. *Nat. Genet.* **2011**, *43*, 1193–1201. [CrossRef] [PubMed]

6. Zhernakova, A.; Withoff, S.; Wijmenga, C. Clinical implications of shared genetics and pathogenesis in autoimmune diseases. *Nat. Rev. Endocrinol.* **2013**, *9*, 646–659. [CrossRef] [PubMed]

7. Trynka, G.; Wijmenga, C.; van Heel, D.A. A genetic perspective on coeliac disease. *Trends Mol. Med.* **2010**, *16*, 537–550. [CrossRef] [PubMed]

8. Kalliomäki, M.; Satokari, R.; Lähteenoja, H.; Vähämiko, S.; Grönlund, J.; Routi, T.; Salminen, S. Expression of microbiota, toll-like receptors, and their regulators in the small intestinal mucosa in celiac disease. *J. Pediatr. Gastroenterol. Nutr.* **2012**, *54*, 727–732. [CrossRef] [PubMed]

9. Kumar, V.; Wijmenga, C.; Withoff, S. From genome-wide association studies to disease mechanisms: Celiac disease as a model for autoimmune diseases. *Semin. Immunopathol.* **2012**, *34*, 567–580. [CrossRef] [PubMed]

10. Elson, C.O.; Cong, Y. Host-microbiota interactions in inflammatory bowel disease. *Gut Microbes* **2012**, *3*, 332–344. [CrossRef] [PubMed]

11. Kalliomäki, M.; Rajala, S.; Elamo, H.; Ashorn, M.; Ruuska, T. Increased expression of CXCL16, a bacterial scavenger receptor, in the colon of children with ulcerative colitis. *J. Crohns Colitis* **2014**, *8*, 1222–1226. [CrossRef] [PubMed]

12. Catassi, C.; Kryszak, D.; Bhatti, B.; Sturgeon, C.; Helzlsouer, K.; Clipp, S.L.; Gelfond, D.; Puppa, E.; Sferruzza, A.; Fasano, A. Natural history of celiac disease autoimmunity in a USA cohort followed since 1974. *Ann. Med.* **2010**, *42*, 530–538. [CrossRef] [PubMed]

13. Sanz, Y.; De Pama, G.; Laparra, M. Unraveling the ties between celiac disease and intestinal microbiota. *Int. Revi. Immunol.* **2011**, *30*, 207–218. [CrossRef] [PubMed]

14. Sandberg-Bennich, S.; Dahlquist, G.; Källén, B. Coeliac disease is associated with intrauterine growth and neonatal infections. *Acta Paediatr.* **2002**, *91*, 30–33. [CrossRef] [PubMed]

15. Ivarsson, A.; Hernell, O.; Stenlund, H.; Persson, L.A. Breast-feeding protects against celiac disease. *Am. J. Clin. Nutr.* **2002**, *75*, 914–921. [PubMed]

16. Sellitto, M.; Bai, G.; Serena, G.; Fricke, W.F.; Sturgeon, C.; Gajer, P.; White, J.R.; Koenig, S.S.K.; Sakamoto, J.; Boothe, D.; *et al.* Proof of concept of microbiome-metabolome analysis and delayed gluten exposure on celiac disease autoimmunity in genetically at-risk infants. *PLoS ONE* **2012**, *7*, e33387. [CrossRef] [PubMed]

17. Mårild, K.; Stephansson, O.; Montgomery, S.; Murray, J.A.; Ludvigsson, J.F. Pregnancy outcome and risk of celiac disease in offspring: A nationwide case-control study. *Gastroenterology* **2012**, *142*, 39–45. [CrossRef] [PubMed]

18. Mårild, K.; Ye, W.; Lebwohl, B.; Green, P.H.R.; Blaser, M.J.; Card, T.; Ludvigsson, J.F. Antibiotic exposure and the development of coeliac disease: A nationwide case-control study. *BMC Gastroenterol.* **2013**, *13*, 109. [CrossRef] [PubMed]

19. Bisgaard, H.; Li, N.; Bonnelykke, K.; Chawes, B.L.K.; Skov, T.; Paludan-Müller, G.; Stokholm, J.; Smith, B.; Krogfelt, K.A. Reduced diversity of the intestinal microbiota during infancy is associated with increased risk of allergic disease at school age. *J. Allergy Clin. Immunol.* **2011**, *128*, 646–652. [CrossRef] [PubMed]

20. Vaahtovuo, J.; Munukka, E.; Korkeamäki, M.; Luukkainen, R.; Toivanen, P. Fecal microbiota in early rheumatoid arthritis. *J. Rheumatol.* **2008**, *35*, 1500–1505. [PubMed]

21. Collado, M.C.; Donat, E.; Ribes-Koninckx, C.; Calabuig, M.; Sanz, Y. Specific duodenal and faecal bacterial groups associated with paediatric coeliac disease. *J. Clin. Pathol.* **2009**, *62*, 264–269. [CrossRef] [PubMed]

22. Collado, M.C.; Donat, E.; Ribes-Koninckx, C.; Calabuig, M.; Sanz, Y. Imbalances in faecal and duodenal bifidobacterium species composition in active and non-active coeliac disease. *BMC Microbiol.* **2008**, *8*, 232. [CrossRef] [PubMed]

23. Morgan, X.C.; Tickle, T.L.; Sokol, H.; Gevers, D.; Devaney, K.L.; Ward, D.V.; Reyes, J.A.; Shah, S.A.; LeLeiko, N.; Snapper, S.B.; *et al.* Dysfunction of the intestinal microbiome in inflammatory bowel disease and treatment. *Genome Biol.* **2012**, *13*, R79. [CrossRef] [PubMed]

24. Wacklin, P.; Kaukinen, K.; Tuovinen, E.; Collin, P.; Lindfors, K.; Partanen, J.; Mäki, M.; Mättö, J. The duodenal microbiota composition of adult celiac disease patients is associated with the clinical manifestation of the disease. *Inflamm. Bowel Dis.* **2013**, *19*, 934–941. [CrossRef] [PubMed]

25. O'Hara, A.M.; Shananhan, F. The gut flora as a forgotten organ. *EMBO Rep.* **2006**, *7*, 688–693. [CrossRef] [PubMed]

26. Ancuta, P.; Kamat, A.; Kunstman, K.J.; Kim, E.-Y.; Autissier, P.; Wurcel, A.; Zaman, T.; Stone, D.; Mefford, M.; Morgello, S.; *et al.* Microbial translocation is associated with increased monocyte activation and dementia in aids patients. *PLoS ONE* **2008**, *3*, e2516. [CrossRef] [PubMed]

27. Hoffmanová, I.; Sánchez, D.; Hábová, V.; Anděl, M.; Tučková, L.; Tlaskalová-Hogenová, H. Serological markers of enterocyte damage and apoptosis in patients with celiac disease, autoimmune diabetes mellitus and diabetes mellitus type 2. *Physiol. Res.* **2014**, in press.

28. Human, T.; Project, M. Structure, function and diversity of the healthy human microbiome. *Nature* **2012**, *486*, 207–214.

29. Kamada, N.; Seo, S.U.; Chen, G.Y.; Nuñez, C. Role of the gut microbiota in immunity and inflammatory disease. *Nat. Rev. Immunol.* **2013**, *13*, 312–335. [CrossRef] [PubMed]

30. Reikvam, D.H.; Erofeev, A.; Sandvik, A.; Grcic, V.; Jahnsen, F.L.; Gaustad, P.; McCoy, K.D.; Macpherson, A.J.; Meza-Zepeda, L.A.; Johansen, F.-E. Depletion of murine intestinal microbiota: Effects on gut mucosa and epithelial gene expression. *PLoS ONE* **2011**, *6*, e17996. [CrossRef] [PubMed]

31. Khoury, K.A.; Floch, M.H.; Hersh, T. Small intestinal mucosal cell proliferation and bacterial flora in the conventionalization of the germfree mouse. *J. Exp. Med.* **1969**, *130*, 659–670. [CrossRef] [PubMed]

32. Okkubo, T.; Tsuda, M.; Tamura, M.; Yamamura, M. Impaired superoxide production in peripheral blood neutrophils of germ-free rats. *Scard. J. Immunol.* **1990**, *32*, 727–729.

33. Mitsuyama, M.; Ohara, R.; Amako, K.; Nomoto, K.; Yokokura, T. Ontogeny of macrophage function to release superoxide anion in conventional and germfree mice. *Infect. Immun.* **1986**, *52*, 236–239. [PubMed]

34. Sanos, S.L.; Bui, V.L.; Mortha, A.; Oberle, K.; Heners, C.; Johner, C.; Diefenbach, A. RORgammat and commensal microflora are required for the differentiation of mucocal interleukin 22-producing NKp46+ cells. *Nat. Immunol.* **2009**, *10*, 83–91. [CrossRef] [PubMed]

35. Round, J.L.; Lee, S.M.; Li, J.; Tran, G.; Jabri, B.; Chatila, T.A.; Mazmanian, S.K. The Toll-like receptor 2 pathway establishes colonization by a commensal of the human microbiota. *Science* **2011**, *332*, 974–977. [CrossRef] [PubMed]

36. Atarashi, K.; Tanoue, T.; Shima, T.; Imaoka, A.; Kuwahara, T.; Momose, Y.; Cheng, G.; Yamasaki, S.; Saito, T.; Ohba, Y.; *et al.* Induction of colonic regulatory T cells by indigenous *Clostridium* species. *Science* **2011**, *331*, 337–341. [CrossRef] [PubMed]

37. Ivanov, I.I.; Atarashi, K.; Manel, N.; Brodie, E.L.; Shima, T.; Karaoz, U.; Wei, D.; Goldfarb, K.C.; Santee, C.A.; Lynch, S.V.; *et al.* Induction of intestinal Th17 cells by segmented filamentous bacteria. *Cell* **2009**, *139*, 485–498. [CrossRef] [PubMed]

38. Schippa, S.; Iebba, V.; Totino, V.; Santangelo, F.; Lepanto, M.; Alessandri, C.; Nuti, F.; Viola, F.; Di Nardo, G.; Cucchiara, S.; *et al.* A potential role of *Escherichia coli* pathobionts in the pathogenesis of pediatric inflammatory bowel disease. *Can. J. Microbiol.* **2012**, *58*, 426–432. [CrossRef] [PubMed]

39. Iebba, V.; Conte, M.P.; Lepanto, M.S.; Di Nardo, G.; Santangelo, F.; Aloi, M.; Totino, V.; Checchi, M.P.; Longhi, C.; Cucchiara, S.; *et al.* Microevolution in fimH gene of mucosa-associated *Escherichia coli* strains isolated from pediatric patients with inflammatory bowel disease. *Infect. Immun.* **2012**, *80*, 1408–1417. [CrossRef] [PubMed]

40. Chassaing, B.; Koren, O.; Carvalho, F.A.; Ley, R.E.; Gewirtz, A.T. Aiec pathobiont instigates chronic colitis in susceptible hosts by altering microbiota composition. *Gut* **2014**, *63*, 1069–1080. [CrossRef] [PubMed]

41. Schippa, S.; Totino, V.; Marazzato, M.; Lepanto, M.; Santangelo, F.; Aleandri, M.; Gagliardi, A.; Longhi, C.; Pantanella, F.; Iebba, V.; *et al.* *Escherichia coli* population-based study in pediatric crohn's disease. *Adv. Microbiol.* **2014**, *4*, 886–889. [CrossRef]

42. Szebeni, B.; Veres, G.; Dezsofi, A.; Rusai, K.; Vannay, A.; Bokodi, G.; Vásárhelyi, B.; Korponay-Szabó, IR.; Tulassay, T.; Arató, A. Increased mucosal expression of Toll-like receptor (TLR)2 and TLR4 in coeliac disease. *J. Pediatr. Gastroenterol. Nutr.* **2007**, *45*, 187–193. [CrossRef] [PubMed]

43. Cheng, J.; Kalliomäki, M.; Heilig, H.G.; Palva, A.; Lähteenoja, H.; de Vos, W.M.; Salojärvi, J.; Satokari, R. Duodenal microbiota composition and mucosal homeostasis in pediatric celiac disease. *BMC Gastroenterol.* **2013**, *13*, 113. [CrossRef] [PubMed]

44. Goodrich, J.K.; Waters, J.L.; Poole, A.C.; Sutter, J.L.; Koren, O.; Blekhman, R.; Beaumont, M.; Van Treuren, W.; Knight, R.; Bell, J.T.; *et al.* Human genetics shape the gut microbiome. *Cell* **2014**, *159*, 789–799. [CrossRef] [PubMed]

45. David, L.A.; Maurice, C.F.; Carmody, R.N.; Gootenberg, D.B.; Button, J.E.; Wolfe, B.E.; Ling, A.V.; Devlin, A.S.; Varma, Y.; Fischbach, M.A.; *et al.* Diet rapidly and reproducibly alters the human gut microbiome. *Nature* **2014**, *505*, 559–563. [CrossRef] [PubMed]

46. Kurashima, Y.; Goto, Y.; Kiyono, H. Mucosal innate immune cells regulate both gut homeostasis and intestinal inflammation. *Eur. J. Immunol.* **2013**, *43*, 3108–3115. [CrossRef] [PubMed]

47. Stewart, J.A.; Chadwick, V.S.; Murray, A. Investigations into the influence of host genetics on the predominant eubacteria in the faecal microflora of children. *J. Med. Microbiol.* **2005**, *54*, 1239–1242. [CrossRef] [PubMed]

48. Makino, H.; Kushiro, A.; Ishikawa, E.; Kubota, H.; Gawad, A.; Sakai, T.; Oishi, K.; Martin, R.; Ben-Amor, K.; Knol, J.; *et al.* Mother-to-infant transmission of intestinal bifidobacterial strains has an impact on the early development of vaginally delivered infant's microbiota. *PLoS ONE* **2013**, *8*, e78331. [CrossRef] [PubMed]

49. Makino, H.; Kushiro, A.; Ishikawa, E.; Muylaert, D.; Kubota, H.; Sakai, T.; Oishi, K.; Martin, R.; Ben Amor, K.; Oozeer, R.; *et al.* Transmission of intestinal bifidobacterium longum subsp. Longum strains from mother to infant, determined by multilocus sequencing typing and amplified fragment length polymorphism. *Appl. Environ. Microbiol.* **2011**, *77*, 6788–6793. [CrossRef] [PubMed]

50. Benson, A.K.; Kelly, S.A.; Legge, R.; Ma, F.; Low, S.J.; Kim, J.; Zhang, M.; Oh, P.L.; Nehrenberg, D.; Hua, K.; *et al.* Individuality in gut microbiota composition is a complex polygenic trait shaped by multiple environmental and host genetic factors. *Proc. Natl. Acad. Sci. USA* **2010**, *107*, 18933–18938. [CrossRef] [PubMed]

51. Khachatryan, Z.A.; Ktsoyan, Z.A.; Manukyan, G.P.; Kelly, D.; Ghazaryan, K.A.; Aminov, R.I. Predominant role of host genetics in controlling the composition of gut microbiota. *PLoS ONE* **2008**, *3*, e3064. [CrossRef] [PubMed]

52. Spor, A.; Koren, O.; Ley, R. Unravelling the effects of the environment and host genotype on the gut microbiome. *Nat. Rev. Microbiol.* **2011**, *9*, 279–290. [CrossRef] [PubMed]

53. Elinav, E.; Strowig, T.; Kau, A.L.; Henao-Mejia, J.; Thaiss, C.A.; Booth, C.J.; Peaper, D.R.; Bertin, J.; Eisenbarth, S.C.; Gordon, J.I.; *et al.* NLRP6 inflammasome regulates colonic microbioal ecology and risk for colitis. *Cell* **2011**, *145*, 745–757. [CrossRef] [PubMed]

54. Wlodarska, M.; Thaiss, C.A.; Nowarski, R.; Henao-Mejia, J.; Zhang, J.-P.; Brown, E.M.; Frankel, G.; Levy, M.; Katz, M.N.; Philbrick, W.M.; *et al.* Nlrp6 inflammasome orchestrates the colonic host-microbial interface by regulating goblet cell mucus secretion. *Cell* **2014**, *156*, 1045–1059. [CrossRef] [PubMed]

55. Thompson, C.L.; Hofer, M.J.; Campbell, I.L.; Holmes, A.J. Community dynamics in the mouse gut microbiota: A possible role for irf9-regulated genes in community homeostasis. *PLoS ONE* **2010**, *5*, e10335. [CrossRef] [PubMed]

56. Sawcer, S.; Hellenthal, G.; Pirinen, M.; Spencer, C.C.A.; Patsopoulos, N.A.; Moutsianas, L.; Dilthey, A.; Su, Z.; Freeman, C.; Hunt, S.E.; *et al.* Genetic risk and a primary role for cell-mediated immune mechanisms in multiple sclerosis. *Nature* **2011**, *476*, 214–219. [CrossRef] [PubMed]

57. Jostins, L.; Ripke, S.; Weersma, R.K.; Duerr, R.H.; McGovern, D.P.; Hui, K.Y.; Lee, J.C.; Schumm, L.P.; Sharma, Y.; Anderson, C.A.; *et al.* Host-microbe interactions have shaped the genetic architecture of inflammatory bowel disease. *Nature* **2012**, *491*, 119–124. [CrossRef] [PubMed]

58. Bevins, C.L.; Salzman, N.H. Paneth cells, antimicrobial peptides and maintenance of intestinal homeostasis. *Nat. Rev. Microbiol.* **2011**, *9*, 356–368. [CrossRef] [PubMed]

59. Knights, D.; Silverberg, M.S.; Weersma, R.K.; Gevers, D.; Dijkstra, G.; Huang, H.; Tyler, A.D.; van Sommeren, S.; Imhann, F.; Stempak, J.M.; *et al.* Complex host genetics influence the microbiome in inflammatory bowel disease. *Genome Med.* **2014**, *6*, 107. [CrossRef] [PubMed]

60. Petnicki-Ocwieja, T.; Hrncir, T.; Liu, Y.-J.; Biswas, A.; Hudcovic, T.; Tlaskalova-Hogenova, H.; Kobayashi, K.S. NOD2 is required for the regulation of commensal microbiota in the intestine. *Proc. Natl. Acad. Sci. USA* **2009**, *106*, 15813–15818. [CrossRef] [PubMed]

61. Frank, D.N.; Robertson, C.E.; Hamm, C.M.; Kpadeh, Z.; Zhang, T.; Chen, H.; Zhu, W.; Sartor, R.B.; Boedeker, E.C.; Harpaz, N.; *et al.* Disease phenotype and genotype are associated with shifts in intestinal-associated microbiota in inflammatory bowel diseases. *Inflamm. Bowel Dis.* **2011**, *17*, 179–184. [CrossRef] [PubMed]

62. Strober, W.; Kitani, A.; Fuss, I.; Asano, N.; Watanabe, T. The molecular basis of NOD2 susceptibility mutations in crohn's disease. *Mucosal Immunol.* **2008**, *1* (Suppl. 1), S5–S9. [CrossRef] [PubMed]

63. Staubach, F.; Künzel, S.; Baines, A.C.; Yee, A.; McGee, B.M.; Bäckhed, F.; Baines, J.F.; Johnsen, J.M. Expression of the blood-group-related glycosyltransferase B4galnt2 influences the intestinal microbiota in mice. *ISME J.* **2012**, *6*, 1345–1355. [CrossRef] [PubMed]

64. Schippa, S.; Iebba, V.; Santangelo, F.; Gagliardi, A.; De Biase, R.V.; Stamato, A.; Bertasi, S.; Lucarelli, M.; Conte, M.P.; Quattrucci, S. Cystic fibrosis transmembrane conductance regulator (CFTR) allelic variants relate to shifts in faecal microbiota of cystic fibrosis patients. *PLoS ONE* **2013**, *8*, e61176. [CrossRef] [PubMed]

65. Quince, C.; Lundin, E.E.; Andreasson, A.N.; Greco, D.; Rafter, J.; Talley, N.J.; Agreus, L.; Andersson, A.F.; Engstrand, L.; D'Amato, M. The impact of crohn's disease genes on healthy human gut microbiota: A pilot study. *Gut* **2013**, *62*, 952–954. [CrossRef] [PubMed]

66. Palma, G.D.; Capilla, A.; Nova, E.; Castillejo, G.; Varea, V.; Pozo, T.; Garrote, J.A.; Polanco, I.; López, A.; Ribes-Koninckx, C.; *et al.* Influence of milk-feeding type and genetic risk of developing coeliac disease on intestinal microbiota of infants: The proficel study. *PLoS ONE* **2012**, *7*, e30791. [CrossRef] [PubMed]

67. Olivares, M.; Neef, A.; Castillejo, G.; Palma, G.D.; Varea, V.; Capilla, A.; Palau, F.; Nova, E.; Marcos, A.; Polanco, I.; *et al.* The HLA-DQ2 genotype selects for early intestinal microbiota composition in infants at high risk of developing coeliac disease. *Gut* **2014**, *64*, 406–417. [CrossRef] [PubMed]

68. Toivanen, P.; Vaahtovuo, J.; Eerola, E. Influence of major histocompatibility complex on bacterial composition of fecal flora. *Infect. Immun.* **2001**, *69*, 2372–2377. [CrossRef] [PubMed]

69. Bolnick, D.I.; Snowberg, L.K.; Caporaso, J.G.; Lauber, C.; Knight, R.; Stutz, W.E. Major histocompatibility complex class iib polymorphism influences gut microbiota composition and diversity. *Mol. Ecol.* **2014**, *23*, 4831–4845. [CrossRef] [PubMed]

70. Fagarasan, S.; Honjo, T. Intestinal iga synthesis: Regulation of front-line body defences. *Nat. Rev. Immunol.* **2003**, *3*, 63–72. [CrossRef] [PubMed]

71. Cebula, A.; Seweryn, M.; Rempala, G.A.; Pabla, S.S.; McIndoe, R.A.; Denning, T.L.; Bry, L.; Kraj, P.; Kisielow, P.; Ignatowicz, L. Thymus-derived regulatory T cells contribute to tolerance to commensal microbiota. *Nature* **2013**, *497*, 258–262. [CrossRef] [PubMed]

72. Rajagopalan, G.; Polich, G.; Sen, M.M.; Singh, M.; Epstein, B.E.; Lytle, A.K.; Rouse, M.S.; Patel, R.; David, C.S. Evaluating the role of HLA-DQ polymorphisms on immune response to bacterial superantigens using transgenic mice. *Tissue Antigens* **2008**, *71*, 135–145. [CrossRef] [PubMed]

73. McGovern, D.P.B.; Jones, M.R.; Taylor, K.D.; Marciante, K.; Yan, X.; Dubinsky, M.; Ippoliti, A.; Vasiliauskas, E.; Berel, D.; Derkowski, C.; *et al.* Fucosyltransferase 2 (FUT2) non-secretor status is associated with Crohn's disease. *Hum. Mol. Genet.* **2010**, *19*, 3468–3476. [CrossRef] [PubMed]

74. Parmar, A.S.; Alakulppi, N.; Paavola-Sakki, P.; Kurppa, K.; Halme, L.; Färkkilä, M.; Turunen, U.; Lappalainen, M.; Kontula, K.; Kaukinen, K.; *et al.* Association study of FUT2 (rs601338) with celiac disease and inflammatory bowel disease in the finnish population. *Tissue Antigens* **2012**, *80*, 488–493. [CrossRef] [PubMed]

75. Weiss, F.U.; Schurmann, C.; Guenther, A.; Ernst, F.; Teumer, A.; Mayerle, J.; Simon, P.; Völzke, H.; Radke, D.; Greinacher, A.; *et al.* Fucosyltransferase 2 (FUT2) non-secretor status and blood group b are associated with elevated serum lipase activity in asymptomatic subjects, and an increased risk for chronic pancreatitis: A genetic association study. *Gut* **2015**, *64*, 646–656. [CrossRef] [PubMed]

76. Ludvigsson, J.F.; Montgomery, S.M.; Ekbom, A. Risk of pancreatitis in 14,000 individuals with celiac disease. *Clin. Gastroenterol. Hepatol.* **2007**, *5*, 1347–1353. [CrossRef] [PubMed]

77. Wacklin, P.; Tuimala, J.; Nikkilä, J.; Tims, S.; Mäkivuokko, H.; Alakulppi, N.; Laine, P.; Rajilic-Stojanovic, M.; Paulin, L.; de Vos, W.M.; *et al.* Faecal microbiota composition in adults is associated with the FUT2 gene determining the secretor status. *PLoS ONE* **2014**, *9*, e94863. [CrossRef] [PubMed]

78. Rausch, P.; Rehman, A.; Künzel, S.; Häsler, R.; Ott, S.J.; Schreiber, S.; Rosenstiel, P.; Franke, A.; Baines, J.F. Colonic mucosa-associated microbiota is influenced by an interaction of crohn disease and FUT2 (secretor) genotype. *Proc. Natl. Acad. Sci. USA* **2011**, *108*, 19030–19035. [CrossRef] [PubMed]

79. Wacklin, P.; Mäkivuokko, H.; Alakulppi, N.; Nikkilä, J.; Tenkanen, H.; Räbinä, J.; Partanen, J.; Aranko, K.; Mättö, J. Secretor genotype (FUT2 gene) is strongly associated with the composition of bifidobacteria in the human intestine. *PLoS ONE* **2011**, *6*, e20113. [CrossRef] [PubMed]

80. Kumar, H.; Lund, R.; Laiho, A.; Lundelin, K.; Ley, R.E.; Isolauri, E.; Salminen, S. Gut microbiota as an epigenetic regulator: Pilot study based on whole-genome methylation analysis. *mBio* **2014**, *5*. [CrossRef] [PubMed]

81. Remely, M.; Aumueller, E.; Merold, C.; Dworzak, S.; Hippe, B.; Zanner, J.; Pointner, A.; Brath, H.; Haslberger, A.G. Effects of short chain fatty acid producing bacteria on epigenetic regulation of FFAR3 in type 2 diabetes and obesity. *Gene* **2014**, *537*, 85–92. [CrossRef] [PubMed]

82. Gonsky, R.; Deem, R.L.; Landers, C.J.; Derkowski, C.A.; Berel, D.; McGovern, D.P.B.; Targan, S.R. Distinct ifng methylation in a subset of ulcerative colitis patients based on reactivity to microbial antigens. *Inflamm. Bowel Dis.* **2011**, *17*, 171–178. [CrossRef] [PubMed]

83. Masotti, A. Interplays between gut microbiota and gene expression regulation by mirnas. *Front. Cell. Infect. Microbiol.* **2012**, *2*, 137. [CrossRef] [PubMed]

84. Dalmasso, G.; Nguyen, H.T.T.; Yan, Y.; Laroui, H.; Charania, M.A.; Ayyadurai, S.; Sitaraman, S.V.; Merlin, D. Microbiota modulate host gene expression via micrornas. *PLoS ONE* **2011**, *6*, e19293. [CrossRef] [PubMed]

85. Singh, N.; Shirdel, E.A.; Waldron, L.; Zhang, R.-H.; Jurisica, I.; Comelli, E.M. The murine caecal microrna signature depends on the presence of the endogenous microbiota. *Int. J. Biol. Sci.* **2012**, *8*, 171–186. [CrossRef] [PubMed]

86. Alenghat, T.; Artis, D. Epigenomic regulation of host-microbiota interactions. *Trends Immunol.* **2014**, *35*, 518–525. [CrossRef] [PubMed]

87. Smith, P.M.; Howitt, M.R.; Panikov, N.; Michaud, M.; Gallini, C.A.; Bohlooly-Y, M.; Glickman, J.N.; Garrett, W.S. The microbial metabolites, short-chain fatty acids, regulate colonic treg cell homeostasis. *Science* **2013**, *341*, 569–573. [CrossRef] [PubMed]

88. De Filippo, C.; Cavalieri, D.; Di Paola, M.; Ramazzotti, M.; Poullet, J.B.; Massart, S.; Collini, S.; Pieraccini, G.; Lionetti, P. Impact of diet in shaping gut microbiota revealed by a comparative study in children from europe and rural africa. *Proc. Natl. Acad. Sci. USA* **2010**, *107*, 14691–14696. [CrossRef] [PubMed]

89. Zimmer, J.; Lange, B.; Frick, J.-S.; Sauer, H.; Zimmermann, K.; Schwiertz, A.; Rusch, K.; Klosterhalfen, S.; Enck, P. A vegan or vegetarian diet substantially alters the human colonic faecal microbiota. *Eur. J. Clin. Nutr.* **2012**, *66*, 53–60. [CrossRef] [PubMed]

90. Wu, G.D.; Chen, J.; Hoffmann, C.; Bittinger, K.; Chen, Y.-Y.; Keilbaugh, S.A.; Bewtra, M.; Knights, D.; Walters, W.A.; Knight, R.; *et al.* Linking long-term dietary patterns with gut microbial enterotypes. *Science* **2011**, *334*, 105–108. [CrossRef] [PubMed]

91. Guaraldi, F.; Salvatori, G. Effect of breast and formula feeding on gut microbiota shaping in newborns. *Front. Cell. Infect. Microbiol.* **2012**, *2*, 94. [CrossRef] [PubMed]

92. Akobeng, A.K.; Ramanan, A.V.; Buchan, I.; Heller, R.F. Effect of breast feeding on risk of coeliac disease: A systematic review and meta-analysis of observational studies. *Arch. Dis. Child.* **2006**, *91*, 39–43. [CrossRef] [PubMed]

93. Aronsson, C.A.; Lee, H.-S.; Liu, E.; Uusitalo, U.; Hummel, S.; Yang, J.; Hummel, M.; Rewers, M.; She, J.-X.; Simell, O.; *et al.* Age at gluten introduction and risk of celiac disease. *Pediatrics* **2015**, *135*, 239–245. [CrossRef] [PubMed]

94. Størdal, K.; White, R.A.; Eggesbø, M. Early feeding and risk of celiac disease in a prospective birth cohort. *Pediatrics* **2013**, *132*, e1202–1209. [CrossRef] [PubMed]

95. Olivares, M.; Albrecht, S.; De Palma, G.; Ferrer, M.D.; Castillejo, G.; Schols, H.A.; Sanz, Y. Human milk composition differs in healthy mothers and mothers with celiac disease. *Eur. J. Nutr.* **2015**, *54*, 119–128. [CrossRef] [PubMed]

96. Ozkan, T.; Ozeke, T.; Meral, A. Gliadin-specific IgA antibodies in breast milk. *J. Int. Med. Res.* **2000**, *28*, 234–240. [CrossRef] [PubMed]

97. Dominguez-Bello, M.G.; Costello, E.K.; Contreras, M.; Magris, M.; Hidalgo, G.; Fierer, N.; Knight, R. Delivery mode shapes the acquisition and structure of the initial microbiota across multiple body habitats in newborns. *Proc. Natl. Acad. Sci. USA* **2010**, *107*, 11971–11975. [CrossRef] [PubMed]

98. Decker, E.; Engelmann, G.; Findeisen, A.; Gerner, P.; Laass, M.; Ney, D.; Posovszky, C.; Hoy, L.; Hornef, M.W. Cesarean delivery is associated with celiac disease but not inflammatory bowel disease in children. *Pediatrics* **2010**, *125*, e1433–e1440. [CrossRef] [PubMed]

99. De Palma, G.; Nadal, I.; Collado, M.C.; Sanz, Y. Effects of a gluten-free diet on gut microbiota and immune function in healthy adult human subjects. *Br. J. Nutr.* **2009**, *102*, 1154–1160. [CrossRef] [PubMed]

100. Zeissig, S.; Blumberg, R.S. Life at the beginning: Perturbation of the microbiota by antibiotics in early life and its role in health and disease. *Nat. Immunol.* **2014**, *15*, 307–310. [CrossRef] [PubMed]

101. Di Cagno, R.; De Angelis, M.; De Pasquale, I.; Ndagijimana, M.; Vernocchi, P.; Ricciuti, P.; Gagliardi, F.; Laghi, L.; Crecchio, C.; Guerzoni, M.E.; *et al.* Duodenal and faecal microbiota of celiac children: Molecular, phenotype and metabolome characterization. *BMC Microbiol.* **2011**, *11*, 219. [CrossRef] [PubMed]

102. Nistal, E.; Caminero, A.; Vivas, S.; Ruiz de Morales, J.M.; Sáenz de Miera, L.E.; Rodríguez-Aparicio, L.B.; Casqueiro, J. Differences in faecal bacteria populations and faecal bacteria metabolism in healthy adults and celiac disease patients. *Biochimie* **2012**, *94*, 1724–1729. [CrossRef] [PubMed]

103. Schippa, S.; Iebba, V.; Barbato, M.; Di Nardo, G.; Totino, V.; Checchi, M.P.; Longhi, C.; Maiella, G.; Cucchiara, S.; Conte, M.P. A distinctive 'microbial signature' in celiac pediatric patients. *BMC Microbiol.* **2010**, *10*, 175. [CrossRef] [PubMed]

104. Ou, G.; Hedberg, M.; Hörstedt, P.; Baranov, V.; Forsberg, G.; Drobni, M.; Sandström, O.; Wai, S.N.; Johansson, I.; Hammarström, M.-L.; *et al.* Proximal small intestinal microbiota and identification of rod-shaped bacteria associated with childhood celiac disease. *Am. J. Gastroenterol.* **2009**, *104*, 3058–3067. [CrossRef] [PubMed]

105. Wacklin, P.; Laurikka, P.; Lindfors, K.; Collin, P.; Salmi, T.; Lähdeaho, M.-L.; Saavalainen, P.; Mäki, M.; Mättö, J.; Kurppa, K.; *et al.* Altered duodenal microbiota composition in celiac disease patients suffering from persistent symptoms on a long-term gluten-free diet. *Am. J. Gastroenterol.* **2014**, *109*, 1933–1941. [CrossRef] [PubMed]

106. Meji, T.G.; Budding, A.E.; Grasman, M.E.; Kneepkens, C.M.; Savelkoul, P.H.; Mearin, M.L. Composition and diversity of the duodenal mucosa-associated microbiome in children with untreated coeliac disease. *Scand. J. Gastroenterol.* **2013**, *48*, 530–536.

107. Sánchez, E.; Nadal, I.; Donat, E.; Ribes-Koninckx, C.; Calabuig, M.; Sanz, Y. Reduced diversity and increased virulence-gene carriage in intestinal enterobacteria of coeliac children. *BMC Gastroenterol.* **2008**, *8*, 50. [CrossRef] [PubMed]

108. Sánchez, E.; Laparra, J.M.; Sanz, Y. Discerning the role of bacteroides fragilis in celiac disease pathogenesis. *Appl. Environ. Microbiol.* **2012**, *78*, 6507–6515. [CrossRef] [PubMed]

109. Fasano, A.; Shea-Donohue, T. Mechanisms of disease: The role of intestinal barrier function in the pathogenesis of gastrointestinal autoimmune diseases. *Nat. Clin. Pract. Gastroenterol. Hepatol.* **2005**, *2*, 416–422. [CrossRef] [PubMed]

110. Sánchez, E.; Ribes-Koninckx, C.; Calabuig, M.; Sanz, Y. Intestinal staphylococcus spp. and virulent features associated with coeliac disease. *J. Clin. Pathol.* **2012**, *65*, 830–834. [CrossRef] [PubMed]

111. Laparra, J.M.; Sanz, Y. Bifidobacteria inhibit the inflammatory response induced by gliadins in intestinal epithelial cells via modifications of toxic peptide generation during digestion. *J. Cell. Biochem.* **2010**, *109*, 801–807. [CrossRef] [PubMed]

112. Cinova, J.; De Palma, G.; Stepankova, R.; Kofronova, O.; Kverka, M.; Sanz, Y.; Tuckova, L. Role of intestinal bacteria in gliadin-induced changes in intestinal mucosa: Study in germ-free rats. *PLoS ONE* **2011**, *6*, e16169. [CrossRef] [PubMed]

113. Orlando, A.; Linsalata, M.; Notarnicola, M.; Tutino, V.; Russo, F. Lactobacillus gg restoration of the gliadin induced epithelial barrier disruption: The role of cellular polyamines. *BMC Microbiol.* **2014**, *14*, 19. [CrossRef] [PubMed]

114. Olivares, M.; Sanz, Y. Intestinal microbiota and Celiac Disease. In *Advances in the Understanding of Gluten Related Pathology and the Evolution of Gluten-Free Foods*; OmniaScience: Barcelona, Spain, 2015; in press.

115. Sjöberg, V.; Sandström, O.; Hedberg, M.; Hammarström, S.; Hernell, O.; Hammarström, M.-L. Intestinal T-cell responses in celiac disease—Impact of celiac disease associated bacteria. *PLoS ONE* **2013**, *8*, e53414. [CrossRef] [PubMed]

116. D'Arienzo, R.; Stefanile, R.; Maurano, F.; Mazzarella, G.; Ricca, E.; Troncone, R.; Auricchio, S.; Rossi, M. Immunomodulatory effects of lactobacillus casei administration in a mouse model of gliadin-sensitive enteropathy. *Scand. J. Immunol.* **2011**, *74*, 335–341. [CrossRef] [PubMed]

117. Laparra, J.M.; Olivares, M.; Gallina, O.; Sanz, Y. Bifidobacterium longum cect 7347 modulates immune responses in a gliadin-induced enteropathy animal model. *PLoS ONE* **2012**, *7*, e30744. [CrossRef] [PubMed]

118. Medina, M.; De Palma, G.; Ribes-Koninckx, C.; Calabuig, M.; Sanz, Y. Bifidobacterium strains suppress *in vitro* the pro-inflammatory milieu triggered by the large intestinal microbiota of coeliac patients. *J. Inflamm. (Lond.)* **2008**, *5*, 19. [CrossRef] [PubMed]

119. De Palma, G.; Kamanova, J.; Cinova, J.; Olivares, M.; Drasarova, H.; Tuckova, L.; Sanz, Y. Modulation of phenotypic and functional maturation of dendritic cells by intestinal bacteria and gliadin: Relevance for celiac disease. *J. Leukoc. Biol.* **2012**, *92*, 1043–1054. [CrossRef] [PubMed]

120. Smecuol, E.; Hwang, H.J.; Sugai, E.; Corso, L.; Cherñavsky, A.C.; Bellavite, F.P.; González, A.; Vodánovich, F.; Moreno, M.L.; Vázquez, H.; *et al.* Exploratory, randomized, double-blind, placebo-controlled study on the effects of bifidobacterium infantis natren life start strain super strain in active celiac disease. *J. Clin. Gastroenterol.* **2013**, *47*, 139–147. [CrossRef] [PubMed]

121. Olivares, M.; Castillejo, G.; Varea, V.; Sanz, Y. Double-blind, randomised, placebo-controlled intervention trial to evaluate the effects of bifidobacterium longum cect 7347 in children with newly diagnosed coeliac disease. *Br. J. Nutr.* **2014**, *112*, 30–40. [CrossRef] [PubMed]

122. Klemenak, M.; Dolinšek, J.; Langerholc, T.; Di Gioia, D.; Mičetić-Turk, D. Administration of Bifidobacterium breve Decreases the Production of TNF-α in Children with Celiac Disease. *Dig. Dis. Sci.* **2015**. [CrossRef] [PubMed]

nutrients

MDPI

Article

Effect of Gliadin on Permeability of Intestinal Biopsy Explants from Celiac Disease Patients and Patients with Non-Celiac Gluten Sensitivity

Justin Hollon [1,*], Elaine Leonard Puppa [2], Bruce Greenwald [3], Eric Goldberg [3], Anthony Guerrerio [4] and Alessio Fasano [5]

1   Department of Pediatric Gastroenterology, Naval Medical Center Portsmouth, 620 John Paul Jones Circle, Portsmouth, VA 23708, USA
2   University of Maryland School of Medicine, Baltimore, MD 21201, USA; eleonard@peds.umaryland.edu
3   Division of Gastroenterology and Hepatology, University of Maryland School of Medicine, Baltimore, MD 21201, USA; bgreenwa@medicine.umaryland.edu (B.G.); egoldber@medicine.umaryland.edu (E.G.)
4   Division of Pediatric Gastroenterology and Nutrition, Johns Hopkins University School of Medicine, Baltimore, MD 21205, USA; aguerrerio@jhmi.edu
5   Center for Celiac Research, Massachusetts General Hospital and Division of Pediatric Gastroenterology and Nutrition, Massachusetts General Hospital for Children, Boston, MA 02114, USA; afasano@partners.org
*   Correspondence: justin.hollon@med.navy.mil; Tel.: +757-953-4529; Fax: +757-953-3293

Received: 28 October 2014; Accepted: 11 February 2015; Published: 27 February 2015

Abstract: Background: Intestinal exposure to gliadin leads to zonulin upregulation and consequent disassembly of intercellular tight junctions and increased intestinal permeability. We aimed to study response to gliadin exposure, in terms of barrier function and cytokine secretion, using intestinal biopsies obtained from four groups: celiac patients with active disease (ACD), celiac patients in remission (RCD), non-celiac patients with gluten sensitivity (GS) and non-celiac controls (NC). Methods: *Ex-vivo* human duodenal biopsies were mounted in microsnapwells and luminally incubated with either gliadin or media alone. Changes in transepithelial electrical resistance were monitored over 120 min. Media was subsequently collected and cytokines quantified. Results: Intestinal explants from all groups (ACD ($n = 6$), RCD ($n = 6$), GS ($n = 6$), and NC ($n = 5$)) demonstrated a greater increase in permeability when exposed to gliadin *vs.* media alone. The increase in permeability in the ACD group was greater than in the RCD and NC groups. There was a greater increase in permeability in the GS group compared to the RCD group. There was no difference in permeability between the ACD and GS groups, between the RCD and NC groups, or between the NC and GS groups. IL-10 was significantly greater in the media of the NC group compared to the RCD and GS groups. Conclusions: Increased intestinal permeability after gliadin exposure occurs in all individuals. Following gliadin exposure, both patients with gluten sensitivity and those with active celiac disease demonstrate a greater increase in intestinal permeability than celiacs in disease remission. A higher concentration of IL-10 was measured in the media exposed to control explants compared to celiac disease in remission or gluten sensitivity.

Keywords: celiac disease; gluten sensitivity; IL-10

1. Introduction

Gluten is recognized as the environmental trigger of celiac disease (CD), an immune-mediated small intestinal enteropathy that has a prevalence in the United States of nearly 1% [1]. In this condition, the reaction to gluten's immunogenic fraction, gliadin, is mediated by T-cell activation and is genetically associated with the human leukocyte antigen (HLA) alleles DQA1*0501/DQB1*0201. Diagnosis of CD is primarily reliant on histologic demonstration of the characteristic enteropathy, with supporting criteria, such as the presence of the celiac-specific antibodies to tissue transglutaminase (tTG) and HLA testing. Treatment of CD is lifelong maintenance of a gluten-free diet (GFD).

It is important to note that symptom alleviation on a GFD alone does not equate to a diagnosis of CD [2]. Along with the increasing awareness of CD has come the emerging recognition that there are individuals who clinically react to gluten-containing food ingestion without demonstration of a T-cell mediated process in the gastrointestinal mucosa. These individuals are classified as having non-celiac gluten sensitivity (GS) [3,4]. The rising awareness of GS is in part responsible for the growing popularity of the GFD, to the point that most people in the United States now on a GFD do not have CD [5]. While the symptoms of GS may mirror that of CD, and these symptoms may resolve on a GFD, these individuals have no histologic evidence of small intestinal enteropathy while on a gluten-containing diet. Moreover, GS carries no association with an elevation of tTG autoantibodies, although several studies have shown a higher frequency of positive anti-gliadin antibodies (AGA) than the general population [6–8]. While the frequency of the HLA DQ2/8 genes is higher in GS than the general population, presence of these genes, unlike in CD, is not a prerequisite [6,8]. Generally established as a "diagnosis of exclusion", defining GS necessitates eliminating CD as the source of symptoms, followed by dietary elimination of gluten and, ultimately, reintroduction of gluten-containing foods in order to establish return of symptoms in association with gluten ingestion. This reintroduction is typically performed as an open challenge, although double-blind placebo controlled re-challenges have been performed [9,10].

The apparent lack of adaptive immune activation in GS raises the hypothesis that the similarities between GS and CD may be more related to a common defect in intestinal barrier function [11]. The intestinal barrier, by limiting uncontrolled access of non-self antigens in the lamina propria, is an integral part of immune surveillance, and impaired barrier function may play a role in a number of immune-mediated diseases, including CD [12–14]. In healthy intestinal epithelium, this intestinal barrier should be impermeable to macromolecules such as gliadin due to competent paracellular tight junctions. However, it has been well-demonstrated that antigenic gliadin peptides, which are inherently resistant to intraluminal digestion, are able to cross the intestinal epithelium of CD patients secondary to the gliadin-mediated, MyD88-dependent release of zonulin and consequent disassembly of the tight junction barrier [15,16]. In this study, we aimed to study whether gliadin causes a similar effect in non-celiac subjects by exposing, to gliadin, intestinal biopsy explants obtained from four different study groups: celiac patients with active disease (ACD), celiac patients in remission (RCD), non-celiac patients with gluten sensitivity (GS) and non-celiac controls (NC).

2. Methods

Biopsy specimens were taken from the second portion of the duodenum from adult subjects undergoing esophagogastroduodenoscopy (EGD) for clinically indicated reasons. All study subjects gave informed consent to undergo additional biopsies for the purpose of this study. This study was approved by the Institutional Review Board of the University of Maryland, Baltimore, and was conducted in accordance with their ethical standards and regulatory requirements.

2.1. Study Group Categorization

Clinically indicated biopsy specimens were submitted to pathology for standard reading by a pathologist with additional training in gastrointestinal pathology and were staged according to the Marsh Oberhuber classification [17]. Study subjects were classified into one of four different study groups: celiac patients with active disease (ACD, regular diet $\geq$ 2 months, $n = 6$), celiac patients in remission (RCD, GFD $\geq$ 12 months, $n = 6$), non-celiac patients with gluten sensitivity (GS, regular diet $\geq$ 2 months, $n = 6$), and non-celiac controls (NC, regular diet, $n = 5$).

For this study, all potential GS subjects were enrolled from the University of Maryland Center for Celiac Research in Baltimore, MD after presenting to clinic with a history of complete resolution of CD-like clinical symptoms after initiation of a GFD, yet no history of a previous EGD with duodenal biopsies while on a gluten-containing diet. To differentiate GS from CD, these patients were instructed to initiate an open (non-blinded) gluten challenge for a minimum of 2 months prior to endoscopy, with instruction to ingest a minimum of 10 grams of gluten daily, or the equivalent of 4 slices of wheat-based bread, and to subsequently proceed to endoscopy only if they experience a return of symptoms. The GS group was ultimately defined by those participants who had return of symptoms upon open gluten re-challenge and both negative CD serology (tTG and/or anti-endomysial antibodies (EMA)) and preserved duodenal villous architecture on histopathology (Marsh stage 0–1) [3]. Conversely, the ACD group was defined according to the modified 2012 criteria of the European Society of Pediatric Gastroenterology, Hepatology and Nutrition, as those participants who, after being on a gluten-containing diet for a minimum of 2 months, had biopsies demonstrating either villous blunting (Marsh 3) or, if accompanied by elevated tTG autoantibodies, crypt hyperplasia and intraepithelial lymphocytosis (Marsh 2) [18]. The RCD group was defined as having a previous biopsy-proven diagnosis of CD, with evidence of complete mucosal healing on the repeat biopsies taken at the time of the study (Marsh 0–1). These participants were maintained on a GFD prior to endoscopy. The NC group was defined as individuals that underwent an upper endoscopy because of dyspeptic symptoms; having demonstrated negative CD serology, Marsh 0–1 on duodenal histology, and no prior history of being on a GFD.

2.2. Transepithelial Electrical Resistance (TEER) Measurements

Intestinal permeability was assessed *ex vivo* by measuring transepithelial electrical resistance (TEER) of biopsy explants using a dual planar electrode (Endohm Evom; World Precision Instruments, Sarasota, FL), expressed in Ω cm^2 and normalized by the baseline resistance values. After their collection, four small-intestine biopsies were oriented on presterilized filter paper with the villi facing upward and mounted onto the modified microsnapwell system as previously described by El Asmar *et al.* [19]. After 30 min incubation at 37 °C, a baseline TEER measurement (time 0) was obtained. Subsequently, a pair of biopsy explants were then luminally exposed to Dulbecco's Modified Eagle's Medium (DMEM) alone and a pair of biopsy explants were exposed to pepsin-trypsin digested gliadin (PT-gliadin), prepared as previously described [20] and suspended in DMEM at a final concentration of 1 mg/mL. TEER values were then monitored at 30 min intervals for a total of 120 min. TEER values for each pair of biopsies were averaged and data was expressed as the fractional change from the baseline TEER.

2.3. Cytokine Quantification

Media was collected from the luminal (apical) and basolateral sides of the microsnapwell system at 120 min and cytokine levels were quantified using the Human ProInflammatory 7-Plex Ultra-Sensitive Kit (Meso Scale Discovery (MSD), Rockville, MD, US) which measures interleukin (IL)-12p70, IL-1β, interferon (IFN)-γ, IL-6, IL-8, IL-10, and tumor necrosis factor (TNF)-α via multiplex electrochemiluminescence detection. MSD plates were analyzed on the MSD MS2400 imager. All standards and samples were measured in duplicate and the assays were performed according to the manufacturer's instructions. Cytokine levels were calculated using the manufacturer's software, given in pg/mL and presented as medians with interquartile ranges. Per the manufacturer's instructions, the lower limit of detection, in pg/mL, for the assay is 0.77 for IL-12p70, 0.58 for IL-1β, 0.8 for IFN-γ, 0.18 for IL-6, 0.10 for IL-8, 0.57 for IL-10, and 0.28 for TNF-α.

2.4. Statistical Analysis

Differences within each group (between explants exposed to media alone and those exposed to PT-gliadin) were assessed by Wilcoxon matched pairs signed rank test; comparisons between groups at a given time point or condition were first assessed by a Kruskal–Wallis (KW) test. For time points showing significance by KW, Mann Whitney tests were performed on all pairs. For cytokine measurements, values and differences less than one half the lower limit of detection were set to one half the lower limit of detection. All data were analyzed and graphed using Prism version 6.0 software (GraphPad Software, La Jolla, CA, USA). A *p* value < 0.05 was considered statistically significant.

3. Results

Comparing within each group (Figure 1), there was a significant increase in permeability in intestinal explants exposed to PT-gliadin as compared to explants exposed to media alone for all time intervals (30, 60, 90 and 120 min) in the ACD group (*p* = 0.002, 0.002, 0.009, 0.04, respectively) and the GS group (*p* = 0.02, 0.009, 0.02, 0.004, respectively). In the NC group, there was a significantly greater increase in permeability in the PT-gliadin exposed explants compared to those exposed to media alone at 30, 60 and 120 min (*p* = 0.008, 0.03, 0.008, respectively). In the RCD group, there was a significantly greater increase in permeability in the PT-gliadin exposed explants compared to those exposed to media alone at 60 min only (*p* = 0.04).

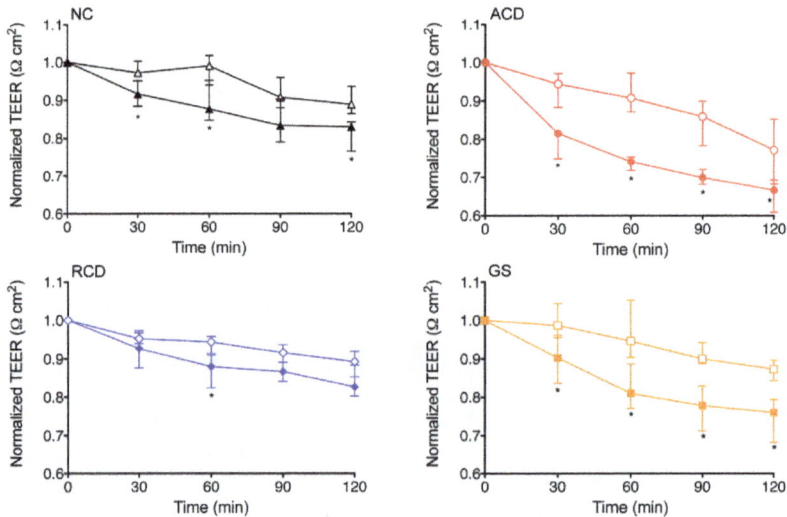

Figure 1. Normalized transepithelial electrical resistance (TEER) changes in human intestinal explants exposed to PT-gliadin or media alone. Explants obtained from non-celiac controls (NC), celiac patients with active disease (ACD), celiac patients in remission (RCD), and non-celiac patients with gluten sensitivity (GS). Explants were exposed to media alone (open symbols) or to PT-gliadin (filled symbols). NC (black triangle) explants demonstrated a greater increase in permeability (decrease in TEER) when exposed to PT-gliadin *vs.* exposure to media alone at 30, 60 and 120 min. RCD (blue diamond) explants demonstrated a greater increase in permeability when exposed to PT-gliadin vs exposure to media alone at 60 and 120 min. ACD (red circle) and GS (gold square) explants demonstrated a greater increase in permeability when exposed to PT-gliadin vs exposure to media alone at 30, 60, 90 and 120 min. Symbol denotes the median. Whiskers denote the 25th to 75th percentile. * *p* < 0.05.

When comparing between groups, intestinal explants incubated in media alone showed no significant difference in permeability except at 30 min between the RCD and NC groups (*p* = 0.03) (Figure 2A). In order to assess for the isolated effect of exposure to PT-gliadin at each measurement interval, exposures to media alone in each study group were used as the baseline TEER values that were subtracted from the corresponding values of the PT-gliadin exposed tissue explants (Figure 2B). As shown in Figure 2B, following gliadin exposure, the increase in permeability over baseline in explants from the ACD group was significantly greater than that of the explants from the RCD group at 30, 60 and 90 min (*p* = 0.004, 0.004, 0.02, respectively). The GS group had a significant increase in permeability over baseline compared to the RCD group at 90 min (p = 0.03). Increase in permeability over baseline in explants from the ACD group was significantly greater than that of the explants from the NC group at 30 min (p = 0.02). There was no significant difference in permeability between explants from the RCD and NC groups, the NC and GS groups, or the GS and ACD groups. There was no significant difference in permeability between explants from the RCD and NC groups, the NC and GS groups, or the GS and ACD groups. Coefficient of variation (mean ± standard deviation) for the TEER measurements were 16% ± 20%, 8.5% ± 6.5%, 2.8% ± 1.3%, and 6.4% ± 5.6% for the GS, ACD, RCD, and NC samples, respectively, in media alone, while it was 11% ± 10%, 17% ± 14%, 5.8% ± 3.6%, and 5.1% ± 3.2%, respectively, in the media plus PT-gliadin samples.

After 2 h, production of the anti-inflammatory cytokine IL-10 was significantly greater for the NC group compared to the GS and RCD groups in media alone (p = 0.01, 0.03) and in PT-gliadin containing media collected from the basolateral side of explants (p = 0.01, 0.03) (Figure 3). There was no significant difference in the change of measured levels of the proinflammatory cytokines IL-12p70, IL-1β, IFN-γ, IL-6, IL-8, or TNF-α on exposure to PT-gliadin in either the luminally or basolaterally exposed media and in IL-10 in the luminally exposed media (data not shown).

4. Discussion

CD is mediated by T-cell activation against gluten's immunogenic fraction, gliadin; specifically, a 33-mer peptide fragment that is resistant to intraluminal proteolysis and serves as the primary antigen for T-cell proliferation [21]. Activation of the adaptive immune response requires specific HLA class II genes and is typically accompanied by specific celiac-associated IgA antibodies; the end result of this inflammatory cascade—the characteristic enteropathy—must be histologically demonstrated for a diagnosis of CD to be made. However, there is an emerging recognition that there are individuals who react to gluten-containing food in a manner symptomatically indistinguishable from CD yet without the typical CD serology or associated histopathology. These individuals are defined as having non-celiac gluten sensitivity (GS) [3,4]. Adverse reactions to gluten outside the gastrointestinal tract, such as dermatitis herpetiformis and gluten ataxia [22], have been well-studied, yet research has only recently begun to clearly define the spectrum of gastrointestinal gluten-related disorders, and there are no objective laboratory markers to-date that are specific for GS. As the absence of an adaptive immune response in GS distinguishes this condition from CD, the aim of this study was to further evaluate the role of the intestinal barrier in these two conditions, both in terms of its barrier function and cytokine secretion.

Due to the integrity of intestinal tight junctions, normal intestinal epithelium should be impermeable to such indigestible macromolecules such as the 33-mer gliadin peptide fragment, yet in CD these antigens are able to pass from the lumen to the lamina propria. Compromised permeability to macromolecules appears to be independent of the enteropathy encountered in CD, with research demonstrating that unaffected first-degree relatives of CD patients similarly have increased intestinal permeability at baseline [23]. The mechanisms of gliadin-induced permeability in CD have been well-studied and include the interaction of specific gliadin peptides with the CXCR3 receptor expressed on the luminal side of enterocytes, paracellular trafficking via zonulin release, and subsequent tight junction disassembly [15,16,24,25]. Enhanced intestinal permeability upon gliadin exposure does not appear to be limited to CD patients. A previous *ex vivo* study conducted by Drago *et al.* using duodenal biopsy explants in a microsnapwell system demonstrated that, following 60 min of PT-gliadin exposure, tissue from both RCD patients and controls demonstrated a significant increase in intestinal permeability as well as a temporally-associated increase in zonulin release [20]. Moreover, a recently published study by Vazquez-Roque *et al.* using lactulose/mannitol (LA/MA) permeability testing in patients with diarrhea-predominant irritable bowel syndrome (IBS) demonstrated higher small bowel permeability in patients randomized to a 4-week gluten-containing diet compared to those randomized to a four-week GFD [26].

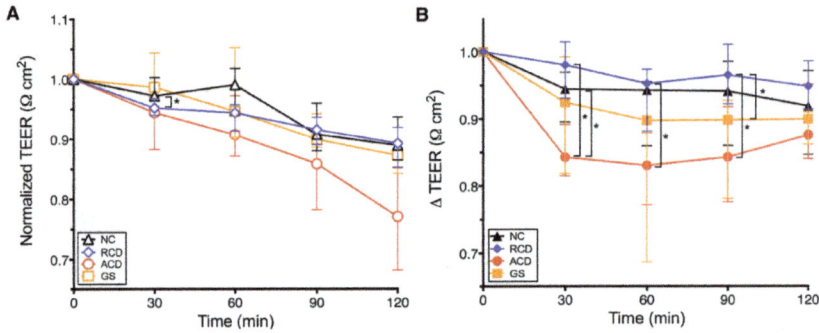

Figure 2. Comparison between groups of gut permeability changes induced by either PT-gliadin or media alone measured as normalized transepithelial electrical resistance changes (Δ TEER) in human intestinal explants. Explants obtained from celiac patients in remission (RCD), non-celiac controls (NC), non-celiac patients with gluten sensitivity (GS), and celiac patients with active disease (ACD). A decrease in TEER indicates increased gut permeability. A. TEER changes of explants exposed to media alone. Explants incubated in media alone demonstrated no significant differences in permeability except between NC (black triangle) and RCD (blue diamond) groups at 30 min. B. TEER of PT-gliadin exposed explants minus TEER of corresponding explants exposed to media alone (Δ TEER). Increases in permeability in explants from the ACD group (red circle) were significantly greater than in explants from the RCD group (blue diamond) at 30, 60 and 90 min, and the NC group (black triangle) at 30 min. Increases in permeability in explants from the GS group (gold square) were significantly greater than in explants from the RCD group at 90 min. There was no significant difference in permeability between explants from the ACD and GS groups, between explants from the RCD and NC groups, or between explants from the NC and GS groups. Symbol denotes the median. Whiskers denote the 25th to 75th percentile. * $p < 0.05$.

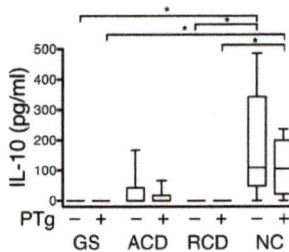

Figure 3. Comparison between groups of IL-10 secretion from the basolateral side of biopsy explants after 120 min, with and without PT-gliadin exposure. Media collected from the basolateral sides of explants obtained from non-celiac patients with gluten sensitivity (GS), celiac patients with active disease (ACD), celiac patients in remission (RCD), and non-celiac controls (NC). The NC group showed concentrations of IL-10 significantly higher than the corresponding media from the GS and RCD group. In the graphs, the box defines the 25th and 75th percentile; center line the median; whiskers the range. * $p < 0.05$.

In order to investigate the role of gut barrier dysfunction in gluten-related disorders, a study conducted by Sapone *et al.* performed LA/MA permeability testing on GS, ACD and dyspeptic (control) patients [8]. The ACD group demonstrated a significantly higher urinary LA/MA ratio (increased intestinal permeability) than the GS group. However there was not an associated increase in the urinary LA/MA ratio when compared to the controls in either the ACD or the GS population. This urinary LA/MA ratio was performed on patients after a period of fasting and, as such, is a marker of baseline permeability. In our *ex vivo* study, this is akin to the baseline, or media-only, TEER study arm shown in Figure 2A. Like the Sapone *et al.* study, our TEER results of the media-only biopsy explants demonstrated no increase in permeability in the GS group compared to the NC group, or in the ACD group compared to the NC group.

Figures 1 and 2B illustrate the effects on intestinal permeability after direct exposure to PT-gliadin. Similar to the previously mentioned study on RCD and control patients conducted by Drago *et al.* we found a statistically significant increase in intestinal permeability upon PT-gliadin exposure across all four study groups (Figure 1). Figure 2B demonstrates that, when comparing between groups, upon PT-gliadin exposure, the GS explants reacted similarly to the ACD explants, with no statistical difference between these groups. The NC explants reacted similarly to the RCD explants, likewise with no statistical difference between these groups. Both the ACD and GS explants had a statistically greater increase in permeability than the RCD explants, and explants from the NC and RCD groups reacted to a lesser degree than those from the ACD group. These results complement those previously reported by Sapone *et al.*; although GS patients have a normal intestinal barrier at baseline, gliadin exposure induces increased intestinal permeability in these patients, with a response that closely resembles that observed in the ACD group and is more pronounced than that observed in the RCD group.

The RCD group demonstrated the smallest degree in permeability change upon exposure to PT-gliadin and the difference reached significance at only 60 min. This is a delay when compared to the other study groups, which all demonstrated an increase in permeability at the first measured interval of 30 min. The RCD group was the only group in our study on a strict GFD prior to endoscopy, suggesting that the gluten-induced activation of the zonulin pathway is comparatively delayed in intestinal tissue that is not routinely exposed to dietary gluten, even in those patients with celiac disease. Similarly, the randomized controlled trial by Vazquez-roque *et al.* demonstrated significantly increased small bowel permeability by (LA/MA) testing in IBS patients randomized to a gluten-containing diet compared to those randomized to 4 weeks of a strict GFD [26]. Given that symptom-onset upon gluten-containing food exposure in the GS population is comparatively faster than in patients with CD, further permeability experiments comparing GS patients on a strict GFD to those with RCD would help contribute to the understanding of the timing of these alterations.

Cytokine quantification from the media collected from the luminal and basolateral sides of the biopsy explants after 120 min of PT-gliadin exposure failed to show any significant difference in the classic inflammatory cytokines, to include IL-6, IL-8, IFN-γ, and TNF-α. The relatively short period of incubation may in part explain the lack of detection of an inflammatory innate response to gluten exposure. Production of the anti-inflammatory cytokine IL-10 was significantly higher in the media collected from the basolateral side of the explants obtained from the NC group as compared to the GS and RCD groups (Figure 3) in both the unexposed media and the media exposed to PT-gliadin. IL-10 is a key mediator for regulating the innate intestinal immune response [27]. A study by Madsen *et al.* in IL-10 deficient mice demonstrated that IL-10 plays a significant role in intestinal permeability and, in fact, deficiencies of IL-10 lead to increased intestinal permeability prior to the development of mucosal inflammation [28]. We do not suggest that patients with GS or CD are IL-10 deficient; however, this degree of IL-10 production in the NC group may be indicative of a more competent innate immune response. Further studies will be needed to help elucidate if this lack of secretion of IL-10 is a primary factor leading to an exaggerated increase in PT-gliadin induced permeability or a secondary marker of a separate defect in innate immunity.

A primary limitation of this study relates to the lack of objective laboratory biomarkers specific for GS. Currently, the diagnosis is based on exclusion criteria; specifically these patients should have negative CD serology (anti-EMA and/or anti-tTG), normal duodenal histopathology, and resolution of CD-like symptoms on a GFD with subsequent return of symptoms upon dietary reintroduction of gluten-containing food [3]. For the purposes of this study, our GS patients had undergone an open gluten challenge and we recognize that such a method could allow for the possibility of patients without true GS being included in the GS group due to placebo-response. While dietary re-challenge in a blinded fashion would have helped avoid the possibility of a placebo effect, the necessity of a gluten-containing diet at biopsy precluded this type of intervention. Similarly, no patients in our control group had previously attempted a GFD; ideally, the control group would have been comprised of those who had already had GS ruled-out by a negative GFD trial. The percentage of patients with IBS who truly have GS may be as high as 30%; given that the indication for duodenal biopsies in our NC group would include the non-specific gastrointestinal symptoms of CD and GS, it is conceivable that some of the NC patients may have undiagnosed GS [9].

5. Conclusions

This study demonstrates that gliadin exposure induces an increase in intestinal permeability in all individuals, regardless of whether or not they have celiac disease. The results of this study suggest that gluten exposure leads to altered barrier function in both ACD and GS, resulting in an exaggerated increase in intestinal permeability when compared to RCD. The intestinal mucosal secretion of IL-10 from the basolateral surface seen in NC subjects in this study was not observed in those with RCD or GS. Specific laboratory markers for GS are still necessary to allow for a more objective definition of GS and further research into GS disorders would benefit from double-blind, placebo-controlled studies.

Acknowledgments: The authors thank Karen Lammers, Rosaria Fiorentino and Stefania Senger (Center for Celiac Research, Boston, MA, USA) for their technical help and expertise. The authors are grateful to Carmen Cuffari (Johns Hopkins Pediatric Gastroenterology Fellowship Program) for his guidance and encouragement. The views expressed in this article are those of the authors and do not necessarily reflect the official policy or position of the United States Department of Defense.

Author Contributions: The authors' responsibilities were as follows—A.F. conceived and designed the study. J.H., E.L. and A.F. contributed to the design of the study and participated in subject recruitment. J.H. conducted the study and was the primary author for the manuscript. B.G. and E.G. participated in the recruitment of the patients and carried out the endoscopy procedures. J.H., T.G. and A.F. were involved in the analysis and interpretation of the data. T.G. and A.F. critically revised the manuscript. All authors approved the final version of the manuscript.

Conflicts of Interest: The authors declare no conflict of interest.

References

1. Fasano, A.; Berti, I.; Gerarduzzi, T.; Not, T.; Colletti, R.B.; Drago, S.; Elitsur, Y.; Green, P.H.; Guandalini, S.; Hill, I.D.; *et al.* Prevalence of celiac disease in at-risk and not-at-risk groups in the United States: A large multicenter study. *Arch. Intern. Med.* **2003**, *163*, 286–292. [CrossRef] [PubMed]

2. Campanella, J.; Biagi, F.; Bianchi, P.I.; Zanellati, G.; Marchese, A.; Corazza, G.R. Clinical response to gluten withdrawal is not an indicator of coeliac disease. *Scand. J. Gastroenterol.* **2008**, *43*, 1311–1314. [CrossRef] [PubMed]

3. Sapone, A.; Bai, J.C.; Ciacci, C.; Dolinsek, J.; Green, P.H.R.; Hadjivassiliou, M.; Kaukinen, K.; Rostami, K.; Sanders, D.S.; Schumann, M.; *et al.* Spectrum of gluten-related disorders: Consensus on new nomenclature and classification. *BMC Med.* **2012**, *10*, 13. [CrossRef] [PubMed]

4. Ludvigsson, J.F.; Leffler, D.A.; Bai, J.C.; Biagi, F.; Fasano, A.; Green, P.H.; Hadjivassiliou, M.; Kaukinen, K.; Kelly, C.P.; Leonard, J.N.; *et al.* The Oslo definitions for coeliac disease and related terms. *Gut* **2012**, *62*, 43–52. [CrossRef] [PubMed]

5. Rubio-Tapia, A.; Ludvigsson, J.F.; Brantner, T.L.; Murray, J.A.; Everhart, J.E. The prevalence of celiac disease in the United States. *Am. J. Gastroenterol.* **2012**, *107*, 1538–1544. [CrossRef] [PubMed]

6. Wahnschaffe, U.; Schulzke, J.D.; Zeitz, M.; Ullrich, R. Predictors of clinical response to gluten-free diet in patients diagnosed with diarrhea-predominant irritable bowel syndrome. *Clin. Gastroenterol. Hepatol.* **2007**, *5*, 844–850. [CrossRef] [PubMed]

7. Volta, U.; Tovoli, F.; Cicola, R.; Parisi, C.; Fabbri, A.; Piscaglia, M.; Fiorini, E.; Caio, G. Serological tests in gluten sensitivity (nonceliac gluten intolerance). *J. Clin. Gastroenterol.* **2012**, *46*, 680–685. [CrossRef] [PubMed]

8. Sapone, A.; Lammers, K.M.; Casolaro, V.; Cammarota, M.; Giuliano, M.T.; de Rosa, M.; Stefanile, R.; Mazzarella, G.; Tolone, C.; Russo, M.I.; *et al.* Divergence of gut permeability and mucosal immune gene expression in two gluten-associated conditions: Celiac disease and gluten sensitivity. *BMC Med.* **2011**, *9*, 23. [CrossRef] [PubMed]

9. Carroccio, A.; Mansueto, P.; Iacono, G.; Soresi, M.; D'Alcamo, A.; Cavataio, F.; Brusca, I.; Florena, A.M.; Ambrosiano, G.; Seidita, A.; *et al.* Non-celiac wheat sensitivity diagnosed by double-blind placebo-controlled challenge: Exploring a new clinical entity. *Am. J. Gastroenterol.* **2012**, *107*, 1898–1906. [CrossRef] [PubMed]

10. Biesiekierski, J.R.; Newnham, E.D.; Irving, P.M.; Barrett, J.S.; Haines, M.; Doecke, J.D.; Shepherd, S.J.; Muir, J.G.; Gibson, P.R. Gluten causes gastrointestinal symptoms in subjects without celiac disease: A double-blind randomized placebo-controlled trial. *Am. J. Gastroenterol.* **2011**, *106*, 508–514. [CrossRef] [PubMed]

11. Verdu, E.F.; Armstrong, D.; Murray, J.A. Between celiac disease and irritable bowel syndrome: The "no man's land" of gluten sensitivity. *Am. J. Gastroenterol.* **2009**, *104*, 1587–1594. [CrossRef] [PubMed]

12. Liu, Z.; Li, N.; Neu, J. Tight junctions, leaky intestines, and pediatric diseases. *Acta Paediatr.* **2005**, *94*, 386–393. [CrossRef] [PubMed]

13. Monsuur, A.J.; Wijmenga, C. Understanding the molecular basis of celiac disease: What genetic studies reveal. *Ann. Med.* **2006**, *38*, 578–591. [CrossRef] [PubMed]

14. Fasano, A.; Shea-Donohue, T. Mechanisms of disease: The role of intestinal barrier function in the pathogenesis of gastrointestinal autoimmune diseases. *Nat. Clin. Pract. Gastroenterol. Hepatol.* **2005**, *2*, 416–422. [CrossRef] [PubMed]

15. Fasano, A.; Not, T.; Wang, W.; Uzzau, S.; Berti, I.; Tommasini, A.; Goldblum, S.E. Zonulin, a newly discovered modulator of intestinal permeability, and its expression in coeliac disease. *Lancet* **2000**, *355*, 1518–1519. [CrossRef] [PubMed]

16. Cummins, A.G.; Thompson, F.M.; Butler, R.N.; Cassidy, J.C.; Gillis, D.; Lorenzetti, M.; Southcott, E.K.; Wilson, P.C. Improvement in intestinal permeability precedes morphometric recovery of the small intestine in coeliac disease. *Clin. Sci. (Lond.)* **2001**, *100*, 379–386. [CrossRef]

17. Marsh, M.N. The natural history of gluten sensitivity: Defining, refining and re-defining. *QJM* **1995**, *88*, 9–13. [PubMed]

18. Husby, S.; Koletzko, S.; Korponay-Szabo, I.R.; Mearin, M.L.; Phillips, A.; Shamir, R.; Troncone, R.; Giersiepen, K.; Branski, D.; Catassi, C.; *et al.* European society for pediatric gastroenterology, hepatology, and nutrition guidelines for the diagnosis of coeliac disease. *J. Pediatr. Gastroenterol. Nutr.* **2012**, *54*, 136–160. [CrossRef] [PubMed]

19. El Asmar, R.; Panigrahi, P.; Bamford, P.; Berti, I.; Not, T.; Coppa, G.V.; Catassi, C.; Fasano, A. Host-dependent zonulin secretion causes the impairment of the small intestine barrier function after bacterial exposure. *Gastroenterology* **2002**, *123*, 1607–1615.

20. Drago, S.; El Asmar, R.; Di Pierro, M.; Grazia Clemente, M.; Tripathi, A.; Sapone, A.; Thakar, M.; Iacono, G.; Carroccio, A.; D'Agate, C.; *et al.* Gliadin, zonulin and gut permeability: Effects on celiac and non-celiac intestinal mucosa and intestinal cell lines. *Scand. J. Gastroenterol.* **2006**, *41*, 408–419. [CrossRef] [PubMed]

21. Shan, L.; Molberg, O.; Parrot, I.; Hausch, F.; Filiz, F.; Gray, G.M.; Sollid, L.M.; Khosla, C. Structural basis for gluten intolerance in celiac sprue. *Science* **2002**, *297*, 2275–2279. [CrossRef] [PubMed]

22. Hadjivassiliou, M.; Sanders, D.S.; Grunewald, R.A.; Woodroofe, N.; Boscolo, S.; Aeschlimann, D. Gluten sensitivity: From gut to brain. *Lancet Neurol.* **2010**, *9*, 318–330. [CrossRef] [PubMed]

23. Van Elburg, R.M.; Uil, J.J.; Mulder, C.J.; Heymans, H.S. Intestinal permeability in patients with coeliac disease and relatives of patients with coeliac disease. *Gut* **1993**, *34*, 354–357.

24. Tripathi, A.; Lammers, K.M.; Goldblum, S.; Shea-Donohue, T.; Netzel-Arnett, S.; Buzza, M.S.; Antalis, T.M.; Vogel, S.N.; Zhao, A.; Yang, S.; *et al.* Identification of human zonulin, a physiological modulator of tight junctions, as prehaptoglobin-2. *Proc. Natl. Acad. Sci. USA* **2009**, *106*, 16799–16804. [CrossRef] [PubMed]

25. Lammers, K.M.; Lu, R.; Brownley, J.; Lu, B.; Gerard, C.; Thomas, K.; Rallabhandi, P.; Shea-Donohue, T.; Tamiz, A.; Alkan, S.; *et al.* Gliadin induces an increase in intestinal permeability and zonulin release by binding to the chemokine receptor CXCR3. *Gastroenterology* **2008**, *135*, 194–204.e3. [CrossRef] [PubMed]

26. Vazquez-Roque, M.I.; Camilleri, M.; Smyrk, T.; Murray, J.A.; Marietta, E.; O'Neill, J.; Carlson, P.; Lamsam, J.; Janzow, D.; Eckert, D.; *et al.* A controlled trial of gluten-free diet in patients with irritable bowel syndrome-diarrhea: Effects on bowel frequency and intestinal function. *Gastroenterology* **2013**, *144*, 903–911.e3. [CrossRef] [PubMed]

27. Moore, K.W.; de Waal Malefyt, R.; Coffman, R.L.; O'Garra, A. Interleukin-10 and the interleukin-10 receptor. *Annu. Rev. Immunol.* **2001**, *19*, 683–765. [CrossRef] [PubMed]

28. Madsen, K.L.; Malfair, D.; Gray, D.; Doyle, J.S.; Jewell, L.D.; Fedorak, R.N. Interleukin-10 gene-deficient mice develop a primary intestinal permeability defect in response to enteric microflora. *Inflamm. Bowel Dis.* **1999**, *5*, 262–270. [CrossRef] [PubMed]

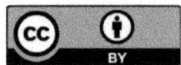

nutrients

MDPI

Review

The Role of Gluten in Celiac Disease and Type 1 Diabetes

Gloria Serena [1,2,†], Stephanie Camhi [1,†], Craig Sturgeon [1,2], Shu Yan [1] and Alessio Fasano [1,*]

[1] Center for Celiac Research, Mucosal Immunology and Biology Research Center, Massachusetts General Hospital and Division of Pediatric Gastroenterology and Nutrition, Massachusetts General Hospital for Children, Boston, MA 02114, USA; gserena@mgh.harvard.edu (G.S.); sscamhi@partners.org (S.C.); csturgeon@mgh.harvard.edu (C.S.); syan4@mgh.harvard.edu (S.Y.)

[2] Graduate Program in Life Sciences, University of Maryland School of Medicine, Baltimore, MD 21201, USA

* Correspondence: afasano@mgh.harvard.edu; Tel.: +1-617-724-4604

† These authors contributed equally to this work.

Received: 26 June 2015; Accepted: 11 August 2015; Published: 26 August 2015

Abstract: Celiac disease (CD) and type 1 diabetes (T1D) are autoimmune conditions in which dietary gluten has been proven or suggested to play a pathogenic role. In CD; gluten is established as the instigator of autoimmunity; the autoimmune process is halted by removing gluten from the diet; which allows for resolution of celiac autoimmune enteropathy and subsequent normalization of serological markers of the disease. However; an analogous causative agent has not yet been identified for T1D. Nevertheless; the role of dietary gluten in development of T1D and the potentially beneficial effect of removing gluten from the diet of patients with T1D are still debated. In this review; we discuss the comorbid occurrence of CD and T1D and explore current evidences for the specific role of gluten in both conditions; specifically focusing on current evidence on the effect of gluten on the immune system and the gut microbiota.

Keywords: celiac disease; type 1 diabetes; gluten

1. Celiac Disease

Celiac disease (CD) is an autoimmune enteropathy caused by the ingestion of gluten in genetically susceptible individuals. It is characterized by the presence of autoimmune antibodies, systemic clinical manifestations, small intestinal enteropathy and genetic predisposition [1]. CD is a T-cell mediated disorder where gliadin derived peptides activate immune cells in the gut lamina propria and recruit infiltrating T lymphocytes, which initiate an adaptive Th1 response and concurrent increase of interferon gamma (IFN-γ) and interleukin-15 (IL-15). This leads to the activation of intraepithelial lymphocyte toxicity which results in profound tissue remodeling.

The etiology of CD is influenced by both environmental and genetic factors. The most characterized genetic contribution to CD is the human leukocyte antigen system (HLA), contributing to 40% of genetic variance [2]. Major histocompatibility coplex (MHC) class II HLA DQ2 and DQ8 confer the greatest disease susceptibility. The majority of patients carry variants of DQ2 (95%) encoded by alleles DQA1*05/DQB*02 and a minority (5%) carries DQ8 encoded by DQA1*03/DQB1*03:02 alleles. In addition, there is evidence for gene dosage effect with increased risk for those with homozygous allotypes [3]. Genome-wide association studies and a recent dense fine mapping study report 57 non HLA loci, which account for 18% of the genetic variance [4]. Of note, HLA and other genetic susceptibility are necessary but not sufficient for disease development. Additionally, environmental causative agents for CD, other than gliadin, have been explored.

Several studies have shown an association between active CD and gastrointestinal dysbiosis characterized by higher amount of *Proteobacteria* and *Bacteroidetes* and associated with a reduced abundance of the phylum *Firmicutes* during the acute phase of the disease [5]. A proof of concept study from our group revealed that genetically predisposed infants present a specific fecal microbiota in which *Bacteroides* are reduced and *Firmicutes* are more abundant before the onset of the disease [6]. Together, these data suggest a possible causative role of dysbiosis in the onset of CD.

Prevalence of CD is between 1% and 2% of the total population in North America, South America, the Middle East and North Africa, and there is preliminary evidence for similar rates in Asian populations [7]. The disease incidence is also increased in first degree family members of those with CD (10%–15%) and in individuals with other autoimmune diseases [8]. Of the affected population, studies suggest that only 10%–15% is actually diagnosed. Despite high estimates of undiagnosed cases, recent studies have also indicated a surprisingly sharp increase in the prevalence of CD over the past decades, with North America and Europe experiencing the highest increase [9].

Classical presentation of CD consists mainly of gastrointestinal symptoms associated with malabsorption including diarrhea, steatorrhea, weight loss, or failure to thrive. Other extra-intestinal symptoms include iron deficiency, recurrent abdominal pain, aphthous stomatitis, chronic fatigue, short stature and reduced bone density [10]. Serum testing is extremely reliable and forms the first line of testing for CD. Patients are first screened for serum IgA anti-tissue transglutaminse antibodies if they are not IgA deficient [11]. In individuals with IgA deficiency, serum IgG anti-tissue transglutamminase antibody levels are measured instead of traditional markers. Recently, IgG anti-deamidated gliadin has emerged as an alternative test, due to its better sensitivity and specificity (capability of discriminating false positives and false negatives) [12]. A more specific, but more expensive and operator dependent, test is sometimes used to confirm borderline results: anti endomysium IgA. While performing the serologic screening, patients should remain on a gluten containing diet in order to maintain high sensitivity of test results. Finally, a confirmed diagnosis requires a small intestinal biopsy. Histological changes should show increased number of intraepithelial lymphocytes, elongated crypts and at least partial villous atrophy [10].

The definitive treatment for CD is complete elimination of the offending gluten. A gluten free diet (GFD) should cause no side effects, since gluten has limited nutritional value, but consumption of certain nutrients, in particular fibers, iron, calcium and folates tends to be lower in the GFD [12]. Strict compliance is necessary when adhering to a GFD as even small amounts of contamination can prove problematic [9]. Maximum contamination has recently been defined as 20 ppm by both the Codex Alimentarius and Food and Drug Administration [13]. Intestinal healing and decrease of serologic markers should begin between 6 and 24 months following the initiation of GFD [12]. Currently, the only available treatment for CD patients is a strict GFD. This therapy, however, fails to induce complete improvement in 7%–30% of patients. Thus, the number of studies evaluating alternative therapeutic strategies for CD, such as genetically modified gluten, inhibitors of zonulin—the regulator of intestinal tight junctions—or supplementary probiotics, have recently increased [14–17].

2. Celiac Disease and Gluten

Gluten is a complex molecule contained in several grains such as wheat, rye and barley [12,18]. The major proteic components that characterize gluten are glutenin polymers and gliadin monomers. Glutenins can be subdivided into low and high molecular weight proteins, while the gliadin protein family contains α-, β-, γ- and ω- types [19]. Both glutenins and gliadins are characterized by a high amount of prolines (20%) and glutamines (40%) that protect them from complete degradation in the gastrointestinal tract and make them difficult to digest [20].

The link between onset of CD and ingestion of gluten containing grains was established around 1950. Since then, the role of gliadin as the environmental factor for CD has been well established [12,18]. Several studies revealed the capability of gliadin peptides to trigger an immune response in CD patients. Castellanos-Rubio and colleagues showed that intestinal biopsies from active CD patients stimulated *in vitro* with gliadin express a vast range of pro-inflammatory cytokines derived from a Th1/Th17 driven adaptive immune response [21]. Furthermore, Palova *et al.* reported that peripheral blood mononuclear cells (PBMC) from CD patients responded to gliadin by secreting interleukin 1 beta (IL-1β) and interleukin-18 (IL-18) [22]. Recently, IL-15 has also been found to be up-regulated in the epithelium and the lamina propria of patients with active CD [23,24].

Presently, the chain of events by which gliadin triggers onset of clinical disease is hypothesized as the following: after oral ingestion, partially digested gliadin peptides interact with the small intestinal mucosa and trigger an innate immune response characterized by release of IL-8 and IL-15 from epithelial cells and lamina propria dendritic cells [25,26]. IL-8 is a potent chemo-attractant and its production leads to the immediate recruitment of neutrophils in the lamina propria, while the release of IL-15 induces enterocyte apopotosis via NKG2D⁺ cells. Specific gliadin peptides interact with CXCR3 receptors expressed on the epithetlium's apical side [27]. This interaction triggers the release of zonulin leading to increase antigen trafficking [28,29]. Gliadin peptides are then translocated into the lamina propria where they are deamidated by transglutaminase 2 [30]. Consequently to the deamidation, the peptides interact with macrophages and dendritic cells of the intestinal submucosa [31]. The following Th1/Th17 driven adaptive immune response is characterized by high production of pro-inflmmatory cytokines IFN-γ, tumor necrosis factor-α (TNF-α) and interleukin-17 (IL-17), which further increase intestinal permeability and provoke damage in the intestinal mucosa [32] (Figure 1).

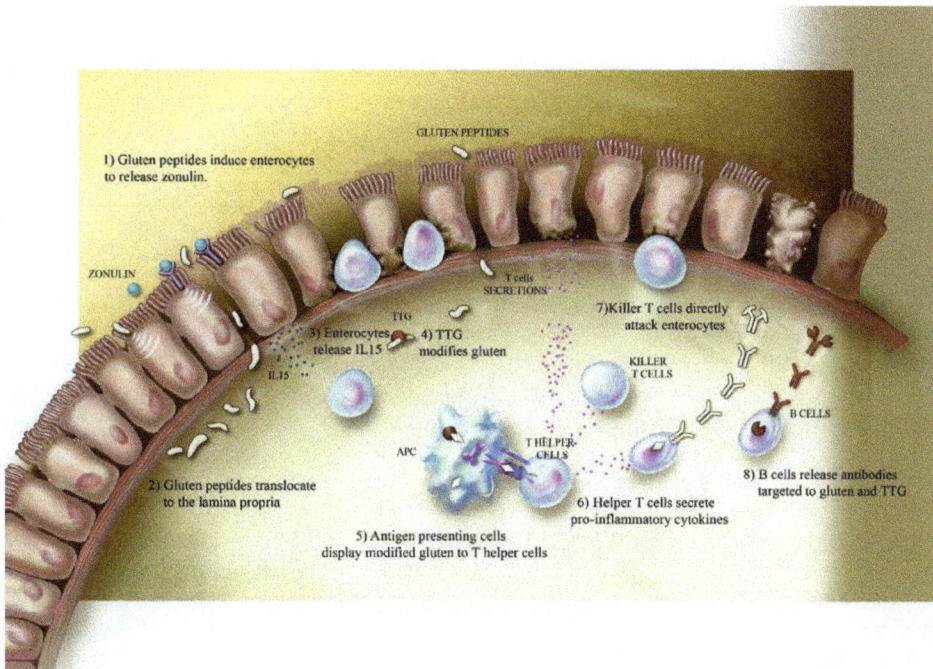

Figure 1. Mechanisms by which ingested gluten triggers celiac disease: digested gluten interacts with epithelial cells in the small intestine and triggers the disruption of tight junctions (1). The consequent increased intestinal permeability leads to the translocation of gluten peptides to the lamina propria (2) where they induce the production of IL-15 (3). In the lamina propria, gluten peptides are modified by tissue transglutaminase enzymes (4) and trigger an adaptive immune response (5–8).

Several studies have focused on the specific components of gluten that play a role in the various steps of disease onset. Many epitopes have been described and associated respectively with increased gut permeability, cytotoxic or immunomodulatory activities [33]. The majority of these epitopes are found in α- and ω-gliadins. The 57-89 peptide (33-mer) α-gliadin fragment has been particularly well studied. It contains most of the epitopes and has been reported to have immunomodulatory effects [34]. Shan *et al.* identified three distinct T cell epitopes within its aminoacidic sequence and they demonstrated its strong proteolitic resistance during digestion. Other known peptides are the cytotoxic peptide, the gut permeating peptides and the IL-8 releasing peptide [35].

As with many other autoimmune diseases, CD has been characterized by an increased worldwide prevalence in recent decades. Rubio-Tapia *et al.* showed that the incidence of CD in the USA has increased five-fold in fifty years [36]; similar results have been reported in Finland, where the overall prevalence of CD increased from 1.05% to 1.99% in 20 years [37]. Catassi *et al.* confirmed the increase in incidence of the disease in the past three decades and demonstrated that the loss of immunological tolerance to gluten can also occur later in adulthood [9].

The reasons behind the increased prevalence of CD in the last 50 years are not fully understood. The rapid change in incidence suggests that this higher prevalence cannot be attributed exclusively to genetic changes in the populations, but rather to environmental factors. The hygiene hypothesis has long been considered as the most plausible explanation for the increased incidence of autoimmune diseases; however, data from developing countries suggest that this may not be the case for CD. Several studies have considered variables that may be related to the increased incidence of CD, focusing mostly on timing of gluten introduction, amount of gluten supplemented to the diet, and the effects of breast feeding.

The introduction of gluten to Man's diet has been reported to occur around 10,000 years ago; since then, its consumption has expanded up to five-fold [38]. Many hypothesize that the increased gluten intake of the last few decades paired with the introduction of a westernized diet in many countries may play a critical role in the increased prevalence of CD worldwide. In the last fifty years, an increase in gluten consumption has been reported in countries like Italy and Sweden. The corresponding increase in prevalence of CD in the same countries suggests that the amount of gluten consumed may be considered a major risk factor for development of CD [39,40]. This hypothesis appears to be corroborated by studies that show the introduction of a small amount of gluten between four and six months of age reduces the risk of the disease [41]. A retrospective analysis study explored whether the increased incidence of CD might be due to an increased gluten content in wheat derived from wheat breeding. Domesticated modern wheat has been shown to significantly differ from wild wheat: modern wheat has larger grains and higher protein content [38]. Interestingly, the author of this study did not find clear evidence to corroborate this hypothesis. Furthermore, the lack of sufficient data regarding the incidence of CD per year made it difficult to determine if the pro capita intake of wheat or gluten might have played a role in the incidence of CD. Another important aspect speculated to be a risk factor for CD is the time of gluten introduction in the infant diet. In the mid-1980s, the Swedish epidemic of symptomatic CD coincided with the new dietary recommendation of not feeding gluten-containing foods to infants until six months of age. Interestingly, the incidence of CD decreased when an earlier introduction of gluten (>4 months) was reintroduced as the standard of care in Sweden [40]. Conversely, two recent studies that followed infants deemed as high risk of CD, due to first degree relation to a CD patient, concluded that the timing of gluten introduction was not a significant factor in determining disease onset, although a later introduction of gluten was shown to be associated with a delayed onset of the disease [3,42]. The same studies also considered the effects of additional biological and environmental factors such as breast feeding and genetic predisposition to CD. Particularly during the first months of life, breast-feeding is well-regarded as the optimal feeding mode for infants. The advantages of breast-feeding in the health of infants have been reported by several studies [43,44]. Human milk aids in growth and supports the child's neural and immunological development. However, the question whether breast-feeding can protect against the development of CD has been a matter of discussion for long time. An analysis of the Swedish CD epidemic reported that the development of CD in children under two years of age was reduced if they were still breast-fed when dietary gluten was introduced and that this "protective effect" of breast-feeding was even more pronounced if the infants were breast-fed also after the introduction of gluten [45]. Lionetti *et al.* showed that breast feeding did not modify the risk of CD among at risk-infants [3]. Similar data were confirmed by another study in which the authors concluded that CD development is not influenced by the duration of breast-feeding or by continuing breast-feeding after introduction of gluten [46].

Several studies have focused on relating intestinal dysbiosis to various diseases, among which CD is included. It has been shown that the dysbiosis characterizing active CD patients is partially reversible and linked to the presence of gluten in the diet. Nadal *et al.* found that the initiation of a GFD normalized the increase of gram-negative bacteria, *Bacteroides* and *E. coli* groups that characterized children with active CD [47]. Similarly, a study from Collado *et al.* reported that the elimination of gluten from the diet of pediatric patients led to a reduction in *E. coli* and *Staphylococcus*, which were found to be in higher abundance during the active state of the disease [5]. The beneficial effects of a GFD on the microflora and its metabolic function seem to be related to diet duration [48].

3. Type-1 Diabetes

T1D is an autoimmune disorder caused by the destruction of the insulin producing β-cells of the pancreas [49]. Although it is widely accepted that adults can also develop T1D, the highest incidence rate is found in adolescents [50–52]. Epidemiological studies have estimated the worldwide prevalence of T1D to be less than 1%. Recent evidences, however, suggest that its incidence has been increasing 3% per year [53]. Some large scale studies, such as The Environmental Determinants of Diabetes in the Young (TEDDY) [54], The Diabetes AutoImmunity Study in the Young (DAISY) [55], and TrialNet [56], have been initiated to identify potential environmental triggers and biomarkers for T1D so that, in the future, intervention may be possible to delay or even prevent the development of this condition.

The disease's first manifestations develop when lack of insulin prevents cells from adequate glucose uptake, which is necessary and vital to cell function. Classic symptoms include polyuria, polydipsia, weight loss, fatigue, and hyperglycemia, which, if left untreated, can lead to a coma and ultimately to death [57]. Diagnosis of diabetes includes fasting blood glucose higher than 126 mg/dL, any blood glucose of 200 mg/dL or an abnormal oral glucose-tolerance test [58]. Since 2009, the American Diabetes Association has modified the guidelines for diabetes diagnosis to include the measurement of glycated hemoglobin levels (A1C). This reflects the amount of blood glucose attached to hemoglobin and it is considered positive if higher than 6.5% on two occasions.

An important serological component that characterizes T1D and distinguishes it from type 2 diabetes is the presence of auto-antibodies against β-cell auto-antigens. Islet cell antibodies (ICA) were the first auto-antibodies described to be associated with the development of T1D [59]. In addition to ICA, more than 90% of T1D patients have auto-antibodies to insulin (IAA) [60], glutamic acid decarboxylase (GADA) [61], and protein tyrosine phosphatase like protein (IA2). These auto-antibodies are also used to identify subjects at high risk of developing the disease, since they are present months to years before symptom onset and can be detected in serum as early as six months of age in genetically susceptible individuals [62].

The exact pathogenesis of T1D is not completely understood, however it is well accepted that both genetic and environmental factors play a role. The genetic locus with the highest association to T1D is the HLA locus, which accounts for about 50% of the genetic load [63]. HLA DQ2 and DQ8 loci are the strongest determinants of diabetes susceptibility and HLA DR4 and DR3 have been shown to be associated with T1D. The heterozygous DR3/DR4 genotype is associated with the highest risk of disease onset, followed by DR3/DR3 and DR4/DR4 homozygosity [64].

Other genes that have also been associated with T1D are IL-2 receptor α [65], cytotoxic T lymphocyte antigen (CTLA4) [66], protein tyrosine phosphatase non-receptor 22 (PTPN22) [67], intercellular adhesion molecule 1 (ICAM1) [68], and the insulin gene (INS) [69]. In addition to genetic components, it is suggested that environmental factors may play a key role in T1D onset. The incidence of diabetes is increasing faster than can be explained by genetics alone, which is likely due to environmental changes.

Although many possible contributing environmental factors have been identified, to date none have been confirmed as a clear causative agent of T1D. The most frequently proposed candidates are viruses, such as enteroviruses [70–73], rotavirus [74,75], and rubella [52]. The potential role of these pathogens in the onset of T1D would corroborate the hygiene hypothesis [76]. In the last decades, changes in microbiome composition has also been suggested to be involved in the development of T1D by either altering intestinal permeability or modifying immune system regulation [77]. Studies in non-obese diabetic (NOD) mice in specific pathogen-free or germ free conditions confirmed the role of the microbiome in the regulation of islet specific autoimmunity [78]. Human studies have shown a correlation between T1D onset and a lower diversity and stability of the intestinal microflora, including a decreased ratio between *Firmicutes* and *Bacteroidetes* [79,80]. Other environmental factors such as climate and nutrition have been shown to be risk factors for T1D, but also in these cases there is no strong evidence that these agents are causative of T1D [81].

4. Type 1 Diabetes and Gluten

Although numerous studies have suggested a potentially pathogenic role of gluten in T1D, the exact mechanisms by which it may play a role in the onset and development of T1D are not yet fully understood (Box 1).

Studies in human samples have reported that upon stimulation with wheat proteins or their components, patients with T1D showed a heightened proliferative T cell response as compared to control patients [82–84]. PBMC from these patients produced significantly more pro-inflammatory cytokines compared to control subjects. Similarly, Klemetti *et al.* found that PBMC from T1D patients proliferated more as compared to controls when stimulated with wheat proteins [85]. This proliferative behavior, however, appeared to depend on the duration of disease. While 24% of patients with newly diagnosed T1D responded to the stimulus, only 15% of patients with longer duration of T1D and 5% of non-disease control subjects showed proliferative behavior. Such observed alterations characterizing the adaptive immune response are not restricted to the periphery. Jejunal biopsies from patients with T1D have increased CD25+ mononuclear cell density as compared to control patients when stimulated with gliadin [83]. Furthermore, observations *in vivo* showed that rectal administration of gluten in T1D patients induced infiltration of CD3 and Tγδ rectal lymphocytes in a subgroup of patients [84]. Dietary gluten has also been shown to affect components of the innate immune system, such as dendritic cells [86].

The use of animal models, such as the NOD mice or BBdp rats, have allowed for a better understanding of the effect of dietary gluten on T1D progression, even as early as during gestation. The cumulative incidence of T1D has been shown to be reduced in offspring of NOD mice fed a GFD during pregnancy [87]. Similarly, it has been found that diabetes onset is delayed in offspring of NOD mice fed a modified diet (in which wheat barley proteins were absent) during gestation [88]. These results do not seem to translate to humans, as Lamb *et al.* found the maternal frequency of ingestion of gluten-containing foods during the final trimester of pregnancy to have no effect on the development of T1D in offspring [89].

A reduced incidence of diabetes was observed in NOD mouse offspring from mothers fed a basal (gluten-containing) diet during gestation but a wheat barley protein-free (WBP) diet at or after weaning [88]. Similarly, offspring from basal fed mothers who started a WBP free diet after weaning had reduced T1D incidence compared to offspring with identical gestational feeding practices but who received a basal diet after weaning. Taken together, these findings suggest that the infant diet during weaning is a stronger modulator of T1D development than maternal feeding practices during gestation. In humans, the effect of timing of gluten introduction on T1D and/or IA development remains controversial. Some studies report a marked increase in risk of IA development and/or T1D incidence in infants introduced to gluten prior to three months of age or later than six months of age [90–93], while others report no effect whatsoever [94,95]. Interestingly, a Swedish group has reported that the introduction of gluten after six months of age increased risk of GADA or IA-2A positivity almost six-fold in children who also were introduced to cow's milk formula before two months of age [93]. This finding therefore suggests a synergistic effect of early exposure to cow's milk formula and late exposure to gluten.

There is strong evidence that removal of gluten from the diet can selectively be protective against development of diabetes [96,97]. Incidence of hypoglycemia is higher in NOD mice maintained on a gluten-containing diet, while a GFD casein-based diet serves to reduce incidence of hypoglycemia, delay onset of T1D, and reduce IA titers [98]. Additionally, incidence of diabetes in NOD mice maintained on a WBP-free diet is reduced as compared to mice maintained on a standard gluten containing diet (51% *versus* 81%), and IA titers are lower in NOD mice maintained on a lifelong WBP diet or a WBP diet following weaning [88]. Hypothesized mechanisms for these advantageous effects of GFD include modification of intestinal permeability and the composition of the gut microbiota. Watts *et al.* found an increase in intraluminal zonulin in BBdp rats just prior to hypoglycemia, which correlated with increased intestinal permeability in the animals [99].

The elimination of gluten from the diet has been shown to be advantageous also by modulating the microbiota composition. Marietta and colleagues observed that NOD mice fed a standard gluten-containing diet had increased *Barnesiella*, *Bifidobacterium*, *Tannerella* and *Turcibacter* microbes, as compared to an increase in *Akkermansia* and *Bacteroides* microbes in GFD NOD mice [96]. In addition, NOD mice fed a GFD were observed to have greater total microbial richness than NOD mice fed a gluten-containing diet. Hansen and colleagues also reported distinct microbial signatures associated with diet and found a marked increase in the bacterial phylum *Verrucomicrobia*, TM7 and *Proteobacteria* in GFD NOD mice [87]. In BBdp animal models, total islet number was increased in rats housed in germ-free *versus* specific pathogen-free (SPF) conditions [98]. In these SPF conditions, beta cell mass was lowest in BBdp animals fed a gluten-containing diet. Taken together, these findings suggest that microbes play an important role in modulating islet and beta cell integrity, which in turn modulates development of T1D.

Box 1. Main findings about the correlation between gluten and the onset of T1D.

- *In vitro* studies:

  - Upon stimulation with wheat proteins T cells from T1D patients show a higher proliferative and pro-inflammatory response than T cells from control subjects [85].
  - Upon stimulation with gliadin, jejunal biopsies from T1D patients show increased CD25+ cell density as compared to control patients [83].

- *In vivo* studies:

  - Incidence of T1D is reduced in offspring of NOD mice fed a GFD during pregnancy [87].
  - Removal of gluten from the diet selectively protects NOD mice from developing T1D [96].
  - FGD casein-based diet reduces incidence of hypoglycemia, delays onset of T1D and reduces IA titers in NOD mice [98].
  - Gluten containing diet alters the composition of the innate immune system in BALB/c and NOD mice and it is correlated with an increased expression of dendritic cells activation markers in NOD mice [86].

- *Human studies:*

  - Introduction of gluten in the diet of infants prior to 3 months of age or later than 6 months is correlated with an increase in risk of IA development and T1D incidence [91,92].
  - Introduction of gluten after 6 months of age increases risk of GADA and IA-2A positivity [93].

Box 1 summarizes the main findings about the correlation between gluten and the onset of T1D.

5. Comorbidity between Celiac Disease and Type-1 Diabetes

The association between CD and T1D was first reported in the late 1960s. The prevalence of CD in patients with T1D is estimated to fall between 1.4% and 19.7% [100–103]. This comorbidity can largely be attributed to overlapping genetic HLA risk loci; in both conditions, the HLA-DQ2 and DQ8 genes have been shown to be important determinants of disease susceptibility. Additionally, some non-HLA genes such as PTPN22 and CTLA4 have been associated with either CD or T1D [67].

Usually, T1D develops prior to diagnosis of CD, though cases exist in which CD develops as the primary disease and T1D develops later in life [104–107]. In the latter case, individuals are significantly older at T1D onset than those who develop it prior to CD. Additionally, individuals who develop CD and T1D tend to be younger at diabetes onset than those with T1D who never go on to develop CD [108].

Because of the high rate of comorbidity between CD and T1D, there is great need for a more efficient, targeted diagnostic approach. Numerous findings suggest that many CD cases in T1D patients would be overlooked by use of a single serological screening at T1D onset. Tsouka and colleagues recently found that 12.2% of patients who eventually came to have dual diagnosis of CD and T1D first presented with at least one negative celiac screen (in serum) after T1D diagnosis [101]. On average, 47.8 months lapsed between the first negative serological test and a positive result suggesting CD autoimmunity (CDA). Additionally, a cohort by Bakker and colleagues found that 42% of T1D patients who came to develop CD were not diagnosed (with CD) until 10 years following T1D onset [106]. It is also important to recognize that serological markers of CD in patients with T1D may not always prove specific or reliable. It has been recently reported that a small subset of T1D children found to have CDA will spontaneously normalize their celiac serology with a median time of 1.3 years and thus will not be diagnosed with overt CD [102,109]. Though the authors did not classify their participants in this way, those found to have transiently elevated or fluctuating levels of anti-tTG IgA are generally termed as having potential CD. In the work of Castellaneta and colleagues, a small group of T1D patients with potential CD were found to have only an infiltrative lesion or entirely normal mucosa upon inspection with upper endoscopy.

The importance of a systematically correct and timely diagnosis is highlighted by the fact that additional autoimmune diseases are often reported to occur secondary to onset of comorbid T1D and CD with autoimmune thyroid disease (ATD) presenting most commonly [105,106]. Furthermore, Shah *et al.* found that children with dual diagnosis are three times more likely to be vitamin D deficient as compared to healthy children without autoimmune conditions [110]. In the cohort, risk of vitamin D deficiency for children with T1D alone was increased over healthy children by only 1.5 times. This raises the question of whether bone health is affected for children diagnosed with both T1D and CD. Joshi and colleagues reported that children with T1D found to have CDA have lower bone mineral density at the whole body and lumbar spine compared to children with T1D alone. In terms of other medical complications that may arise due to dual diagnosis of CD and T1D, findings are mixed regarding whether individuals with dual diagnosis are at greater risk of retinopathy or nephropathy compared to those with T1D alone (Table 1) [111].

It has been suggested that symptoms associated with CD are more difficult to control in patients that have also T1D. Mackinder *et al.* showed that levels of tTG (IgA) took longer to normalize for children with dual diagnosis compared to children diagnosed with CD alone [100]. Another group found the majority of T1D children diagnosed with concomitant CD presented with gastrointestinal symptoms, all of which resolved with adoption of the gluten free diet. In addition to this, BMI and weight SDS improved significantly in these children, and a trend was observed towards an increase in insulin requirement only for children who were compliant with the gluten free diet [107]. However, it remains to be elucidated whether metabolic control improves for T1D patients with underlying concomitant CD after adoption of the GFD. Two different studies reported higher HbA1c levels and more frequent hypoglycemic episodes in T1D children found to have CDA as compared to children with T1D alone [107,111]. Conversely, others have reported no difference in insulin requirement or growth status between dual diagnosis individuals and individuals with T1D alone [106].

A growing body of evidence suggests that the beneficial effects of a GFD (for patients with concomitant CD) may actually protect against development of further T1D-related complications. Compared to T1D patients without CD, Bakker and colleagues found a lower prevalence of retinopathy and lower total cholesterol in adult T1D patients with concomitant CD. Warncke *et al.*, similarly, reported lower absolute systolic blood pressure in T1D patients with CD as compared to those without CD, suggesting that this modulatory effect is attributed to the GFD [108]. In the same cohort, patients with dual diagnosis had significantly lower levels of HDL cholesterol as compared to individuals with T1D alone; after institution of a GFD, these levels increased significantly and the difference between groups disappeared. It is possible that these improvements in cholesterol level could be due to the normalization of the intestinal mucosa with adoption of a GFD, demonstrating a beneficial effect of adhering to the diet.

Table 1. Main features of celiac disease and type 1 diabetes.

Feature	Celiac Disease	Type 1 Diabetes
Wordwide incidence	0.6% *–1%	<1%
Contribution of HLA genes	HLA DQ2 (**DQA1*05-DQB1*02**) HLA DQ8 (**DQA1*03-DQB1*03:02**)	HLADQ2 and/or DQ8 (**DRB1*0401-DQB1*03:02** and **DRB1*0301-DQB1*0201**)
Non-HLA candidate genes	CTLA4, PTPN22,CD28, ICOS, MYO9B	CTLA4, PTPN22, MIC-A
Symptoms	Diarrhea, steatorrhea, weight loss, failure to thrive, iron deficiency, abdominal pain, reduced bone density, chronic fatigue, growth failure.	Polyuria, polydipsia, extensive hunger, weight loss, chronic fatigue, reduced bone density, growth failure, hyperglycemia.
Diagnosis	Small intestinal biopsy, generally with supporting serological testing.Serologic tests: IgA anti-tTG, IgG anti-tTG, IgA anti-EMA, IgG DGP.	Blood test: Fasting blood glucose level, oral glucose tolerance test, A1C. Serologic tests: ICA, IAA, GADA, IA2 antibodies
Comorbidities	Type 1 diabetes, Down syndrome, Turner syndrome, William's syndrome, vitiligo, Addison's disease, hyperparathyroidism, neuropathy, IgA nephropathy, psoriasis.	Celiac disease, Grave's disease, Hashimoto's disease, Addison disease, vitiligo, autoimmune thyroid disease.
Pathogenesis	Enteropathy is due to dysregulation of the innate and adaptive immune system. Alteration of intestinal permeability.	Autoimmune destruction of pancreatic insulin-producing β-cells by an adaptive and innate immune response. Alteration of intestinal permeability.

6. Conclusions

In this review, we focused on the role of gluten as an important player in the pathogenesis of CD and T1D. The high rate of comorbidity between these two autoimmune diseases and their rapidly increasing prevalence in the last few decades underscore the importance of screening in high risk patients and the need to further explore and detail the contributory role of environmental factors that may be involved.

Conflicts of Interest: The authors declare no conflict of interest.

References

1. Castillo, N.E.; Theethira, T.G.; Leffler, D.A. The present and the future in the diagnosis and management of celiac disease. *Gastroenterol. Rep.* **2015**, *3*, 3–11. [CrossRef] [PubMed]
2. Lundin, K.E.; Sollid, L.M. Advances in coeliac disease. *Curr. Opin. Gastroenterol.* **2014**, *30*, 154–162. [CrossRef] [PubMed]

3. Lionetti, E.; Castellaneta, S.; Francavilla, R.; Pulvirenti, A.; Tonutti, E.; Amarri, S.; Barbato, M.; Barbera, C.; Barera, G.; Bellantoni, A.; *et al.* Introduction of gluten, HLA status, and the risk of celiac disease in children. *N. Engl. J. Med.* **2014**, *371*, 1295–1303. [CrossRef] [PubMed]

4. Gutierrez-Achury, J.; Zhernakova, A.; Pulit, S.L.; Trynka, G.; Hunt, K.A.; Romanos, J.; Raychaudhuri, S.; van Heel, D.A.; Wijmenga, C.; de Bakker, P.I. Fine mapping in the MHC region accounts for 18% additional genetic risk for celiac disease. *Nat. Genet.* **2015**, *47*, 577–578. [CrossRef] [PubMed]

5. Collado, M.C.; Donat, E.; Ribes-Koninckx, C.; Calabuig, M.; Sanz, Y. Specific duodenal and faecal bacterial groups associated with paediatric coeliac disease. *J. Clin. Pathol.* **2009**, *62*, 264–269. [CrossRef] [PubMed]

6. Sellitto, M.; Bai, G.; Serena, G.; Fricke, W.F.; Sturgeon, C.; Gajer, P.; White, J.R.; Koenig, S.S.; Sakamoto, J.; Boothe, D.; *et al.* Proof of concept of microbiome-metabolome analysis and delayed gluten exposure on celiac disease autoimmunity in genetically at-risk infants. *PLoS ONE* **2012**, *7*, e33387. [CrossRef] [PubMed]

7. Yap, T.W.; Chan, W.K.; Leow, A.H.; Azmi, A.N.; Loke, M.F.; Vadivelu, J.; Goh, K.L. Prevalence of serum celiac antibodies in a multiracial Asian population—A first study in the young Asian adult population of Malaysia. *PLoS ONE* **2015**, *10*, e0121908. [CrossRef] [PubMed]

8. Emilsson, L.; Wijmenga, C.; Murray, J.A.; Ludvigsson, J.F. Autoimmune Disease in First-Degree Relatives and Spouses of Individuals With Celiac Disease. *Clin. Gastroenterol. Hepatol. Off. Clin. Pract. J. Am. Gastroenterol. Assoc.* **2015**, *13*, 1271–1277. [CrossRef] [PubMed]

9. Catassi, C.; Kryszak, D.; Bhatti, B.; Sturgeon, C.; Helzlsouer, K.; Clipp, S.L.; Gelfond, D.; Puppa, E.; Sferruzza, A.; Fasano, A. Natural history of celiac disease autoimmunity in a USA cohort followed since 1974. *Ann. Med.* **2010**, *42*, 530–538. [CrossRef] [PubMed]

10. Kelly, C.P.; Bai, J.C.; Liu, E.; Leffler, D.A. Advances in diagnosis and management of celiac disease. *Gastroenterology* **2015**, *148*, 1175–1186. [CrossRef] [PubMed]

11. Dieterich, W.; Ehnis, T.; Bauer, M.; Donner, P.; Volta, U.; Riecken, E.O.; Schuppan, D. Identification of tissue transglutaminase as the autoantigen of celiac disease. *Nat. Med.* **1997**, *3*, 797–801. [CrossRef] [PubMed]

12. Fasano, A.; Catassi, C. Clinical practice: Celiac disease. *N. Engl. J. Med.* **2012**, *367*, 2419–2426. [CrossRef] [PubMed]

13. Lee, H.J.; Andreson, Z.; Ryu, D. Gluten free contamination in foods labeles "Gluten free" in United States. *J. Food Prot.* **2014**, *77*, 1830–1833. [CrossRef] [PubMed]

14. Fasano, A.; Not, T.; Wang, W.; Uzzau, S.; Berti, I.; Tommasini, A.; Goldblum, S.E. Zonulin, a newly discovered modulator of intestinal permeability, and its expression in coeliac disease. *Lancet* **2000**, *355*, 1518–1519. [CrossRef]

15. Fasano, A. Surprises from celiac disease. *Sci. Am.* **2009**, *301*, 54–61. [CrossRef] [PubMed]

16. Maiuri, L.; Ciacci, C.; Ricciardelli, I.; Vacca, L.; Raia, V.; Rispo, A.; Griffin, M.; Issekutz, T.; Quaratino, S.; Londei, M. Unexpected role of surface transglutaminase type II in celiac disease. *Gastroenterology* **2005**, *129*, 1400–1413. [CrossRef] [PubMed]

17. Gianfrani, C.; Siciliano, R.A.; Facchiano, A.M.; Camarca, A.; Mazzeo, M.F.; Costantini, S.; Salvati, V.M.; Maurano, F.; Mazzarella, G.; Iaquinto, G.; *et al.* Transamidation of wheat flour inhibits the response to gliadin of intestinal T cells in celiac disease. *Gastroenterology* **2007**, *133*, 780–789. [CrossRef] [PubMed]

18. Meresse, B.; Ripoche, J.; Heyman, M.; Cerf-Bensussan, N. Celiac disease: From oral tolerance to intestinal inflammation, autoimmunity and lymphomagenesis. *Mucosal Immunol.* **2009**, *2*, 8–23. [CrossRef] [PubMed]

19. Nikulina, M.; Habich, C.; Flohe, S.B.; Scott, F.W.; Kolb, H. Wheat gluten causes dendritic cell maturation and chemokine secretion. *J. Immunol.* **2004**, *173*, 1925–1933. [CrossRef] [PubMed]

20. Skovbjerg, H.; Koch, C.; Anthonsen, D.; Sjostrom, H. Deamidation and cross-linking of gliadin peptides by transglutaminases and the relation to celiac disease. *Biochim. Biophys. Acta* **2004**, *1690*, 220–230. [CrossRef] [PubMed]

21. Castellanos-Rubio, A.; Santin, I.; Irastorza, I.; Castano, L.; Carlos Vitoria, J.; Ramon Bilbao, J. TH17 (and TH1) signatures of intestinal biopsies of CD patients in response to gliadin. *Autoimmunity* **2009**, *42*, 69–73. [CrossRef] [PubMed]

22. Palova-Jelinkova, L.; Danova, K.; Drasarova, H.; Dvorak, M.; Funda, D.P.; Fundova, P.; Kotrbova-Kozak, A.; Cerna, M.; Kamanova, J.; Martin, S.F.; *et al.* Pepsin digest of wheat gliadin fraction increases production of IL-1β via TLR4/MyD88/TRIF/MAPK/NF-κB signaling pathway and an NLRP3 inflammasome activation. *PLoS ONE* **2013**, *8*, e62426. [CrossRef] [PubMed]

Nutrients **2015**, *7*, 7143–7162

23. Di Sabatino, A.; Ciccocioppo, R.; Cupelli, F.; Cinque, B.; Millimaggi, D.; Clarkson, M.M.; Paulli, M.; Cifone, M.G.; Corazza, G.R. Epithelium derived interleukin 15 regulates intraepithelial lymphocyte Th1 cytokine production, cytotoxicity, and survival in coeliac disease. *Gut* **2006**, *55*, 469–477. [CrossRef] [PubMed]

24. Harris, K.M.; Fasano, A.; Mann, D.L. Monocytes differentiated with IL-15 support Th17 and Th1 responses to wheat gliadin: Implications for celiac disease. *Clin. Immunol.* **2010**, *135*, 430–439. [CrossRef] [PubMed]

25. De Nitto, D.; Monteleone, I.; Franze, E.; Pallone, F.; Monteleone, G. Involvement of interleukin-15 and interleukin-21, two γ-chain-related cytokines, in celiac disease. *World J. Gastroenterol.* **2009**, *15*, 4609–4614. [CrossRef] [PubMed]

26. Lammers, K.M.; Lu, R.; Brownley, J.; Lu, B.; Gerard, C.; Thomas, K.; Rallabhandi, P.; Shea-Donohue, T.; Tamiz, A.; Alkan, S.; *et al.* Gliadin induces an increase in intestinal permeability and zonulin release by binding to the chemokine receptor CXCR3. *Gastroenterology* **2008**, *135*, 194–204. [CrossRef] [PubMed]

27. Lammers, K.M.; Khandelwal, S.; Chaudhry, F.; Kryszak, D.; Puppa, E.L.; Casolaro, V.; Fasano, A. Identification of a novel immunomodulatory gliadin peptide that causes interleukin-8 release in a chemokine receptor CXCR3-dependent manner only in patients with coeliac disease. *Immunology* **2011**, *132*, 432–440. [CrossRef] [PubMed]

28. Drago, S.; El Asmar, R.; di Pierro, M.; Grazia Clemente, M.; Tripathi, A.; Sapone, A.; Thakar, M.; Iacono, G.; Carroccio, A.; D'Agate, C.; *et al.* Gliadin, zonulin and gut permeability: Effects on celiac and non-celiac intestinal mucosa and intestinal cell lines. *Scand. J. Gastroenterol.* **2006**, *41*, 408–419. [CrossRef] [PubMed]

29. Fasano, A. Zonulin and its regulation of intestinal barrier function: The biological door to inflammation, autoimmunity, and cancer. *Physiol. Rev.* **2011**, *91*, 151–175. [CrossRef] [PubMed]

30. Garrote, J.A.; Gomez-Gonzalez, E.; Bernardo, D.; Arranz, E.; Chirdo, F. Celiac disease pathogenesis: The proinflammatory cytokine network. *J. Pediatr. Gastroenterol. Nutr.* **2008**, *47* (Suppl. 1), S27–S32. [CrossRef] [PubMed]

31. Thomas, K.E.; Sapone, A.; Fasano, A.; Vogel, S.N. Gliadin stimulation of murine macrophage inflammatory gene expression and intestinal permeability are MyD88-dependent: Role of the innate immune response in Celiac disease. *J. Immunol.* **2006**, *176*, 2512–2521. [CrossRef] [PubMed]

32. Ortega, C.; Fernandez, S.; Estevez, O.A.; Aguado, R.; Molina, I.J.; Santamaria, M. IL-17 producing T cells in celiac disease: Angels or devils? *Int. Rev. Immunol.* **2013**, *32*, 534–543. [CrossRef] [PubMed]

33. Anderson, R.P.; Degano, P.; Godkin, A.J.; Jewell, D.P.; Hill, A.V. *In vivo* antigen challenge in celiac disease identifies a single transglutaminase-modified peptide as the dominant A-gliadin T-cell epitope. *Nat. Med.* **2000**, *6*, 337–342. [CrossRef] [PubMed]

34. Shan, L.; Molberg, O.; Parrot, I.; Hausch, F.; Filiz, F.; Gray, G.M.; Sollid, L.M.; Khosla, C. Structural basis for gluten intolerance in celiac sprue. *Science* **2002**, *297*, 2275–2279. [CrossRef] [PubMed]

35. Camarca, M.E.; Mozzillo, E.; Nugnes, R.; Zito, E.; Falco, M.; Fattorusso, V.; Mobilia, S.; Buono, P.; Valerio, G.; Troncone, R.; *et al.* Celiac disease in type 1 diabetes mellitus. *Ital. J. Pediatr.* **2012**, *38*, 10. [CrossRef] [PubMed]

36. Rubio-Tapia, A.; Kyle, R.A.; Kaplan, E.L.; Johnson, D.R.; Page, W.; Erdtmann, F.; Brantner, T.L.; Kim, W.R.; Phelps, T.K.; Lahr, B.D.; *et al.* Increased prevalence and mortality in undiagnosed celiac disease. *Gastroenterology* **2009**, *137*, 88–93. [CrossRef] [PubMed]

37. Vilppula, A.; Kaukinen, K.; Luostarinen, L.; Krekela, I.; Patrikainen, H.; Valve, R.; Maki, M.; Collin, P. Increasing prevalence and high incidence of celiac disease in elderly people: A population-based study. *BMC Gastroenterol.* **2009**, *9*, 49. [CrossRef] [PubMed]

38. Kasarda, D.D. Can an increase in celiac disease be attributed to an increase in the gluten content of wheat as a consequence of wheat breeding? *J. Agric. Food Chem.* **2013**, *61*, 1155–1159. [CrossRef] [PubMed]

39. Hogberg, L.; Falth-Magnusson, K.; Grodzinsky, E.; Stenhammar, L. Familial prevalence of coeliac disease: A twenty-year follow-up study. *Scand. J. Gastroenterol.* **2003**, *38*, 61–65. [CrossRef] [PubMed]

40. Ivarsson, A.; Persson, L.A.; Nystrom, L.; Ascher, H.; Cavell, B.; Danielsson, L.; Dannaeus, A.; Lindberg, T.; Lindquist, B.; Stenhammar, L.; *et al.* Epidemic of coeliac disease in Swedish children. *Acta Paediatr.* **2000**, *89*, 165–171. [CrossRef] [PubMed]

41. Ivarsson, A.; Myleus, A.; Norstrom, F.; van der Pals, M.; Rosen, A.; Hogberg, L.; Danielsson, L.; Halvarsson, B.; Hammarroth, S.; Hernell, O.; *et al.* Prevalence of childhood celiac disease and changes in infant feeding. *Pediatrics* **2013**, *131*, e687–e694. [CrossRef] [PubMed]

42. Liu, E.; Lee, H.S.; Aronsson, C.A.; Hagopian, W.A.; Koletzko, S.; Rewers, M.J.; Eisenbarth, G.S.; Bingley, P.J.; Bonifacio, E.; Simell, V.; *et al.* Risk of pediatric celiac disease according to HLA haplotype and country. *N. Engl. J. Med.* **2014**, *371*, 42–49. [CrossRef] [PubMed]

43. Hosea Blewett, H.J.; Cicalo, M.C.; Holland, C.D.; Field, C.J. The immunological components of human milk. *Adv. Food Nutr. Res.* **2008**, *54*, 45–80. [PubMed]

44. Newburg, D.S.; Walker, W.A. Protection of the neonate by the innate immune system of developing gut and of human milk. *Pediatr. Res.* **2007**, *61*, 2–8. [CrossRef] [PubMed]

45. Ivarsson, A.; Hernell, O.; Stenlund, H.; Persson, L.A. Breast-feeding protects against celiac disease. *Am. J. Clin. Nutr.* **2002**, *75*, 914–921. [PubMed]

46. Vriezinga, S.L.; Auricchio, R.; Bravi, E.; Castillejo, G.; Chmielewska, A.; Crespo Escobar, P.; Kolacek, S.; Koletzko, S.; Korponay-Szabo, I.R.; Mummert, E.; *et al.* Randomized feeding intervention in infants at high risk for celiac disease. *N. Engl. J. Med.* **2014**, *371*, 1304–1315. [CrossRef] [PubMed]

47. Nadal, I.; Donat, E.; Ribes-Koninckx, C.; Calabuig, M.; Sanz, Y. Imbalance in the composition of the duodenal microbiota of children with coeliac disease. *J. Med. Microbiol.* **2007**, *56*, 1669–1674. [CrossRef] [PubMed]

48. Tjellstrom, B.; Hogberg, L.; Stenhammar, L.; Falth-Magnusson, K.; Magnusson, K.E.; Norin, E.; Sundqvist, T.; Midtvedt, T. Faecal short-chain fatty acid pattern in childhood coeliac disease is normalised after more than one year's gluten-free diet. *Microb. Ecol. Health Dis.* **2013**, *24*. [CrossRef] [PubMed]

49. Krumbhaar, E.B. Spontaneous Diabetes in a Dog. *J. Exp. Med.* **1916**, *24*, 361–365. [CrossRef] [PubMed]

50. Patterson, C.C.; Gyurus, E.; Rosenbauer, J.; Cinek, O.; Neu, A.; Schober, E.; Parslow, R.C.; Joner, G.; Svensson, J.; Castell, C.; *et al.* Trends in childhood type 1 diabetes incidence in Europe during 1989–2008: Evidence of non-uniformity over time in rates of increase. *Diabetologia* **2012**, *55*, 2142–2147. [CrossRef] [PubMed]

51. Patterson, C.C.; Dahlquist, G.G.; Gyurus, E.; Green, A.; Soltesz, G.; Group, E.S. Incidence trends for childhood type 1 diabetes in Europe during 1989–2003 and predicted new cases 2005–20: A multicentre prospective registration study. *Lancet* **2009**, *373*, 2027–2033. [CrossRef]

52. Harjutsalo, V.; Sjoberg, L.; Tuomilehto, J. Time trends in the incidence of type 1 diabetes in Finnish children: A cohort study. *Lancet* **2008**, *371*, 1777–1782. [CrossRef]

53. Tuomilehto, J. The emerging global epidemic of type 1 diabetes. *Curr. Diab. Rep.* **2013**, *13*, 795–804. [CrossRef] [PubMed]

54. Hagopian, W.A.; Lernmark, A.; Rewers, M.J.; Simell, O.G.; She, J.X.; Ziegler, A.G.; Krischer, J.P.; Akolkar, B. TEDDY—The Environmental Determinants of Diabetes in the Young: An observational clinical trial. *Ann. N. Y. Acad. Sci.* **2006**, *1079*, 320–326. [CrossRef] [PubMed]

55. Rewers, M.; Bugawan, T.L.; Norris, J.M.; Blair, A.; Beaty, B.; Hoffman, M.; McDuffie, R.S., Jr.; Hamman, R.F.; Klingensmith, G.; Eisenbarth, G.S.; *et al.* Newborn screening for HLA markers associated with IDDM: Diabetes autoimmunity study in the young (DAISY). *Diabetologia* **1996**, *39*, 807–812. [CrossRef] [PubMed]

56. Skyler, J.S.; Greenbaum, C.J.; Lachin, J.M.; Leschek, E.; Rafkin-Mervis, L.; Savage, P.; Spain, L.; Type 1 Diabetes TrialNet Study Group. Type 1 Diabetes TrialNet—An international collaborative clinical trials network. *Ann. N. Y. Acad. Sci.* **2008**, *1150*, 14–24. [CrossRef] [PubMed]

57. Foster, B. Diabetic Coma: Acetonaemia. *Br. Med. J.* **1878**, *1*, 78–81. [CrossRef] [PubMed]

58. American Diabetes Association. Standards of medical care in diabetes—2012. *Diabetes Care* **2012**, *35* (Suppl. S1), S11–S63.

59. Bottazzo, G.F.; Florin-Christensen, A.; Doniach, D. Islet-cell antibodies in diabetes mellitus with autoimmune polyendocrine deficiencies. *Lancet* **1974**, *2*, 1279–1283. [CrossRef]

60. Palmer, J.P.; Asplin, C.M.; Clemons, P.; Lyen, K.; Tatpati, O.; Raghu, P.K.; Paquette, T.L. Insulin antibodies in insulin-dependent diabetics before insulin treatment. *Science* **1983**, *222*, 1337–1339. [CrossRef] [PubMed]

61. Baekkeskov, S.; Aanstoot, H.J.; Christgau, S.; Reetz, A.; Solimena, M.; Cascalho, M.; Folli, F.; Richter-Olesen, H.; de Camilli, P. Identification of the 64K autoantigen in insulin-dependent diabetes as the GABA-synthesizing enzyme glutamic acid decarboxylase. *Nature* **1990**, *347*, 151–156. [CrossRef] [PubMed]

62. Atkinson, M.A.; Eisenbarth, G.S.; Michels, A.W. Type 1 diabetes. *Lancet* **2014**, *383*, 69–82. [CrossRef]

63. Stankov, K.; Benc, D.; Draskovic, D. Genetic and epigenetic factors in etiology of diabetes mellitus type 1. *Pediatrics* **2013**, *132*, 1112–1122. [CrossRef] [PubMed]

64. Svejgaard, A.; Ryder, L.P. HLA and insulin-dependent diabetes: An overview. *Genet. Epidemiol.* **1989**, *6*, 1–14. [CrossRef] [PubMed]

65. Vella, A.; Cooper, J.D.; Lowe, C.E.; Walker, N.; Nutland, S.; Widmer, B.; Jones, R.; Ring, S.M.; McArdle, W.; Pembrey, M.E.; *et al.* Localization of a type 1 diabetes locus in the IL2RA/CD25 region by use of tag single-nucleotide polymorphisms. *Am. J. Hum. Genet.* **2005**, *76*, 773–779. [CrossRef] [PubMed]

66. Nistico, L.; Buzzetti, R.; Pritchard, L.E.; van der Auwera, B.; Giovannini, C.; Bosi, E.; Larrad, M.T.; Rios, M.S.; Chow, C.C.; Cockram, C.S.; *et al.* The CTLA-4 gene region of chromosome 2q33 is linked to, and associated with, type 1 diabetes. Belgian Diabetes Registry. *Hum. Mol. Genet.* **1996**, *5*, 1075–1080. [CrossRef] [PubMed]

67. Bottini, N.; Musumeci, L.; Alonso, A.; Rahmouni, S.; Nika, K.; Rostamkhani, M.; MacMurray, J.; Meloni, G.F.; Lucarelli, P.; Pellecchia, M.; *et al.* A functional variant of lymphoid tyrosine phosphatase is associated with type I diabetes. *Nat. Genet.* **2004**, *36*, 337–338. [CrossRef] [PubMed]

68. Nishimura, M.; Obayashi, H.; Maruya, E.; Ohta, M.; Tegoshi, H.; Fukui, M.; Hasegawa, G.; Shigeta, H.; Kitagawa, Y.; Nakano, K.; *et al.* Association between type 1 diabetes age-at-onset and intercellular adhesion molecule-1 (ICAM-1) gene polymorphism. *Hum. Immunol.* **2000**, *61*, 507–510. [CrossRef]

69. Bell, G.I.; Horita, S.; Karam, J.H. A polymorphic locus near the human insulin gene is associated with insulin-dependent diabetes mellitus. *Diabetes* **1984**, *33*, 176–183. [CrossRef] [PubMed]

70. Sadeharju, K.; Hamalainen, A.M.; Knip, M.; Lonnrot, M.; Koskela, P.; Virtanen, S.M.; Ilonen, J.; Akerblom, H.K.; Hyoty, H.; Finnish, T.S.G. Enterovirus infections as a risk factor for type I diabetes: Virus analyses in a dietary intervention trial. *Clin. Exp. Immunol.* **2003**, *132*, 271–277. [CrossRef] [PubMed]

71. Lonnrot, M.; Knip, M.; Roivainen, M.; Koskela, P.; Akerblom, H.K.; Hyoty, H. Onset of type 1 diabetes mellitus in infancy after enterovirus infections. *Diabet. Med.* **1998**, *15*, 431–434. [CrossRef]

72. Hyoty, H.; Hiltunen, M.; Knip, M.; Laakkonen, M.; Vahasalo, P.; Karjalainen, J.; Koskela, P.; Roivainen, M.; Leinikki, P.; Hovi, T.; *et al.* A prospective study of the role of coxsackie B and other enterovirus infections in the pathogenesis of IDDM. *Diabetes* **1995**, *44*, 652–657. [CrossRef] [PubMed]

73. Muir, P.; Singh, N.B.; Banatvala, J.E. Enterovirus-specific serum IgA antibody responses in patients with acute infections, chronic cardiac disease, and recently diagnosed insulin-dependent diabetes mellitus. *J. Med. Virol.* **1990**, *32*, 236–242. [CrossRef] [PubMed]

74. Honeyman, M.C.; Stone, N.L.; Harrison, L.C. T-cell epitopes in type 1 diabetes autoantigen tyrosine phosphatase IA-2: Potential for mimicry with rotavirus and other environmental agents. *Mol. Med.* **1998**, *4*, 231–239. [PubMed]

75. Honeyman, M.C.; Coulson, B.S.; Stone, N.L.; Gellert, S.A.; Goldwater, P.N.; Steele, C.E.; Couper, J.J.; Tait, B.D.; Colman, P.G.; Harrison, L.C. Association between rotavirus infection and pancreatic islet autoimmunity in children at risk of developing type 1 diabetes. *Diabetes* **2000**, *49*, 1319–1324. [CrossRef] [PubMed]

76. Okada, H.; Kuhn, C.; Feillet, H.; Bach, J.F. The "hygiene hypothesis" for autoimmune and allergic diseases: An update. *Clin. Exp. Immunol.* **2010**, *160*, 1–9. [CrossRef] [PubMed]

77. Hu, C.; Wong, F.S.; Wen, L. Type 1 diabetes and gut microbiota: Friend or foe? *Pharmacol. Res.* **2015**, *98*, 9–15. [CrossRef] [PubMed]

78. Wen, L.; Ley, R.E.; Volchkov, P.Y.; Stranges, P.B.; Avanesyan, L.; Stonebraker, A.C.; Hu, C.; Wong, F.S.; Szot, G.L.; Bluestone, J.A.; *et al.* Innate immunity and intestinal microbiota in the development of Type 1 diabetes. *Nature* **2008**, *455*, 1109–1113. [CrossRef] [PubMed]

79. De Goffau, M.C.; Fuentes, S.; van den Bogert, B.; Honkanen, H.; de vos, W.M.; Welling, G.W.; Hyoty, H.; Harmsen, H.J. Aberrant gut microbiota composition at the onset of type 1 diabetes in young children. *Diabetologia* **2014**, *57*, 1569–1577. [CrossRef] [PubMed]

80. De Goffau, M.C.; Luopajarvi, K.; Knip, M.; Ilonen, J.; Ruohtula, T.; Harkonen, T.; Orivuori, L.; Hakala, S.; Welling, G.W.; Harmsen, H.J.; *et al.* Fecal microbiota composition differs between children with β-cell autoimmunity and those without. *Diabetes* **2013**, *62*, 1238–1244. [CrossRef] [PubMed]

81. Simmons, K.M.; Michels, A.W. Type 1 diabetes: A predictable disease. *World J. Diabetes* **2015**, *6*, 380–390. [CrossRef] [PubMed]

82. Mojibian, M.; Chakir, H.; Lefebvre, D.E.; Crookshank, J.A.; Sonier, B.; Keely, E.; Scott, F.W. Diabetes-specific HLA-DR-restricted proinflammatory T-cell response to wheat polypeptides in tissue transglutaminase antibody-negative patients with type 1 diabetes. *Diabetes* **2009**, *58*, 1789–1796. [CrossRef] [PubMed]

83. Auricchio, R.; Paparo, F.; Maglio, M.; Franzese, A.; Lombardi, F.; Valerio, G.; Nardone, G.; Percopo, S.; Greco, L.; Troncone, R. *In vitro*-deranged intestinal immune response to gliadin in type 1 diabetes. *Diabetes* **2004**, *53*, 1680–1683. [CrossRef] [PubMed]

84. Troncone, R.; Franzese, A.; Mazzarella, G.; Paparo, F.; Auricchio, R.; Coto, I.; Mayer, M.; Greco, L. Gluten sensitivity in a subset of children with insulin dependent diabetes mellitus. *Am. J. Gastroenterol.* **2003**, *98*, 590–595. [CrossRef] [PubMed]

85. Klemetti, P.; Savilahti, E.; Ilonen, J.; Akerblom, H.K.; Vaarala, O. T-cell reactivity to wheat gluten in patients with insulin-dependent diabetes mellitus. *Scand. J. Immunol.* **1998**, *47*, 48–53. [CrossRef] [PubMed]

86. Larsen, J.; Weile, C.; Antvorskov, J.C.; Engkilde, K.; Nielsen, S.M.; Josefsen, K.; Buschard, K. Effect of dietary gluten on dendritic cells and innate immune subsets in BALB/c and NOD mice. *PLoS ONE* **2015**, *10*, e0118618. [CrossRef] [PubMed]

87. Hansen, C.H.; Krych, L.; Buschard, K.; Metzdorff, S.B.; Nellemann, C.; Hansen, L.H.; Nielsen, D.S.; Frokiaer, H.; Skov, S.; Hansen, A.K. A maternal gluten-free diet reduces inflammation and diabetes incidence in the offspring of NOD mice. *Diabetes* **2014**, *63*, 2821–2832. [CrossRef] [PubMed]

88. Schmid, S.; Koczwara, K.; Schwinghammer, S.; Lampasona, V.; Ziegler, A.G.; Bonifacio, E. Delayed exposure to wheat and barley proteins reduces diabetes incidence in non-obese diabetic mice. *Clin. Immunol.* **2004**, *111*, 108–118. [CrossRef] [PubMed]

89. Lamb, M.M.; Myers, M.A.; Barriga, K.; Zimmet, P.Z.; Rewers, M.; Norris, J.M. Maternal diet during pregnancy and islet autoimmunity in offspring. *Pediatr. Diabetes* **2008**, *9*, 135–141. [CrossRef] [PubMed]

90. Chmiel, R.; Beyerlein, A.; Knopff, A.; Hummel, S.; Ziegler, A.G.; Winkler, C. Early infant feeding and risk of developing islet autoimmunity and type 1 diabetes. *Acta Diabetol.* **2014**, *52*, 621–624. [CrossRef] [PubMed]

91. Ziegler, A.G.; Schmid, S.; Huber, D.; Hummel, M.; Bonifacio, E. Early infant feeding and risk of developing type 1 diabetes-associated autoantibodies. *JAMA* **2003**, *290*, 1721–1728. [CrossRef] [PubMed]

92. Elenberg, Y.; Shaoul, R. The role of infant nutrition in the prevention of future disease. *Front. Pediatr.* **2014**, *2*, 73. [CrossRef] [PubMed]

93. Wahlberg, J.; Vaarala, O.; Ludvigsson, J.; ABIS-Study Group. Dietary risk factors for the emergence of type 1 diabetes-related autoantibodies in 21/2 year-old Swedish children. *Br. J. Nutr.* **2006**, *95*, 603–608. [CrossRef] [PubMed]

94. Hummel, S.; Pfluger, M.; Hummel, M.; Bonifacio, E.; Ziegler, A.G. Primary dietary intervention study to reduce the risk of islet autoimmunity in children at increased risk for type 1 diabetes: The BABYDIET study. *Diabetes Care* **2011**, *34*, 1301–1305. [CrossRef] [PubMed]

95. Lamb, M.M.; Simpson, M.D.; Seifert, J.; Scott, F.W.; Rewers, M.; Norris, J.M. The association between IgG4 antibodies to dietary factors, islet autoimmunity and type 1 diabetes: The Diabetes Autoimmunity Study in the Young. *PLoS ONE* **2013**, *8*, e57936. [CrossRef] [PubMed]

96. Marietta, E.V.; Gomez, A.M.; Yeoman, C.; Tilahun, A.Y.; Clark, C.R.; Luckey, D.H.; Murray, J.A.; White, B.A.; Kudva, Y.C.; Rajagopalan, G. Low incidence of spontaneous type 1 diabetes in non-obese diabetic mice raised on gluten-free diets is associated with changes in the intestinal microbiome. *PLoS ONE* **2013**, *8*, e78687. [CrossRef] [PubMed]

97. Sildorf, S.M.; Fredheim, S.; Svensson, J.; Buschard, K. Remission without insulin therapy on gluten-free diet in a 6-year old boy with type 1 diabetes mellitus. *BMJ Case Rep* **2012**, *2012*. [CrossRef] [PubMed]

98. Patrick, C.; Wang, G.S.; Lefebvre, D.E.; Crookshank, J.A.; Sonier, B.; Eberhard, C.; Mojibian, M.; Kennedy, C.R.; Brooks, S.P.; Kalmokoff, M.L.; *et al.* Promotion of autoimmune diabetes by cereal diet in the presence or absence of microbes associated with gut immune activation, regulatory imbalance, and altered cathelicidin antimicrobial Peptide. *Diabetes* **2013**, *62*, 2036–2047. [CrossRef] [PubMed]

99. Watts, T.; Berti, I.; Sapone, A.; Gerarduzzi, T.; Not, T.; Zielke, R.; Fasano, A. Role of the intestinal tight junction modulator zonulin in the pathogenesis of type I diabetes in BB diabetic-prone rats. *Proc. Natl. Acad. Sci. USA* **2005**, *102*, 2916–2921. [CrossRef] [PubMed]

100. Mackinder, M.; Allison, G.; Svolos, V.; Buchanan, E.; Johnston, A.; Cardigan, T.; Laird, N.; Duncan, H.; Fraser, K.; Edwards, C.A.; *et al.* Nutritional status, growth and disease management in children with single and dual diagnosis of type 1 diabetes mellitus and coeliac disease. *BMC Gastroenterol.* **2014**, *14*, 99. [CrossRef] [PubMed]

101. Tsouka, A.; Mahmud, F.H.; Marcon, M.A. Celiac Disease Associated with Type 1 Diabetes and Celiac Disease Alone: Are these patients different? *J. Pediatr. Gastroenterol. Nutr.* **2015**. [CrossRef] [PubMed]

102. Castellaneta, S.; Piccinno, E.; Oliva, M.; Cristofori, F.; Vendemiale, M.; Ortolani, F.; Papadia, F.; Catassi, C.; Cavallo, L.; Francavilla, R. High rate of spontaneous normalization of celiac serology in a cohort of 446 children with type 1 diabetes: A prospective study. *Diabetes Care* **2015**, *38*, 760–766. [CrossRef] [PubMed]

103. Rohrer, T.R.; Wolf, J.; Liptay, S.; Zimmer, K.P.; Frohlich-Reiterer, E.; Scheuing, N.; Marg, W.; Stern, M.; Kapellen, T.M.; Hauffa, B.P.; *et al.* Microvascular Complications in Childhood-Onset Type 1 Diabetes and Celiac Disease: A Multicenter Longitudinal Analysis of 56,514 Patients From the German-Austrian DPV Database. *Diabetes Care* **2015**, *38*, 801–807. [CrossRef] [PubMed]

104. Larizza, D.; Calcaterra, V.; Klersy, C.; Badulli, C.; Caramagna, C.; Ricci, A.; Brambilla, P.; Salvaneschi, L.; Martinetti, M. Common immunogenetic profile in children with multiple autoimmune diseases: The signature of HLA-DQ pleiotropic genes. *Autoimmunity* **2012**, *45*, 470–475. [CrossRef] [PubMed]

105. Bakker, S.F.; Tushuizen, M.E.; Stokvis-Brantsma, W.H.; Aanstoot, H.J.; Winterdijk, P.; van Setten, P.A.; von Blomberg, B.M.; Mulder, C.J.; Simsek, S. Frequent delay of coeliac disease diagnosis in symptomatic patients with type 1 diabetes mellitus: Clinical and genetic characteristics. *Eur. J. Intern. Med.* **2013**, *24*, 456–460. [CrossRef] [PubMed]

106. Bakker, S.F.; Tushuizen, M.E.; von Blomberg, M.E.; Mulder, C.J.; Simsek, S. Type 1 diabetes and celiac disease in adults: Glycemic control and diabetic complications. *Acta Diabetol.* **2013**, *50*, 319–324. [CrossRef] [PubMed]

107. Narula, P.; Porter, L.; Langton, J.; Rao, V.; Davies, P.; Cummins, C.; Kirk, J.; Barrett, T.; Protheroe, S. Gastrointestinal symptoms in children with type 1 diabetes screened for celiac disease. *Pediatrics* **2009**, *124*, e489–e495. [CrossRef] [PubMed]

108. Warncke, K.; Liptay, S.; Frohlich-Reiterer, E.; Scheuing, N.; Schebek, M.; Wolf, J.; Rohrer, T.R.; Meissner, T.; Holl, R.W. Vascular risk factors in children, adolescents, and young adults with type 1 diabetes complicated by celiac disease: Results from the DPV initiative. *Pediatr. Diabetes* **2015**. [CrossRef] [PubMed]

109. Adlercreutz, E.H.; Wingren, C.J.; Vincente, R.P.; Merlo, J.; Agardh, D. Perinatal risk factors increase the risk of being affected by both type 1 diabetes and coeliac disease. *Acta Paediatr.* **2015**, *104*, 178–184. [CrossRef] [PubMed]

110. Setty-Shah, N.; Maranda, L.; Nwosu, B.U. Increased risk for vitamin d deficiency in obese children with both celiac disease and type 1 diabetes. *Gastroenterol. Res. Pract.* **2014**, *2014*. [CrossRef] [PubMed]

111. Joshi, A.S.; Varthakavi, P.K.; Bhagwat, N.M.; Chadha, M.D.; Mittal, S.S. Coeliac autoimmunity in type I diabetes mellitus. *Arab. J. Gastroenterol.* **2014**, *15*, 53–57. [CrossRef] [PubMed]

nutrients

Article

Increased Intraepithelial Vα24 Invariant NKT Cells in the Celiac Duodenum

Enrique Montalvillo [1], David Bernardo [2,3], Beatriz Martínez-Abad [1], Yessica Allegretti [4], Luis Fernández-Salazar [5], Carmen Calvo [6], Fernando G. Chirdo [4], José A. Garrote [1,7,†] and Eduardo Arranz [1,†,*]

[1] Mucosal Immunology Lab, IBGM, University of Valladolid-CSIC, Sanz y Forés 3, 47003 Valladolid, Spain; emontalvillo@gmail.com (E.M.); beamaraba@gmail.com (B.M.A.); jagarrote@saludcastillayleon.es (J.A.G.)

[2] Antigen Presentation Research Group, Imperial College London, Northwick Park & St Mark's Campus, Level 7W, St Mark's Building Watford Road Harrow HA1 3UJ, UK; d.bernardo.ordiz@gmail.com

[3] Gastroenterology Unit, Hospital Universitario de La Princesa and Instituto de Investigación Sanitaria Princesa (IIS-IP), Centro de Investigación Biomédica en Red de Enfermedades Hepáticas y Digestivas (CIBEREHD), Madrid 28006, Spain

[4] Laboratorio de Investigación en el Sistema Inmune –LISIN, Departamento de Ciencias Biológicas, Facultad de Ciencias Exactas, Universidad Nacional de La Plata, 115, La Plata 1900, Buenos Aires, Argentina; yallegretti@gmail.com (Y.A.); fchirdo@biol.unlp.edu.ar (F.G.C.)

[5] Gastroenterology Unit, Hospital Clínico Universitario; Ramón y Cajal 3, Valladolid 47005, Spain; luisfernsal@gmail.com

[6] Paediatric Unit, Hospital Clínico Universitario; Ramón y Cajal 3, Valladolid 47005, Spain; carmencalvoromero@gmail.com

[7] Medical Laboratory Service, Hospital Universitario Río Hortega; Dulzaina 2, Valladolid 47012, Spain

[*] Correspondence: earranz@med.uva.es; Tel.: +34-983-184-843

[†] These authors contributed equally to this work.

Received: 23 July 2015; Accepted: 21 October 2015; Published: 30 October 2015

Abstract: Celiac Disease (CD) is an interferon (IFN)γ-mediated duodenal hypersensitivity to wheat gluten occurring in genetically predisposed individuals. Gluten-free diet (GFD) leads to a complete remission of the disease. Vα24-restricted invariant NKT (iNKT) cells are important to maintain immune homeostasis in the gut mucosa because of their unique capacity to rapidly produce large quantities of both T-helper (Th)1 and Th2 cytokines upon stimulation. We studied the presence of these cells in the CD duodenum. Duodenal biopsies were obtained from 45 untreated-CD patients (uCD), 15 Gluten Free Diet-CD patients (GFD-CD), 44 non-inflamed non-CD controls (C-controls) and 15 inflamed non-CD controls (I-controls). Two populations from Spain and Argentina were recruited. Messenger RNA (mRNA) expression of Vα24-Jα18 (*invariant* TCRα chain of human iNKT cells), IFNγ and intracellular transcription factor Forkhead Box P3 (Foxp3), and flow cytometry intraepithelial lymphocyte (IEL) profile were determined. Both uCD and GFD-CD patients had higher Vα24-Jα18 mRNA levels than non-CD controls (I and C-controls). The expression of Vα24-Jα18 correlated with Marsh score for the severity of mucosal lesion and also with increased mRNA IFNγ levels. uCD and GFD-CD patients had decreased mRNA expression of FoxP3 but increased expression of Vα24-Jα18, which revealed a CD-like molecular profile. Increased numbers of iNKT cells were confirmed by flow cytometry within the intraepithelial lymphocyte compartment of uCD and GFD-CD patients and correlated with Vα24-Jα18 mRNA expression. In conclusion, we have found an increased number of iNKT cells in the duodenum from both uCD and GFD-CD patients, irrespective of the mucosal status. A CD-like molecular profile, defined by an increased mRNA expression of Vα24-Jα18 together with a decreased expression of FoxP3, may represent a pro-inflammatory signature of the CD duodenum.

Keywords: Celiac Disease; Intraepithelial Lymphocytes; iNKT; Vα24-Jα18; IFNγ; Celiac Disease-like molecular profile

Nutrients **2015**, *7*, 8960–8976

1. Introduction

Celiac disease (CD) is an inflammatory disorder of the small intestine induced by wheat gluten and other prolamins from rye, barley and some varieties of oats [1] in genetically susceptible individuals. It is characterized by an interferon (IFN)-γ mediated type I cytokine profile [2]. CD manifestation is characterized by an increased number of intraepithelial and lamina propria lymphocytes, villous atrophy, tissue remodeling and the presence of anti-transglutaminase antibodies [3]. At present, the only treatment for CD is a life-long strict gluten-free diet (GFD), which normally leads to a complete remission of the disease [4].

Gut intraepithelial lymphocytes (IEL) comprise a heterogeneous population of cells outside the normal circulation. In addition to conventional T lymphocytes (CD3$^+$ TCRαβ$^+$, either CD4$^+$ or CD8$^+$) with an outstanding CD3$^+$ CD8$^+$ prevalence, Natural Killer (NK) cells and unconventional IEL populations such as CD8αα, TCRγδ$^+$ cells, CD3$^+$CD4$^-$CD8$^-$ cells and NKT lymphocytes are widely represented [5,6].

Increased total numbers of IEL CD3$^+$ (both classical and TCRγδ$^+$) and decreased IEL non-T cells (CD3$^-$, CD103$^+$) have been consistently reported in CD [7–9]. A direct cytolytic effect of conventional CD3$^+$αβ$^+$CD8$^+$ cytotoxic IEL on adjacent enterocytes is undisputed [10,11] and related to villous atrophy [7]. However, the role of IEL TCRγδ$^+$ in CD pathogenesis remains elusive, although they may have a key role in oral tolerance as supported by the identification of a subset of regulatory TCRγδ$^+$ IEL population capable of limiting the cytotoxicity of IEL in CD treated on a GFD [12].

Classical regulatory Tcells (Tregs; CD3$^+$, CD4$^+$, CD25$^+$ and intracellular transcription factor Forkhead Box P3$^+$ (FoxP3$^+$)) and non-classical interleukin (IL)-10 producing regulatory cells (Tr1: CD3$^+$, CD4$^+$, CD25$^-$ and intracellular FoxP3$^-$) are the main regulatory T-cells found in the intestine [13]. Tregs elicit their function by suppressing IL-2 production and T-cell proliferation [14], while Tr1 cells are the main source of IL-10 in the intestinal lamina propria since they are chronically stimulated and limit the production of pro-inflammatory cytokine by controlling inflammatory responses to dietary antigens. Compared to Tregs, the finding of larger numbers of Tr1 in the intestinal lamina propria suggests that these cells have an important regulatory capacity [15,16].

Invariant NKT cells (iNKT; CD3$^+$, TCR Vα24$^+$Vβ11$^+$) are also important to maintain immune homeostasis [13]. Human iNKT cells express classical NK cell markers as well as an *invariant* TCRα chain (iNKTα) (Vα24-Jα18 in humans) paired to "semi-invariant" TCRβ chains (iNKTβ), which recognizes antigens presented by the major histocompatibility complex (MHC) class I-like molecule CD1d [17,18]. For all iNKT-cell TCRs, binding to CD1d is primarily mediated by the Vα-Jα rearranged *invariant* CDR3α loop [19]. Therefore, the anti-Vα24-Jα18 is the standard method used to detect human iNKT cells [20,21]. These cells can be sub-divided into CD4$^+$ and CD4$^-$ (most of these CD4$^-$CD8$^-$) cells. CD4$^-$CD8$^-$ iNKT cells produce predominantly T-helper (Th)1 cytokines (IFNγ and TNFα whereas CD4$^+$ iNKT cells can produce both Th1 and Th2 (IL-4 and IL-13) cytokines [13]. Because of their unique capacity to rapidly produce large quantities of both Th1 (IFNγ) and Th2 (IL-4) cytokines upon stimulation [22], iNKT cells may have a key role in protection against tumors or in preventing autoimmune disease [23]. Despite low numbers, iNKT cells have a central role in intestinal homeostasis [17,24,25] and are essential for the development of oral tolerance [26,27]. Nevertheless, their number within the intraepithelial and lamina propria compartments and their specific role in CD pathogenesis remains elusive.

In this manuscript, we aimed to study whether changes in the number of iNKT cells may be altered in the duodenum of CD patients. To these aim we assessed the mRNA expression of Vα24-Jα18 and the proportion of iNKT cells within the intraepithelial compartment to reveal an increased number of these cells in the CD mucosa.

2. Materials and Methods

2.1. Patients and Biopsy Samples

Duodenal samples were collected from two independent populations in Spain (Hospital Clínico Universitario de Valladolid) and Argentina (Biobank from the LISIN, La Plata). The Spanish population included 25 untreated celiac patients (uCD, mean age 28.9 years; range 5–76 years; 42% males) (Table S1), 15 CD patients treated with GFD (GFD-CD; mean age 34.2 years; range 4-71 years; 34% males) (Table S2), 15 non-CD patients with other inflamed conditions (I-controls, mean age 42.1 years; range 15–78 years; 56% males) (Table S3) and 25 non-inflamed non-CD controls (C-controls; mean age 38.3 years; range 6–81 years; 30% males) (Table S4). The Argentinian population included 20 uCD patients (mean age 24.8 years; range 4-56 years; 28% males) (Table S5) and 19 C-controls (mean age 31.4 years; range 6–62 years; 52% males) (Table S6). Regarding age and gender, no statistically differences were found between Spanish and Argentinian patients. Clinical data from patient groups included in the study are shown in Table 1. The experiments were conducted with the understanding and the written consent of the adult participants, or the next of kin, caretakers, or guardians on behalf of the minors/children enrolled in this study. The study and the written consent procedure were approved by the Ethics committees from Hospital Clínico Universitario of Valladolid and Biobank from the LISIN, La Plata.

Table 1. Clinical data from patient groups included in the study.

	Study Patients	*n*	Mean age (Range)	Gender	HLA DQ2/DQ8	IgA anti-tTG/EMA	Marsh Criteria at Diagnosis	GFD
Celiac Patients	uCD	45	27.1 (4–76)	36% males	+	+	II-III	No
	GFD-CD	15	34.2 (4–71)	34% males	+	-	II-III	Yes
Non Celiac Patients	I-controls	15	42.1 (15–78)	56% males	+/-	- (*A)	0-I (M.M)	No
	C-controls	44	35.3 (6–81)	41% males	- (*B)	- (*A)	0	No

uCD (untreated celiac patients), GFD-CD (celiac patients treated with gluten free diet), I-controls (non celiac patients with other inflamed conditions) and C-controls (non-celiac disease patients without other inflamed conditions). IgA anti-tTG (Anti-tissue transglutaminase antibodies), EMA (Endomysium antibodies), GFD (Gluten free diet). M.M (mild mucosal alterations non compatibles with celiac disease). *A Serological test were performed only in genetically susceptible patients. *B Two patients had positive genetic susceptibility markers.

At diagnosis, all CD patients had CD-compatible symptoms, positive anti-endomysium and/or anti-transglutaminase IgA antibodies, CD-associated risk alleles (HLA-DQ2 and DQ8), and duodenal biopsy with histopathological changes. No differences in clinical markers were found between Spanish and Argentinian CD individuals. Patients on a GFD showed an improvement of the histological lesion (Marsh 0-I), and negative serum anti-transglutaminase antibodies for at least one year. Control groups were collected from patients referred to the gastroenterology clinics for diagnostic investigations due to clinical suspicion of intestinal disease (chronic diarrhea, gastritis by Helicobacter pylori, hiatus hernia, *etc.*). Similar symptoms were observed in both populations. Some of these cases showed duodenal inflammation (I-controls) while lack of mucosal affection was found in C-controls. None of them had a final diagnosis of CD.

2.2. Quantitative PCR

Duodenal biopsies from the Spanish (40 CD patients (25 uCD and 15 GFD-CD), 25 C-controls and 15 I-controls) and the Argentinian population (20 uCD and 19 C-controls) were submerged in 0.5 mL of RNALater® solution (Ambion Inc, Austin, Texas, USA) and stored at −20 °C immediately after sample taking. Total RNA was isolated using the TRI-Reagent® Solution according to manufacturer instructions (Ambion Inc, Austin, Texas, USA). In parallel, 15 duodenal samples from each group of patients from the Spanish population were also analyzed by flow cytometry as described below to determine the phenotype of lymphocytes and iNKT cells.

Reverse transcription was carried out by using the SuperScript® First-Strand Synthesis System for reverse transcriptase (RT)-PCR Kit (Applied Biosystems, Carlsbad, CA, USA) with random hexamers as primers. Reactions were performed using the FastStart SYBR Green MasterMix (Roche Applied Science, Mannheim, Germany) with thermolabile Uracil DNA Glycosylase to prevent carry-over contamination. Messenger RNA levels (βactin, IFNγ, Vα24-Jα18 and FoxP3) were measured by quantitative PCR (qPCR) on a LightCycler® instrument (Roche Applied Science, Mannheim, Germany) after extrapolation to an external curve. Primer sets and PCR conditions are described in Table 2. Levels of mRNA are expressed as the ratio molecule/βactin in arbitrary units (AU).

Table 2. Primer sequences for quantitative-PCR.

Molecule	Primers Sequence	NCBI Locus	Annealing T
βactin	fw: 5′ - ATG GGT CAG AAG GAT TCC TAT GTG - 3′ rv: 5′ - CTT CAT GAG GTA GTC AGT CAG GTC - 3′	NM_001101.3	60
IFNγ	fw: 5′ - TGG AAA GAG GAG AGT GAC AG - 3′ rv: 5′ - ATT CAT GTC TTC CTT GAT GG - 3′	NM_000619.2	60
Vα24-Jα18	fw: 5′ - CTG GAG GGA AAG AAC TGC - 3′ rv: 5′ - TGT CAG GGA AAC AGG ACC - 3′	NC_000014.9	65
FoxP3	fw: 5′ - CAG CAC ATT CCC AGA GTT CCT C - 3′ rv: 5′ - GCG TGT GAA CCA GTG GTA GAT C - 3′	NM_014009.3	60

Primer sequences used for quantitative-PCR. NCBI locus and annealing temperature point (annealing T). IFNγ (interferon-γ), Vα24-Jα18 (*invariant* TCRα chain of human iNKT cells), FoxP3 (intracellular transcription factor Forkhead Box P3).

2.3. Isolation of Intraepithelial Lymphocytes and Lamina Propria Mononuclear Cells

Biopsy samples from 15 uCD, 15 GFD, 15 non-inflamed non-CD controls (C-controls) and 15 inflamed non-CD controls (I-controls) were collected from the Spanish population. Samples were kept in ice-chilled physiologic phosphate buffered saline (PBS) and processed within an hour as previously described [28,29]. Briefly, IEL and epithelial cells were released from the mucosal specimens by incubation for 1 hour under gentle agitation with 1 mM ethylenediaminetetraacetic acid (EDTA) and 1 mM dithiothreitol (DTT) in RPMI 1640 medium (GibcoBRL Life Technologies, Vienna, Austria) supplemented with 10% fetal calf serum, 2mM L-glutamine, 100U/mL penicillin, 100 µg/mL streptomycin and 0.25 µg/mL amphotericin (GibcoBRL Life Technologies, Vienna, Austria). Following DTT and EDTA incubation IEL were released into the medium and collected by centrifugation, washed twice in PBS (Lonza, Braine-l'Alleud, Belgium) and stained with fluorochrome-conjugated monoclonal antibodies (mAbs).

The remaining tissue was incubated in moderated rotation at 37 °C for 90–120 min. with 1 mg/mL of collagenase D in RPMI 1640 medium (GibcoBRL Life Technologies, Vienna, Austria) supplemented with 10% fetal calf serum and antibiotics until the biopsies have been completely degraded. Single cell suspensions were filtered (70 µm Nylon Filter, BD Biosciences, San Diego, CA, USA) to remove non-cellular fibers, and the lamina propria mononuclear cells (LPMC) suspension was washed twice in PBS.

2.4. Antibody Labeling and Flow Cytometry Analysis

A total of 100,000 isolated cells (IEL or LPMC) were labeled with fluorochrome-conjugated monoclonal antibodies (mAbs) and their appropriate isotype-matched control antibodies from the same manufacturers. The fluorochrome-conjugated mAbs were: FITC Mouse anti-human CD103 (clone Ber-ACT8), PE Mouse anti-human Vα24-Jα18 (clone 6B11, specifically recognizing all T cells expressing the conserved CDR3 region of the Vα24Jα18 invariant TCRα rearrangement), PE Mouse anti-human TCR$\gamma\delta$ (clone B1), APC Mouse anti-human CD3 (clone HIT3a), APC Mouse anti-human CD25 (clone M-A251), PE-Cy7 Mouse anti-human CD8 (clone RPA-T8) and PE-Cy7 Mouse anti-human CD45 (clone HI30) from BD Pharmingen (San Diego, CA, USA); PE Mouse anti-human FoxP3 (clone PCH101) from eBioscience (San Diego, CA, USA); FITC Mouse anti-human CD4 (clone 13B8.2) and PE Mouse anti-human CD8 (clone B9.11) from Beckman Coulter (Brea , CA, USA). Cells were labeled in phosphate-buffered saline containing 1 mM EDTA and 0.02% sodium azide (fluorescent-activated cell sorting (FACS) buffer). Labeling was performed on ice and in the dark for 20 min. Cells were washed twice in FACS buffer, fixed with 1% paraformaldehyde in 0.85% saline, and stored at 4 °C before acquisition on the flow cytometer within 24 h. For FoxP3 intracellular staining, cells were fixed with Leucoperm A following surface staining and permeabilized with Leucoperm B (Bio-Rad, UK) before adding antibody for intracellular labeling. After incubation cells were washed in FACS buffer, fixed, and acquired as previously reported.

Cells were acquired in a Beckman Coulter FC500 flow cytometer and data processed with Cell BC software (Beckman Coulter, Brea, CA, USA). All IEL and lamina propria lymphocyte (LPL) cells were identified as CD45$^+$ (leukocyte pan-marker) and IELs were also identified as CD103$^+$. Non-T cells (CD3$^-$), TCR$\gamma\delta$ cells (CD3$^+$TCR$\gamma\delta^+$), TCR$\alpha\beta$ cells (CD3$^+$TCR$\gamma\delta^-$) (Figure 1A), iNKT cells (CD3$^+$Vα24-Jα18$^+$) (Figure 1B) and Treg cells (CD3$^+$CD4$^+$CD25$^+$FoxP3$^+$ or CD3$^+$CD4$^+$FoxP3$^+$) were identified by flow cytometry within the intraepithelial and the lamina propria compartments. Numbers of cells were expressed as percentages.

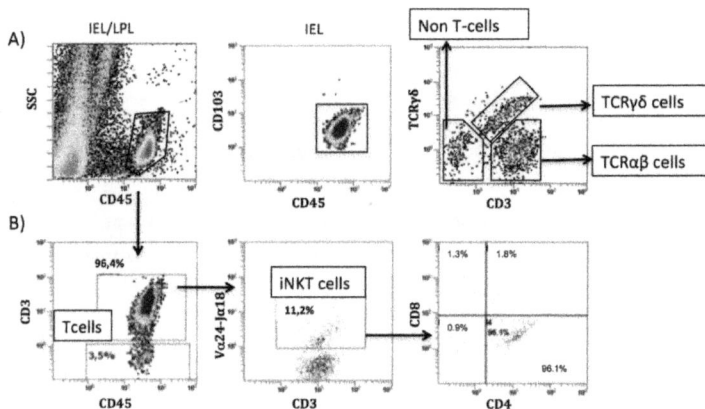

Figure 1. Identification of intraepithelial and lamina propria lymphocytes by flow cytometry. Example of characterization of intraepithelial lymphocytes (IELs)/lamina propria lymphocytes (LPL) in an untreated celiac disease donor. Lamina propria (CD45$^+$) and IEL (CD45$^+$CD103$^+$) were identified and percentages of TCR$\alpha\beta$ cells, TCR$\gamma\delta$ cells and non-T cells determined (**A**). Example of characterization of invariant NKT (iNKT) cells in an untreated celiac disease donor: CD45$^+$CD3$^+$Vα24-Jα18$^+$ cells within the total of CD45$^+$CD3$^+$ cells, iNKT (CD45$^+$CD3$^+$Vα24-Jα18$^+$) phenotype according to the expression of CD4 and/or CD8 within the total of iNKTs (**B**).

2.5. Statistical Analysis

Correlation analyses and two-tailed non-parametric statistical analyses were performed using the Kruskal-Wallis one way analysis of variance test, the Mann-Whitney U test and the non-parametric Spearman's correlation. $p < 0.05$ was considered significant. Flow cytometry results were expressed as percentages and analysed by the two-tailed non-parametric Mann-Whitney U test. $p < 0.05$ was considered significant. Reference values of the IEL subpopulations for each patient's group were expressed as median percentages with the interquartile range (IQR).

3. Results

3.1. Increased Duodenal Vα24-Jα18 mRNA Expression in Celiac Disease Patients

Due to the low numbers of iNKT cells both in blood [21] and tissue samples [22] we first studied the proportion of iNKT cells in duodenal biopsies by assessing the mRNA expression or their restrictive invariant Vα24-Jα18 chain in complete biopsy explants [20,21].

Untreated-CD patients (uCD) had increased Vα24-Jα18 mRNA levels compared to both inflamed non-CD (I-controls) ($p < 0.05$) and non-inflamed non-CD controls (C-controls) ($p < 0.001$) (Figure 2A). Gluten Free Diet-CD patients (GFD-CD) had increased Vα24-Jα18 mRNA levels compared to C-controls ($p < 0.001$). No differences were found between uCD and GFD-CD patients, which suggests an increased load of iNKT cells in duodenal biopsies from both groups of patients irrespectively of the disease status (Figure 2A). We also analyzed duodenal expression of Vα24-Jα18 mRNA in an independent population from Argentina. Figure 2B confirms that CD patients show increased duodenal Vα24-Jα18 mRNA levels compared to non-inflamed non-CD controls ($p < 0.001$), irrespectively of the origin of the samples. No statistically significant differences in Vα24-Jα18 mRNA levels were found between the Spanish and the Argentinian populations, neither within the control nor the untreated CD patient groups.

Samples from GFD-CD patients showed a Marsh score for the severity of the mucosal lesion between 0 and I, and no differences were found in these sub-groups regarding Vα24-Jα18 mRNA expression. Untreated CD patients had a Marsh score rating from I to IIIc, and in these patients, Vα24-Jα18 mRNA levels correlated with the Marsh score (Spearman's $r = 0.063$, $p < 0.05$) (Figure 2C).

3.2. Correlation between Duodenal Vα24-Jα18 and IFNγ mRNA Expression in Celiac Disease

Duodenal samples from CD patients (either treated and untreated) had increased IFNγ mRNA expression compared with non-inflamed non-CD controls both in the Spanish (GFD-CD, $p < 0.05$; uCD, $p < 0.001$) (Figure 3A) and the Argentinian populations (uCD, $p < 0.05$) (Figure 3B) as previously described [30,31]. Since both mRNA levels of IFNγ [2,30] and Vα24-Jα18 (Figure 2C) correlated with the Marsh score for the severity of the mucosal lesion, we studied if the expression of IFNγ and Vα24-Jα18 was related. A correlation was found between the mRNA levels of IFNγ and Vα24-Jα18 in treated and untreated CD samples in both the Spanish (C-controls: Spearman's $r = 0.3115$, p value = n.s; I-controls: Spearman's $r = 0.4265$, p value = n.s; GFD-CD: Spearman's $r = 0.5393$, $p < 0.05$; uCD: Spearman's $r = 0.4323$, $p < 0.05$) and the Argentinian populations (C-controls: Spearman's $r = 0.5895$, $p < 0.05$; uCD: Spearman's $r = 0.6917$, $p < 0.001$) (Figure 3C,D).

3.3. Duodenal Vα24-Jα18 and FoxP3 mRNA Levels Reveal a Celiac Disease Molecular Profile

We next studied FoxP3 mRNA expression in the duodenum as an indirect way of quantifying Treg cells in tissue. CD samples (both uCD and GFD-CD) had decreased FoxP3 expression compared with non-inflamed non-CD-controls (C-controls) (uCD, $p < 0.001$; GFD-CD, $p < 0.001$) (Figure 4A). Similar results were found on a second independent analysis of the Argentinian population (uCD, $p < 0.001$) (Figure 4B). Because CD samples were characterized by increased duodenal mRNA expression of Vα24-Jα18 (Figure 2A,B) and decreased expression of FoxP3 (Figure 4A,B), we studied whether the joint analysis of these two molecules could help us to identify a CD-like molecular profile.

No differences were found between samples from controls or uCD patients in any of the molecules studied in both populations (Spanish and Argentinian). Similar results were also obtained when Vα24-Jα18 and FoxP3 duodenal mRNA expression were independently analysed. Therefore, both populations were merged to increase the sample size of uCD and C-control groups. The joint analysis of both duodenal FoxP3 and Vα24-Jα18 mRNA levels allowed us to discriminate between CD (treated and untreated), and non-CD samples (inflamed or non-inflamed) with a sensibility and sensitivity of 92%, revealing a CD-like molecular profile (C-controls: Spearman's $r = 0.3495$, $p < 0.05$; I-controls: Spearman's $r = -0.4577$, p value = n.s; GFD-CD: Spearman's $r = -0.4858$, $p < 0.05$; uCD: Spearman's $r = -0.056$, p value = n.s) (Figure 4C).

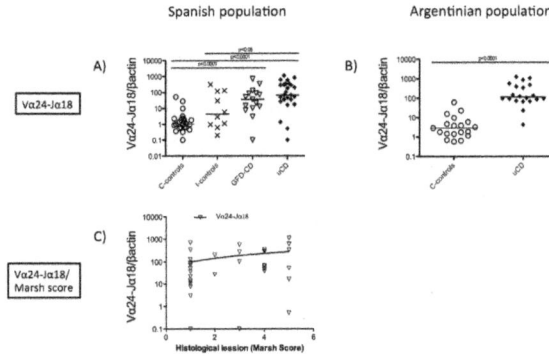

Figure 2. Increased duodenal Vα24-Jα18 mRNA expression in untreated and treated celiac disease patients. Expression levels of Vα24-Jα18 mRNA in duodenal biopsies indicated by the ratio Vα24-Jα18/βactin in arbitrary units (AU), in untreated Celiac Disease (uCD), Gluten Free Diet-CD patients (GFD-CD), inflamed non-CD controls (I-controls) and non-inflamed non-CD controls (C-controls) in the Spanish population (**A**) and in uCD and C-controls in the Argentinian population (**B**). Statistically significant differences are shown (two tailed Mann-Whitney U test; Krustall-Wallis test). Horizontal bars are median values. Correlation between the degree of histological lesion (Marsh score) and the expression level of Vα24-Jα18 mRNA in CD patients. (1: Marsh 0-I, 2: Marsh II, 3: Marsh IIIa, 4: Marsh IIIb, 5: Marsh IIIc) There was an increased of Vα24-Jα18 expression and the duodenal increased level of atrophy (Spearman *r* = 0.063, *p* < 0.05). GFD-CD patients show a Marsh 0-I, uCD show duodenal atrophy Marsh II to IIIc (**C**).

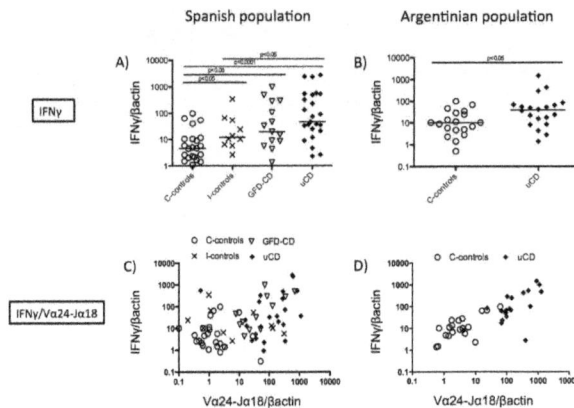

Figure 3. Correlation between duodenal mRNA expression of Vα24-Jα18 and IFNγ. Expression levels of IFNγ mRNA in duodenal biopsies indicated as the ratio IFNγ/βactin, in arbitrary units (AU), in untreated Celiac Disease (uCD), Gluten Free Diet-CD patients (GFD-CD), inflamed non-CD controls (I-controls) and non-inflamed non-CD controls (C-controls) in the Spanish population (**A**) and in uCD and C-controls in the Argentinian population (**B**). Statistically significant differences are shown (two tailed Mann-Whitney U test; Krustall-Wallis test). Horizontal bars are median values. Correlation between the expression of IFNγ and Vα24-Jα18 mRNA, in arbitrary units (AU) in the Spanish population (**C**) (C-controls: Spearman *r* = 0.3115, *p* value = n.s; I-controls: Spearman *r* = 0.4265, *p* value = n.s; GFD-CD: Spearman *r* = 0.5393, *p* value < 0.05; uCD: Spearman *r* = 0.4323, *p* value < 0.05) and in the Argentinian population (**D**) (C-controls: Spearman *r* = 0.5895, *p* value < 0.05; uCD: Spearman *r* = 0.6917, *p* value < 0.001).

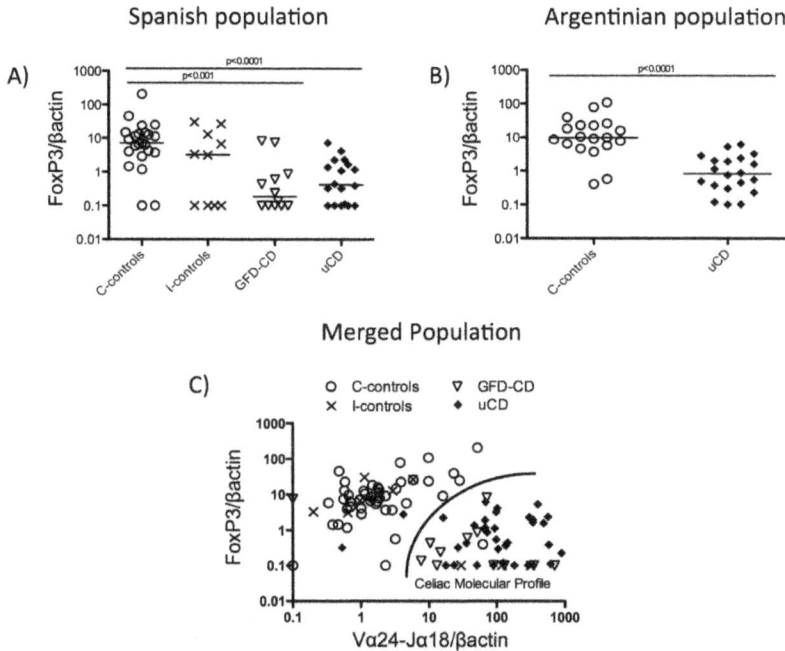

Figure 4. Duodenal mRNA levels of Vα24-Jα18 and FoxP3 reveal a celiac disease molecular profile. Expression levels of FoxP3 mRNA in duodenal biopsies indicated as the ratio FoxP3/βactin, in arbitrary units (AU) in untreated Celiac Disease (uCD), Gluten Free Diet-CD patients (GFD-CD), inflamed non-CD controls (I-controls) and non-inflamed non-CD controls (C-controls) in the Spanish population (**A**) and in uCD and C-controls in the Argentinian population (**B**). Statistical differences are shown (two tailed Mann-Whitney U test; Krustall-Wallis test). Horizontal bars are median values. *Duodenal molecular profile*: Correlation between expression levels of FoxP3 and Vα24-Jα18 mRNA, in arbitrary units (AU) (C-controls: Spearman $r = 0.3495$, p value < 0.05; I-controls: Spearman $r = -0.4577$, p value = n.s; GFD-CD: Spearman $r = -0.4858$, p value < 0.05; uCD: Spearman $r = -0.056$, p value = n.s) (**C**).

All together, our findings suggest an increase of iNKT cells in the CD duodenum as determined by molecular approaches. Therefore, we next studied the number of iNKT cells within the intraepithelial and lamina propria compartments by flow cytometry. To that end, the IEL profile was first analyzed and compared with previous reports before determining the number of iNKT cells in the CD duodenum.

3.4. Intraepithelial Lymphocytes in the Duodenum from Celiac Disease Patients

Total IELs (CD103$^+$CD45$^+$), non-T cells (CD103$^+$CD45$^+$CD3$^-$), TCRγδ$^+$ cells (CD103$^+$CD45$^+$CD3$^+$TCRγδ$^+$) and TCRαβ$^+$ cells (CD103$^+$CD45$^+$CD3$^+$TCRγδ$^-$) were studied within the intraepithelial compartment (as characterized in Figure 1A) given their relevance as biomarkers in CD diagnosis [9,32]. Untreated CD patients had increased numbers of total IELs (median/IQR; 16.80%/4.80) (Figure 5A,E) together with decreased numbers of non-T cells (3.10%/4.00) (Figure 5B,E). The latter was also true in GFD-CD patients although the total number of IELs did not increase (GFD-CD, 10.40%/4.11) (Figure 5A,E). Within the CD3$^+$ subpopulation, both uCD and GFD-CD patients showed higher numbers of TCRγδ$^+$ cells (uCD, 35.78%/11.13; GFD-CD, 32.50%/8.90) (Figure 5C,E), previously described as a distinctive feature of CD patients [9,32]. In support of this, inflamed non-CD controls did not have increased numbers of TCRγδ$^+$ cells (I-controls, 7.51%/2.60) (Figure 5C,E) despite the decreased percentage of non-T cells compared with non-inflamed non-CD controls (I-controls, 16.30%/8.12; C-controls, 28.90%/15.75) (Figure 5B,E). However, these patients had increased numbers of TCRαβ+ cells (I-controls, 76.20%/8.20) compared with the remainder patient groups (uCD, 59.30%/15.6; GFD-CD, 58.80%/10.90; C-controls, 62.10%/14.5) (Figure 5D,E).

Within the intraepithelial compartment, a decreased number of non-T cells together with increased TCRγδ+ cells represent a distinctive pattern of CD patients irrespectively of the disease status [32,33]. Reference values of the IEL subpopulations for each patient's group were expressed as median percentages with the interquartile range (IQR) in Table 3.

Table 3. Specificity of intraepithelial lymphocytes profiling in the diagnosis of celiac disease.

	uCD Median (IQR)	GFD-CD Median (IQR)	I-controls Median (IQR)	C-controls Median (IQR)
Total IELs	16.80% (4.80)	10.40% (4.11)	10.70% (3.70)	8.50% (2.60)
Non-T cells	3.10% (4.00)	9.34% (3.34)	16.30% (8.12)	28.90% (15.75)
TCRγδ+cells	35.78% (11.13)	32.50% (8.90)	7.51% (2.60)	6.44% (2.38)
TCRαβ+cells	59.30% (15,6)	58.80% (10,9)	76.20% (8,9)	62.10% (14,5)

Percentages of duodenal Intraepithelial lymphocyte (IEL) populations in untreated Celiac Disease (uCD), Gluten Free Diet-CD patients (GFD-CD), inflamed non-CD controls (I-controls) and non-inflamed non-CD controls (C-controls) expressed as median percentages with the interquartile range (IQR).

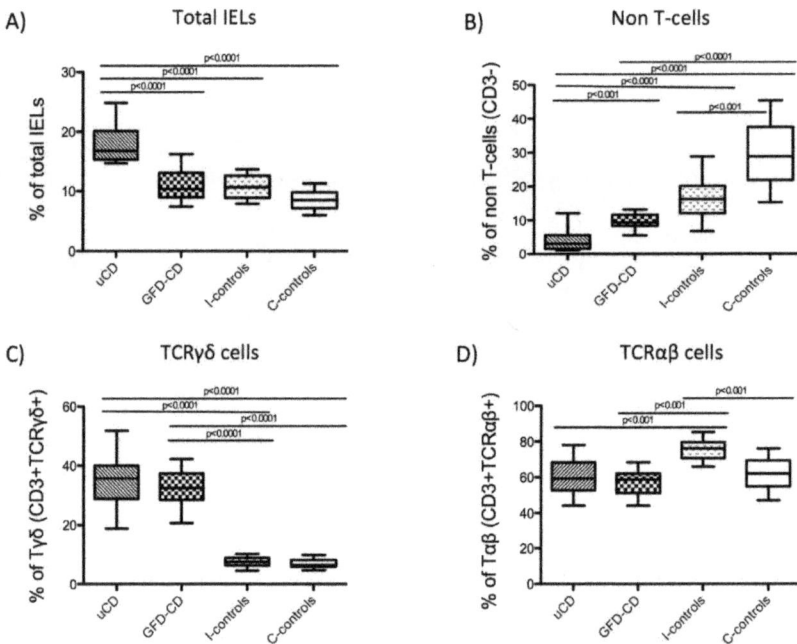

Figure 5. *Cont.*

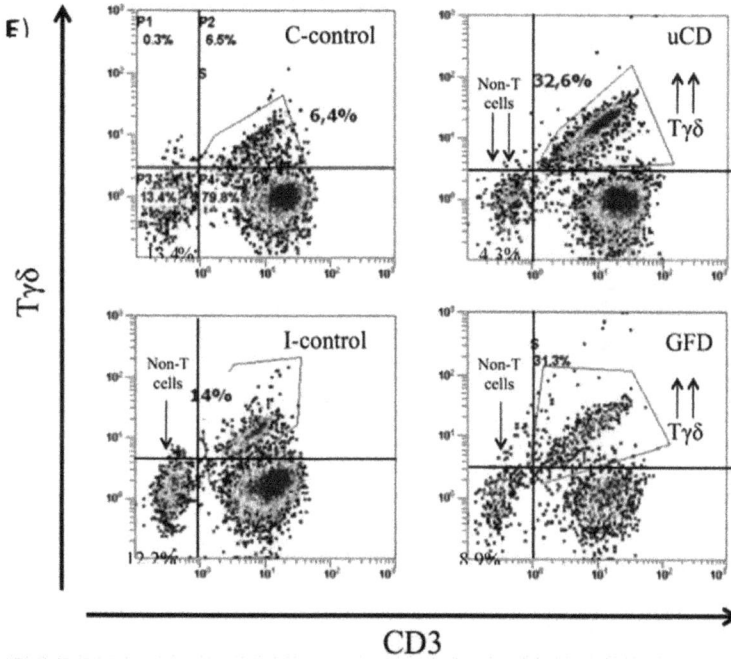

Figure 5. Phenotype of intraepithelial lymphocytes in the duodenum from celiac patients. Phenotype of IELs in untreated Celiac Disease (uCD), Gluten Free Diet-CD patients (GFD-CD), inflamed non-CD controls (I-controls) and non-inflamed non-CD controls (C-controls), analyzed by flow cytometry: Percentage of total IELs (CD103$^+$CD45$^+$) referred to the total of epithelial cells (**A**). Percentage of non-T cells (CD103$^+$CD45$^+$CD3$^-$) (**B**), Tγδ cells (CD103$^+$CD45$^+$CD3$^+$TCRγδ$^+$) (**C**) and Tαβ cells (CD103$^+$CD45$^+$CD3$^+$TCRγδ$^-$) (**D**) referred to the total of IELs. Horizontal bar are median values. Statistically significant differences are shown (two tailed Mann Whitney U test; $p < 0.05$). Representative flow cytometry analysis data of IEL subpopulations (Tγδ, Tαβ and non-T cells) in uCD, GFD-CD, I-controls and C-controls (**E**).

After characterizing the duodenal IEL profile in CD patients and controls, we finally assessed whether the percentage of iNKT cells was increased in the CD duodenum, as suggested by molecular studies.

3.5. Increased Intraepithelial iNKT Cells in Celiac Disease Patients and Correlation with
Vα24-Jα18 mRNA Expression

As suggested by molecular studies (Figure 2A,B), iNKT cells (as characterized in Figure 1B) were increased within the IEL compartment from CD patients (in both, uCD: 7.4%/3.9 and GFD-CD: 6.1%/5.7) compared with non-CD groups (C-controls: 1.9%/0.8 and I-controls: 2.9%/1.5) (Figure 6A).

There were also differences in the phenotype of intraepithelial iNKT cells since CD patients had a higher proportion of CD4$^+$ iNKT cells (uCD: 82.9%/11.4, GFD-CD: 70.0%/10.5, I-controls: 51.8%/14.5, C-controls: 30.2%/15.1) (Figure 6B). However, the number of iNKT cells from the lamina propria did not differ in number in any of the groups (Figure 6C).

As previously shown, the mRNA expression of Vα24-Jα18 was analyzed by qPCR in all of these duodenal biopsies (Figure 2A). For that reason, we studied whether the increased Vα24-Jα18 mRNA expression could be used as a marker of the increased number of intraepithelial iNKT cells found by flow cytometry (Figure 6A). As shown in Figure 6D, the percentage of iNKT cells correlated with Vα24-Jα18 mRNA levels (C-controls: Spearman's $r = 0.8603$, $p < 0.001$; I-controls: Spearman's $r = -0.9455$, $p < 0.001$; GFD-CD: Spearman's $r = -0.9297$, $p < 0.001$; uCD: Spearman's $r = 0.8287$, $p = 0.001$), which confirms our findings, but also that the study of Vα24-Jα18 mRNA levels may be a valid approach to characterize the density of iNKT cells in complex tissues.

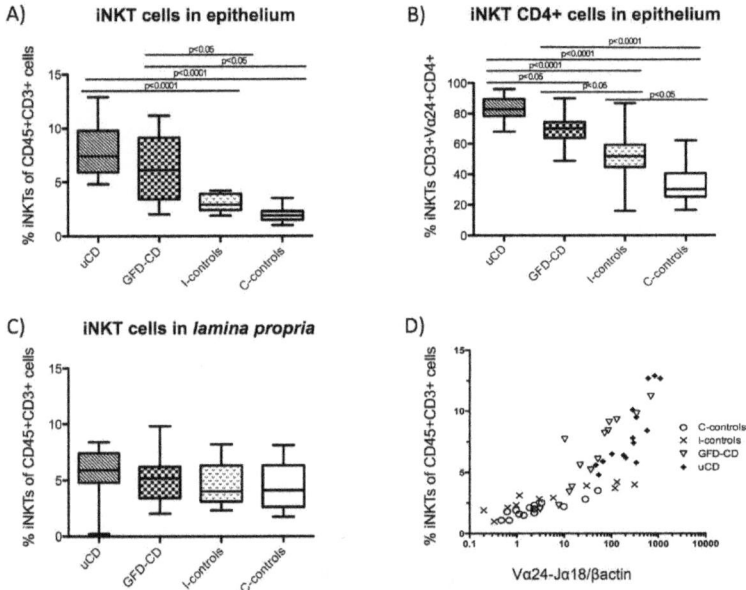

Figure 6. Increased intraepithelial iNKT cells in celiac disease patients and correlation with Vα24-Jα18 mRNA expression. Percentage of iNKT cells (CD45$^+$CD3$^+$Vα24-Jα18$^+$) among the total number of Intraepithelial Lymphocytes (IELs) in untreated Celiac Disease (uCD), Gluten Free Diet-CD patients (GFD-CD), inflamed non-CD controls (I-controls) and non-inflamed non-CD controls (C-controls) (**A**). Percentage of Intraepithelial CD4$^+$ iNKT cells among the total number of iNKT cells in aCD, GFD-CD, I-controls and C-controls (**B**). Percentage of iNKT cells among the total number of Lamina Propria Lymphocytes (LPLs) in aCD, GFD-CD, I-controls and C controls (**C**). Horizontal bars are median values. Statistically significant differences are shown (two tailed Mann Whitney U test; $p < 0.05$). Correlation between Vα24-Jα18 mRNA expression, in arbitrary units (AU) and the percentage of iNKT cells among the total number of IELs in aCD, GFD-CD, I-controls and C controls (C-controls: Spearman $r = 0.8603$, p value<0.001; I-controls: Spearman $r = -0.9455$, p value < 0.0001; GFD-CD: Spearman $r = -0.9297$, p value < 0.0001; uCD: Spearman $r = 0.8287$, p value = 0.001) (**D**).

4. Discussion

Despite their low numbers, iNKT cells may have an essential role for the immune homeostasis in the gastrointestinal tract [17,34]. Here, we studied intestinal iNKT cells in the context of celiac disease by molecular and cellular approaches, and found higher numbers of both total and CD4$^+$ iNKT cells in the intraepithelial compartment of CD patients. We also found a correlation between the mRNA expression of Vα24-Jα18 and (i) the severity of the mucosal lesion, and (ii) the mRNA expression of IFNγ. Finally, the mRNA expression of both Vα24-Jα18 and FoxP3 might define an mRNA CD-like molecular profile. Altogether our findings suggest that the number of duodenal intraepithelial iNKT cells is increased in CD patients.

Invariant NKT cells have a key role in the mechanism of oral tolerance [26,34], and their hepatic depletion leads to the inability of developing oral tolerance in a mouse model [35]. These cells may have an effect in the development of tolerogenic dendritic cells, which are responsible for the proliferation of regulatory T cells [13]. Because of the innate and adaptive features of these cells, and the ability to produce high levels of IL-4 and IFNγ [17], a role for iNKT cells has been suggested in inflammatory bowel disease [36] and in CD [37]. Some studies have characterized circulating numbers of iNKT cells in CD patients, often with contradictory results [21,37,38], but few have reported the number of these cells in the duodenum [37,39,40].

Profiling IEL subpopulations has been used as a tool in the diagnostic work out of CD [9,32,41,42]. Using flow cytometry, a method previously validated by Camarero *et al.* [5,9], we have found similar percentages of IEL subpopulations than previous reports using similar [9,32] and different methods [43], therefore reassuring that we have successfully identified iNKT within IELs. However, these results are opposed to those from Calleja *et al.* [39] who did not find increased total IELs, as it has been previously described [9]. Moreover, neither Calleja *et al.* [39] nor Dunne *et al.* [40] found an increased numbers of iNKT cells in the intraepithelial compartment of CD patients using a similar method. Unfortunately, the nature of these differences between the results reported by these authors and our study remains elusive. However, our finding of a strong correlation between iNKT cells within the intraepithelial compartment and tissue mRNA expression of Vα24-Jα18 confirms a higher density of iNKT cells in the CD duodenum.

A very interesting question is whether the increased numbers of iNKT cells found in the intraepithelial compartment of these patients correlates with similar changes in the number of circulating iNKT cells. However, the study of circulating iNKT cells was not the aim of this research and hence blood samples had not been obtained from patients as we had performed in a previous study [21]. Future analysis will address this issue including the characterization (e.g., homing profile) of circulating iNKT cells in CD patients.

Grose *et al.* consistently reported reduced numbers of intestinal iNKT cells in CD as determined by qPCR [37,44] and by immunofluorescence [37], although in the later study the authors did not discriminate between intraepithelial and lamina propria cells [37]. However, we found increased numbers of iNKT cells in the intraepithelial compartment, but not in the lamina propria. Our findings were also correlated with mRNA expression levels of Vα24-Jα18 despite our qPCR results are not in agreement with the former studies [37,44]. Such discrepancy might be explained because duodenal Vα24-Jα18 mRNA expression varies between different populations. Our results have been confirmed in two different sets of samples from individuals from different continents. Besides, the increased Vα24-Jα18 mRNA expression found in the duodenum of CD patients also correlated with the percentage of intraepithelial iNKT cells by flow cytometry, with the Marsh score for the severity of the lesion, and with the mRNA expression of IFNγ, giving further consistency to our results. We are aware that the expression of the TCR Vα24 chain is not exclusive of iNKT cells and therefore we may be identifying other cell types (by flow cytometry and qPCR).However, the analysis of the Vα24-Jα18 molecule is more restrictive than Vβ11 [21,38]. In fact, the identification of iNKT cells by mRNA expression has been recently proposed as a more reliable alternative than the previously used co-expression of CD3[+] and CD161[+], because T cells (non-NKT) may induce CD161[+] expression after activation [45]. Moreover, we have found a direct correlation between Vα24-Jα18 mRNA expression and the total numbers of Vα24-Jα18[+] cells (representative of pure iNKT cells) in the intraepithelial compartment as determined by flow cytometry. Therefore, we are confident that Vα24-Jα18 mRNA expression is representative of the total numbers of iNKT cells in the duodenal mucosa.

Intraepithelial lymphocytes are an heterogeneous population of T cells and non-T cells, mainly composed of cytotoxic CD8[+] T cells, whose main role is the maintenance of the epithelial integrity by eliminating stressed cells and promoting epithelial repair [6]. Some authors have tried to identify the nature of non-T cells within the IEL compartment, which have been characterized as mainly NK cells, but also T cell precursors [46,47]. Dysregulated activation and increased IEL T cell numbers is a hallmark of CD and this is critically involved in epithelial cell destruction and subsequent development of villous atrophy [7,10]. The mechanisms underlying the massive expansion of IFNγ–producing intraepithelial cytotoxic T lymphocytes (CTLs) and the destruction of the epithelial cells lining the small intestine of CD patients is the focus of current research. Meresse *et al.* [10] reported an oligoclonal expansion of CTLs in CD that exhibits profound genetic reprogramming of NK cell functions. These CTLs expressed aberrant cytolytic NK lineage receptors, such as NKG2C, NKp44, and NKp46, which associated with adaptor molecules bearing immunoreceptor tyrosine-based activation motifs, induce ZAP-70 phosphorylation, cytokine secretion, and proliferation independently of TCR signalling as well as downregulation of the TCR. All of these features are characteristic of the iNKT population [48,49] though we cannot conclude that they really perform these functions in the CD duodenum and are responsible of tissue damage in CD.

IFNγ is mainly produced by the gluten-specific Th1 cells and is essential in CD pathogenesis. Recent studies also suggest that IELs are an important source of IFNγ, and the production of IFNγ persists even after GFD [8]. Our results show a correlation between the increased mRNA expression of IFNγ in CD patients (both treated and untreated) and the mRNA expression of Vα24-Jα18. These results together with the correlation between the mRNA expression of Vα24-Jα18, the Marsh score for the severity of the mucosal lesion and the total number of intraepithelial iNKT cells might suggest that the increased of IFNγ in the CD duodenum might be favoring an increased recruitment of iNKT cells. However, this requires further studies, which may be difficult to perform given the low number of iNKT cells. At present, it is considered that the natural ligands of iNKT cells are glycolipids from the cytoplasm of enterocytes, released to the extracellular matrix after apoptosis or necrosis [18,50,51], favoured by an environment rich in IFNγ and IL-15 characteristic in CD [52,53], and IL-15 plays a central role in the biological function of iNKT cells [54]. This proinflammatory environment may be relevant for the increase and activation of intraepithelial iNKT cells which, in turn, may be also a source of IFNγ.

We also studied FoxP3 mRNA expression as an indirect measurement of Treg and found a lower expression in the CD duodenum. However, we were unable to identify T cells expressing intracellular FoxP3 neither in the duodenal lamina propria nor in the intraepithelial compartment by flow cytometry (data not shown). A possible explanation might be that FoxP3 expression in humans is transient, dependent on the environment and not restricted to T-cells with a *Treg* phenotype [55,56]. In addition, and opposed to murine models [57], there is evidence suggesting that FoxP3 can be also expressed in cells without regulatory function, such as epithelial and tumor cells [58–60]. Therefore it is likely that we were not identifying T cells expressing FoxP3 by qPCR but other non-T cell types which have remained elusive by flow cytometry. Nonetheless, a CD-like molecular profile based on the mRNA expression of Vα24-Jα18 and FoxP3, which is also observed in GFD-CD patients, might be used as a useful diagnostic biomarker.

In conclusion, we have found an increased number of iNKT cells in the duodenum from both uCD and GFD-CD patients, irrespective of the mucosal status. Increased mRNA levels of Vα24-Jα18 correlated with the severity of the mucosal lesion and with the mRNA levels of IFNγ. A CD-like molecular profile, defined by an increased mRNA expression of Vα24-Jα18 together with a decreased expression of FoxP3, may represent a pro-inflammatory signature of the CD duodenum.

Supplementary Materials: Supplementary materials can be accessed at: http://www.mdpi.com/2072-6643/7/11/5444/s1.

Acknowledgments: We are grateful to Garbiñe Roy and Ana Andrés (Servicio de Inmunología, Hospital Ramón y Cajal, Madrid, Spain) for their technical help, and Eduardo Cueto Rua and Luciana Guzman (Hospital Sor Maria Ludovica, La Plata, Argentina), and Nestor Chopita (Hospital San Martin, La Plata, Argentina) for the evaluation and follow-up of the Argentinian patients. This work was supported by grants (to E A) from *Instituto de Salud Carlos III-FEDER (PI070244, PI10/01647); (to J A G) Junta de Castilla y León (SAN673/VA22-08)* and (to E M) *Beca FPI-Junta de Castilla y León/Fondo Social Europeo.*

Author Contributions: E.M., D.B., J.A.G., and E.A. conceived the study. E.M., D.B. and B.M.A. conducted the experiments. E.M., D.B., F.G.C., J.A.G. and E.A. provided intellectual input and data analyses and wrote the manuscript. L.F.S., C.C. and Y.A. provided the human samples.

Conflicts of Interest: The authors declared no conflict of interest.

References

1. Comino, I.; Real, A.; de Lorenzo, L.; Cornell, H.; Lopez-Casado, M.A.; Barro, F.; Lorite, P.; Torres, M.I.; Cebolla, A.; Sousa, C. Diversity in oat potential immunogenicity: Basis for the selection of oat varieties with no toxicity in coeliac disease. *Gut* **2011**, *60*, 915–922. [CrossRef] [PubMed]

2. Leon, A.J.; Gomez, E.; Garrote, J.A.; Arranz, E. The pattern of cytokine expression determines the degree of mucosal damage. *Gut* **2007**, *56*, 441–443. [CrossRef] [PubMed]

3. Abadie, V.; Sollid, L.M.; Barreiro, L.B.; Jabri, B. Integration of genetic and immunological insights into a model of celiac disease pathogenesis. *Annu. Rev. Immunol.* **2011**, *29*, 493–525. [CrossRef] [PubMed]

4. Sollid, L.M.; Lundin, K.E. Diagnosis and treatment of celiac disease. *Mucosal Immunol.* **2009**, *2*, 3–7. [CrossRef] [PubMed]

5. Camarero, C.; Leon, F.; Sanchez, L.; Asensio, A.; Roy, G. Age-related variation of intraepithelial lymphocytes subsets in normal human duodenal mucosa. *Dig. Dis. Sci.* **2007**, *52*, 685–691. [CrossRef] [PubMed]

6. Cheroutre, H.; Lambolez, F.; Mucida, D. The light and dark sides of intestinal intraepithelial lymphocytes. *Nat. Rev. Immunol.* **2011**, *11*, 445–456. [CrossRef] [PubMed]

7. Abadie, V.; Discepolo, V.; Jabri, B. Intraepithelial lymphocytes in celiac disease immunopathology. *Semin. Immunopathol.* **2012**, *34*, 551–566. [CrossRef] [PubMed]

8. Meresse, B.; Malamut, G.; Cerf-Bensussan, N. Celiac disease: An immunological jigsaw. *Immunity* **2012**, *36*, 907–919. [CrossRef] [PubMed]

9. Camarero, C.; Eiras, P.; Asensio, A.; Leon, F.; Olivares, F.; Escobar, H.; Roy, G. Intraepithelial lymphocytes and coeliac disease: Permanent changes in CD3-/CD7+ and T cell receptor gammadelta subsets studied by flow cytometry. *Acta Paediatr.* **2000**, *89*, 285–290. [PubMed]

10. Meresse, B.; Curran, S.A.; Ciszewski, C.; Orbelyan, G.; Setty, M.; Bhagat, G.; Lee, L.; Tretiakova, M.; Semrad, C.; Kistner, E.; *et al.* Reprogramming of CTLS into natural killer-like cells in celiac disease. *J. Exp. Med.* **2006**, *203*, 1343–1355. [CrossRef] [PubMed]

11. Hue, S.; Mention, J.J.; Monteiro, R.C.; Zhang, S.; Cellier, C.; Schmitz, J.; Verkarre, V.; Fodil, N.; Bahram, S.; Cerf-Bensussan, N.; *et al.* A direct role for NKG2D/MICA interaction in villous atrophy during celiac disease. *Immunity* **2004**, *21*, 367–377. [CrossRef] [PubMed]

12. Bhagat, G.; Naiyer, A.J.; Shah, J.G.; Harper, J.; Jabri, B.; Wang, T.C.; Green, P.H.; Manavalan, J.S. Small intestinal CD8+TCRGAMMADELTA+NKG2a+ intraepithelial lymphocytes have attributes of regulatory cells in patients with celiac disease. *J. Clin. Investig.* **2008**, *118*, 281–293. [CrossRef] [PubMed]

13. La Cava, A.; van Kaer, L.; Fu Dong, S. CD4+CD25+ TREGS and NKT cells: Regulators regulating regulators. *Trends Immunol.* **2006**, *27*, 322–327. [CrossRef] [PubMed]

14. Vignali, D.A.; Collison, L.W.; Workman, C.J. How regulatory T cells work. *Nat. Rev. Immunol.* **2008**, *8*, 523–532. [CrossRef] [PubMed]

15. Gianfrani, C.; Levings, M.K.; Sartirana, C.; Mazzarella, G.; Barba, G.; Zanzi, D.; Camarca, A.; Iaquinto, G.; Giardullo, N.; Auricchio, S.; *et al.* Gliadin-specific type 1 regulatory T cells from the intestinal mucosa of treated celiac patients inhibit pathogenic T cells. *J. Immunol.* **2006**, *177*, 4178–4186. [CrossRef] [PubMed]

16. O'Garra, A.; Vieira, P. T(h)1 cells control themselves by producing interleukin-10. *Nat. Rev. Immunol.* **2007**, *7*, 425–428. [CrossRef] [PubMed]

17. Middendorp, S.; Nieuwenhuis, E.E. NKT cells in mucosal immunity. *Mucosal. Immunol.* **2009**, *2*, 393–402. [CrossRef] [PubMed]

18. Brennan, P.J.; Tatituri, R.V.; Brigl, M.; Kim, E.Y.; Tuli, A.; Sanderson, J.P.; Gadola, S.D.; Hsu, F.F.; Besra, G.S.; Brenner, M.B. Invariant natural killer T cells recognize lipid self antigen induced by microbial danger signals. *Nat. Immunol.* **2011**, *12*, 1202–1211. [CrossRef] [PubMed]

19. Sanderson, J.P.; Waldburger-Hauri, K.; Garzon, D.; Matulis, G.; Mansour, S.; Pumphrey, N.J.; Lissin, N.; Villiger, P.M.; Jakobsen, B.; Faraldo-Gomez, J.D.; *et al.* Natural variations at position 93 of the invariant Vα24-Jα18 α chain of human INKT-cell tcrs strongly impact on CD1D binding. *Eur. J. Immunol.* **2012**, *42*, 248–255. [CrossRef] [PubMed]

20. Veldt, B.J.; van der Vliet, H.J.; von Blomberg, B.M.; van Vlierberghe, H.; Gerken, G.; Nishi, N.; Hayashi, K.; Scheper, R.J.; de Knegt, R.J.; van den Eertwegh, A.J.; *et al.* Randomized placebo controlled phase I/II trial of α-galactosylceramide for the treatment of chronic hepatitis C. *J. Hepatol.* **2007**, *47*, 356–365. [CrossRef] [PubMed]

21. Bernardo, D.; van Hoogstraten, I.M.; Verbeek, W.H.; Pena, A.S.; Mearin, M.L.; Arranz, E.; Garrote, J.A.; Scheper, R.J.; Schreurs, M.W.; Bontkes, H.J.; *et al.* Decreased circulating INKT cell numbers in refractory coeliac disease. *Clin. Immunol.* **2008**, *126*, 172–179. [CrossRef] [PubMed]

22. Zeissig, S.; Kaser, A.; Dougan, S.K.; Nieuwenhuis, E.E.; Blumberg, R.S. Role of NKT cells in the digestive system. III. Role of NKT cells in intestinal immunity. *Am. J. Physiol. Gastrointest. Liver Physiol.* **2007**, *293*, G1101–G1105. [CrossRef] [PubMed]

23. Molling, J.W.; Langius, J.A.; Langendijk, J.A.; Leemans, C.R.; Bontkes, H.J.; van der Vliet, H.J.; von Blomberg, B.M.; Scheper, R.J.; van den Eertwegh, A.J. Low levels of circulating invariant natural killer T cells predict poor clinical outcome in patients with head and neck squamous cell carcinoma. *J. Clin. Oncol.* **2007**, *25*, 862–868. [CrossRef] [PubMed]

24. Van der Vliet, H.J.; Molling, J.W.; von Blomberg, B.M.; Nishi, N.; Kolgen, W.; van den Eertwegh, A.J.; Pinedo, H.M.; Giaccone, G.; Scheper, R.J. The immunoregulatory role of CD1D-restricted natural killer T cells in disease. *Clin. Immunol.* **2004**, *112*, 8–23. [CrossRef] [PubMed]

25. Dowds, C.M.; Blumberg, R.S.; Zeissig, S. Control of intestinal homeostasis through crosstalk between natural killer T cells and the intestinal microbiota. *Clin. Immunol.* **2015**, *159*, 128–133. [CrossRef] [PubMed]

26. Kim, H.J.; Hwang, S.J.; Kim, B.K.; Jung, K.C.; Chung, D.H. NKT cells play critical roles in the induction of oral tolerance by inducing regulatory T cells producing IL-10 and transforming growth factor beta, and by clonally deleting antigen-specific t cells. *Immunology* **2006**, *118*, 101–111. [CrossRef] [PubMed]

27. Chang, J.H.; Lee, J.M.; Youn, H.J.; Lee, K.A.; Chung, Y.; Lee, A.Y.; Kweon, M.N.; Kim, H.Y.; Taniguchi, M.; Kang, C.Y. Functional maturation of lamina propria dendritic cells by activation of NKT cells mediates the abrogation of oral tolerance. *Eur. J. Immunol.* **2008**, *38*, 2727–2739. [CrossRef] [PubMed]

28. Madrigal, L.; Lynch, S.; Feighery, C.; Weir, D.; Kelleher, D.; O'Farrelly, C. Flow cytometric analysis of surface major histocompatibility complex class II expression on human epithelial cells prepared from small intestinal biopsies. *J. Immunol. Methods* **1993**, *158*, 207–214. [CrossRef]

29. Aarsaether, N.; Nilsen, B.M. Nucleotide excision repair in human cells. Biochemistry and implications in diseases. *Tidsskr. Nor. Laegeforen.* **1995**, *115*, 2786–2789. [PubMed]

30. Leon, F.; Sanchez, L.; Camarero, C.; Roy, G. Cytokine production by intestinal intraepithelial lymphocyte subsets in celiac disease. *Dig. Dis. Sci.* **2005**, *50*, 593–600. [CrossRef] [PubMed]

31. Garrote, J.A.; Gomez-Gonzalez, E.; Bernardo, D.; Arranz, E.; Chirdo, F. Celiac disease pathogenesis: The proinflammatory cytokine network. *J. Pediatr. Gastroenterol. Nutr.* **2008**, *47* (Suppl. 1), S27–S32. [CrossRef] [PubMed]

32. Leon, F.; Camarero, C.; Eiras, P.; Roy, G. Specificity of IEL profiling in the diagnosis of celiac disease. *Am. J. Gastroenterol.* **2004**, *99*, 958. [CrossRef] [PubMed]

33. Arranz, E.; Bode, J.; Kingstone, K.; Ferguson, A. Intestinal antibody pattern of coeliac disease: Association with gamma/delta T cell receptor expression by intraepithelial lymphocytes, and other indices of potential coeliac disease. *Gut* **1994**, *35*, 476–482. [CrossRef] [PubMed]

34. Van Dieren, J.M.; van der Woude, C.J.; Kuipers, E.J.; Escher, J.C.; Samsom, J.N.; Blumberg, R.S.; Nieuwenhuis, E.E. Roles of CD1D-restricted NKT cells in the intestine. *Inflamm. Bowel Dis.* **2007**, *13*, 1146–1152. [CrossRef] [PubMed]

35. Cardell, S.L. The natural killer T lymphocyte: A player in the complex regulation of autoimmune diabetes in non-obese diabetic mice. *Clin. Exp. Immunol.* **2006**, *143*, 194–202. [CrossRef] [PubMed]

36. Grose, R.H.; Thompson, F.M.; Baxter, A.G.; Pellicci, D.G.; Cummins, A.G. Deficiency of invariant NKT cells in crohn's disease and ulcerative colitis. *Dig. Dis. Sci.* **2007**, *52*, 1415–1422. [CrossRef] [PubMed]

37. Grose, R.H.; Cummins, A.G.; Thompson, F.M. Deficiency of invariant natural killer T cells in coeliac disease. *Gut* **2007**, *56*, 790–795. [CrossRef] [PubMed]

38. Van der Vliet, H.J.; von Blomberg, B.M.; Nishi, N.; Reijm, M.; Voskuyl, A.E.; van Bodegraven, A.A.; Polman, C.H.; Rustemeyer, T.; Lips, P.; van den Eertwegh, A.J.; *et al.* Circulating Vα24⁺ Vβ11⁺ NKT cell numbers are decreased in a wide variety of diseases that are characterized by autoreactive tissue damage. *Clin. Immunol.* **2001**, *100*, 144–148. [CrossRef] [PubMed]

39. Calleja, S.; Vivas, S.; Santiuste, M.; Arias, L.; Hernando, M.; Nistal, E.; Casqueiro, J.; Ruiz de Morales, J.G. Dynamics of non-conventional intraepithelial lymphocytes-NK, NKT, and gammadelta T-in celiac disease: Relationship with age, diet, and histopathology. *Dig. Dis. Sci.* **2011**, *56*, 2042–2049. [CrossRef] [PubMed]

40. Dunne, M.R.; Elliott, L.; Hussey, S.; Mahmud, N.; Kelly, J.; Doherty, D.G.; Feighery, C.F. Persistent changes in circulating and intestinal gammadelta T cell subsets, invariant natural killer T cells and mucosal-associated invariant T cells in children and adults with coeliac disease. *PLoS ONE* **2013**, *8*, e76008. [CrossRef] [PubMed]

41. Leon, F.; Eiras, P.; Roy, G.; Camarero, C. Intestinal intraepithelial lymphocytes and anti-transglutaminase in a screening algorithm for coeliac disease. *Gut* **2002**, *50*, 740–741. [CrossRef] [PubMed]

42. Fernandez-Banares, F.; Carrasco, A.; Garcia-Puig, R.; Rosinach, M.; Gonzalez, C.; Alsina, M.; Loras, C.; Salas, A.; Viver, J.M.; Esteve, M. Intestinal intraepithelial lymphocyte cytometric pattern is more accurate than subepithelial deposits of anti-tissue transglutaminase iga for the diagnosis of celiac disease in lymphocytic enteritis. *PLoS ONE* **2014**, *9*, e101249. [CrossRef] [PubMed]

43. Walker, M.M.; Murray, J.A. An update in the diagnosis of coeliac disease. *Histopathology* **2011**, *59*, 166–179. [CrossRef] [PubMed]

44. Grose, R.H.; Thompson, F.M.; Cummins, A.G. Deficiency of 6b11+ invariant NKT-cells in celiac disease. *Dig. Dis. Sci.* **2008**, *53*, 1846–1851. [CrossRef] [PubMed]

45. Wingender, G.; Kronenberg, M. Role of NKT cells in the digestive system. Iv. The role of canonical natural killer T cells in mucosal immunity and inflammation. *Am. J. Physiol. Gastrointest. Liver Physiol.* **2008**, *294*, G1–G8. [CrossRef] [PubMed]

46. Eiras, P.; Roldan, E.; Camarero, C.; Olivares, F.; Bootello, A.; Roy, G. Flow cytometry description of a novel CD3-/CD7+ intraepithelial lymphocyte subset in human duodenal biopsies: Potential diagnostic value in coeliac disease. *Cytometry* **1998**, *34*, 95–102. [CrossRef]

47. Eiras, P.; Leon, F.; Camarero, C.; Lombardia, M.; Roldan, E.; Bootello, A.; Roy, G. Intestinal intraepithelial lymphocytes contain a CD3- CD7+ subset expressing natural killer markers and a singular pattern of adhesion molecules. *Scand. J. Immunol.* **2000**, *52*, 1–6. [CrossRef] [PubMed]

48. Yu, K.O.; Porcelli, S.A. The diverse functions of CD1D-restricted NKT cells and their potential for immunotherapy. *Immunol. Lett.* **2005**, *100*, 42–55. [CrossRef] [PubMed]

49. Shimizu, K.; Shinga, J.; Yamasaki, S.; Kawamura, M.; Dorrie, J.; Schaft, N.; Sato, Y.; Iyoda, T.; Fujii, S. Transfer of mRNA encoding invariant NKT cell receptors imparts glycolipid specific responses to T cells and gammadeltat cells. *PLoS ONE* **2015**, *10*, e0131477. [CrossRef] [PubMed]

50. O'Keeffe, J.; Podbielska, M.; Hogan, E.L. Invariant natural killer T cells and their ligands: Focus on multiple sclerosis. *Immunology* **2015**, *145*, 468–475. [CrossRef] [PubMed]

51. Schrumpf, E.; Tan, C.; Karlsen, T.H.; Sponheim, J.; Bjorkstrom, N.K.; Sundnes, O.; Alfsnes, K.; Kaser, A.; Jefferson, D.M.; Ueno, Y.; *et al.* The biliary epithelium presents antigens to and activates natural killer T cells. *Hepatology* **2015**, *62*, 1249–1259. [CrossRef] [PubMed]

52. Sarra, M.; Cupi, M.L.; Monteleone, I.; Franze, E.; Ronchetti, G.; Di Sabatino, A.; Gentileschi, P.; Franceschilli, L.; Sileri, P.; Sica, G.; *et al.* IL-15 positively regulates IL-21 production in celiac disease mucosa. *Mucosal Immunol.* **2013**, *6*, 244–255. [CrossRef] [PubMed]

53. Van Bergen, J.; Mulder, C.J.; Mearin, M.L.; Koning, F. Local communication among mucosal immune cells in patients with celiac disease. *Gastroenterology* **2015**, *148*, 1187–1194. [CrossRef] [PubMed]

54. Gill, N.; Rosenthal, K.L.; Ashkar, A.A. Nk and nkt cell-independent contribution of interleukin-15 to innate protection against mucosal viral infection. *J. Virol.* **2005**, *79*, 4470–4478. [CrossRef] [PubMed]

55. Pillai, V.; Ortega, S.B.; Wang, C.K.; Karandikar, N.J. Transient regulatory T-cells: A state attained by all activated human T-cells. *Clin. Immunol.* **2007**, *123*, 18–29. [CrossRef] [PubMed]

56. Bernardo, D.; Al-Hassi, H.O.; Mann, E.R.; Tee, C.T.; Murugananthan, A.U.; Peake, S.T.; Hart, A.L.; Knight, S.C. T-cell proliferation and forkhead box p3 expression in human T cells are dependent on T-cell density: Physics of a confined space? *Hum. Immunol.* **2012**, *73*, 223–231. [CrossRef] [PubMed]

57. Gibbons, D.L.; Spencer, J. Mouse and human intestinal immunity: Same ballpark, different players; different rules, same score. *Mucosal Immunol.* **2011**, *4*, 148–157. [CrossRef] [PubMed]

58. Ebert, L.M.; Tan, B.S.; Browning, J.; Svobodova, S.; Russell, S.E.; Kirkpatrick, N.; Gedye, C.; Moss, D.; Ng, S.P.; MacGregor, D.; *et al.* The regulatory T cell-associated transcription factor FoxP3 is expressed by tumor cells. *Cancer Res.* **2008**, *68*, 3001–3009. [CrossRef] [PubMed]

59. Morgan, M.E.; van Bilsen, J.H.; Bakker, A.M.; Heemskerk, B.; Schilham, M.W.; Hartgers, F.C.; Elferink, B.G.; van der Zanden, L.; de Vries, R.R.; Huizinga, T.W.; *et al.* Expression of FoxP3 mRNA is not confined to CD4$^+$CD25$^+$ T regulatory cells in humans. *Hum. Immunol.* **2005**, *66*, 13–20. [CrossRef] [PubMed]

60. Chen, G.Y.; Chen, C.; Wang, L.; Chang, X.; Zheng, P.; Liu, Y. Cutting edge: Broad expression of the FoxP3 locus in epithelial cells: A caution against early interpretation of fatal inflammatory diseases following *in vivo* depletion of FoxP3-expressing cells. *J. Immunol.* **2008**, *180*, 5163–5166. [CrossRef] [PubMed]

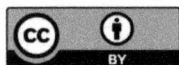

nutrients

MDPI

Review

Gliadin-Specific T-Cells Mobilized in the Peripheral Blood of Coeliac Patients by Short Oral Gluten Challenge: Clinical Applications

Stefania Picascia [1], Roberta Mandile [2], Renata Auricchio [2,3], Riccardo Troncone [2,3] and Carmen Gianfrani [1,3,*]

[1] Institute of Protein Biochemistry-CNR, Via Pietro Castellino 111, Naples 80131, Italy; s.picascia@ibp.cnr.it
[2] Department of Translational Medical Science (DISMET), Section of Pediatrics, University of Naples Federico II, Via S Pansini 5, Naples 80131, Italy; ro.mandile@libero.it (R.M.); r.auricchio@unina.it (R.A.); troncone@unina.it (R.T.)
[3] European Laboratory for the Investigation of Food-Induced Diseases (ELFID), University of Naples Federico II, Via S Pansini 5, Naples 80131, Italy
* Correspondence: c.gianfrani@ibp.cnr.it; Tel.: +39-081-613-2265; Fax: +39-081-613-2277

Received: 14 September 2015; Accepted: 26 November 2015; Published: 2 December 2015

Abstract: Celiac disease (CD) is a common lifelong food intolerance triggered by dietary gluten affecting 1% of the general population. Gliadin-specific T-cell lines and T-cell clones obtained from intestinal biopsies have provided great support in the investigation of immuno-pathogenesis of CD. In the early 2000 a new *in vivo*, less invasive, approach was established aimed to evaluate the adaptive gliadin-specific T-cell response in peripheral blood of celiac patients on a gluten free diet. In fact, it has been demonstrated that three days of ingestion of wheat-containing food induces the mobilization of memory T lymphocytes reactive against gliadin from gut-associated lymphoid tissue into peripheral blood of CD patients. Such antigen-specific T-cells releasing interferon-γ can be transiently detected by using the enzyme-linked immunospot (ELISPOT) assays or by flow cytometry tetramer technology. This paper discusses the suitability of this *in vivo* tool to investigate the repertoire of gluten pathogenic peptides, to support CD diagnosis, and to assess the efficacy of novel therapeutic strategies. A systematic review of all potential applications of short oral gluten challenge is provided.

Keywords: celiac disease; gluten challenge; interferon-γ; ELISPOT

1. Introduction

Celiac Disease (CD) is one of the most common food intolerances affecting almost 1% of worldwide population [1]. The disease develops in genetically predisposed subjects as a consequence of an abnormal immune response to wheat gluten and related prolamines of rye and barley. A decisive role in the pathogenesis is played by intestinal gliadin-specific T-cells whose presence seems to be specific of CD patients. Though the causative factor is a dietary protein, CD is considered a chronic inflammatory disorder characterized by autoimmune features. In fact, virtually all subjects with CD produce antibodies against the tissue transglutaminase (tTG) of IgA type which are the disease hallmark with diagnostic relevance [2].

For decades, CD has been considered prevalently an intestinal disease, and the enteropathy the main clinical and histological outcome. Accordingly, the evaluation of small intestinal histology has been for many years the only diagnostic tool in CD [3]. However, the high specificity and sensitivity of tTG IgA antibodies has recently led to a revision of the diagnostic criteria, especially for pediatric subjects. Based on these new guidelines from the ESPGHAN (The European Society for Paediatric Gastroenterology Hepatology and Nutrition), the evaluation of intestinal mucosa should be no more necessary to make a diagnosis of CD in the presence of clear symptoms, genetics, and high anti-tTG titers [4]. Although subjects with overt CD also have a high level of antibodies against gliadin, either for native (AGA) and deamidated (DGP) gliadin peptides, the AGA are not recommended in the diagnosis of CD due to their low sensitivity and specificity. By contrast, the DGP-IgG have a higher specificity and are recommended for the CD diagnosis in case of IgA deficiency, or in patients with both anti-tTG and anti-endomysium (EMA) negative serology. Furthermore, the use of DGP is suggested especially for patients younger than two years. Notwithstanding, a diagnostic challenge is still posed for those patients deliberately on gluten-free diets to which the intestinal histology and serum antibodies are not helpful. For these specific cases, and for other situations of diagnostic uncertainty, there is still a demand of novel approaches to make a clear and undoubted diagnosis of CD.

For both diagnostic purposes, and to study the mechanisms leading to CD, the demonstration and characterization of gliadin-specific, pathogenic T-cell response is mandatory. In the early 2000s, Anderson and co-workers established an *in vivo* approach to detect in peripheral blood the gluten-specific T-cells of intestinal origin by using the sensitive enzyme-linked immunospot (ELISPOT) assay, widely and successfully used to study antigen-specific T cells secreting cytokines, as well as antibody-producing B cells, particularly in infectious diseases [5]. The procedure developed by Anderson and co-workers requires the oral administration of wheat bread for three days to celiac patients on strict gluten free diet (GFD) and the collection of blood samples soon before and six days after the challenge started [6]. Since its first application, several studies have shown that the short gluten challenge (SGC) quickly mobilizes T-cells in the blood of celiac patients on GFD that can be revealed by interferon-γ ELISPOT assays, or flow cytometry tetramers technology, thus suggesting its great clinical potentiality. In general, the clinical symptoms are not severe, and the serum levels of CD-associated antibodies are unchanged, though in some patients morphological changes can occur after three days of the gluten challenge [7–10].

2. Genetic Susceptibility, Clinical Spectrum, and Pathogenesis

The susceptibility to develop celiac disease is strongly influenced by inherited factors. The Human Leukocyte Antigen (HLA) class II genes encoding for DQ2.5 (DQA1*05 and DQB1*02 alleles) and for DQ8 heterodimers (DQA1*03 and DQB1*0301 alleles) are the main risk factors [11]. Although more than 90% of patients with celiac disease have the DQ2.5 genotype, and the remaining ones carry either the DQ2.2 or the DQ8 genes, HLA class II account for about 40% of the genetic risk in CD [12–14]. Genome wide association studies (GWAS) have recently identified two genes, the B08 and B39 of the HLA class I locus, and a large number of non-HLA genes associated to CD, almost all of them involved in the inflammatory pathways [15].

In CD patients the dietary ingestion of wheat gluten activates a strong immune response characterized by the lymphocytic infiltration in the proximal part of the small bowel [11]. Gluten-activated T lymphocytes populate both the epithelium and lamina propria, and play a key role in damaging the intestinal mucosa [11,16]. The consequence is the villous atrophy and crypt hyperplasia that occurs within a variable window of time after the first gluten consumption. The intestinal damage can range from very mild, showing little or absent histological intestinal lesions, to a complete villous flattening, according to Marsh-Oberhuber classification [17]. From the clinical point of view, CD can present in different forms [18]. In the "classical" form, the ingestion of gluten induces an enteropathy mainly characterized by signs of malabsorption with different degrees of villous atrophy. Most common in adult age, CD may have a "non-classical" form, with no weight loss, nor classical symptoms. The disease may even be "subclinical", with no symptoms albeit in the presence of a villous atrophy. In addition, there are genetically predisposed individuals who have high anti-tTG titers, but normal small bowel mucosa. It has been reported that almost one third of these individuals with "potential celiac disease" will develop the overt disease within nine years [19].

Recent evidence has highlighted that the number of gluten-reactive T cells both in peripheral blood and in the small intestinal biopsy of CD patients positively correlated with the degree of histological intestinal damage. Similarly, the serum anti-TG IgA antibody levels have been found to significantly correlate to the Marsh grade of mucosal damage [16,20].

Furthermore, it is well known that T lymphocytes reacting to specific gluten peptides and releasing inflammatory cytokines, such as IFN-γ and IL-21, reside in the intestinal mucosa of subjects with CD but not in healthy controls [21]. These cells, mainly CD4+T lymphocytes, react to long fragments (up to 30–40 amino acid residues) of gluten resistant to gastrointestinal enzymatic degradation. These gluten peptides pass through the epithelial barrier via transcellular [22] or paracellular transport [23,24], this latter favored by an increased epithelial permeability mediated by the release of zonulin, an intestinal peptide that is involved in the tight junction regulation [25]. When in the *lamina propria* compartment, the gluten peptides become substrate for the enzyme tissue transglutaminase type 2 (tTG2) [26]. In particular stress conditions, the tTG2 is released in the extracellular matrix, and acquires an open active form [27]. After the activation, tTG2 specifically converts glutamine residues (neutrally charged) in glutamic acid (negatively charged) residues. The deamidated peptides fit the binding pockets of both DQ2 and DQ8 molecules, having a strong affinity for negative charged peptides [28]. As a consequence, the complex gluten peptide-HLA DQ2/DQ8 is specifically recognized by CD4+ T lymphocytes bearing the α/β T-cell receptor (TCR) and activating the inflammatory cascade.

The great heterogeneity of gluten proteins accounts for the large diversity of T-cell epitopes found to be active in celiac patients [29,30]. The identification of a complete repertoire of gluten immunogenic sequences is mandatory to better understand either CD pathogenesis, and to provide the bases for specific disease-targeted immuno-modulatory treatments. Among the several immunogenic sequences, three peptides were found the most active: the 33-mer from the α-gliadin (containing the DQ2.5-glia-α1a, DQ2.5-glia-α2 epitopes); the 17-mer from ω-gliadin (containing the DQ2.5-glia-ω-1, DQ2.5-glia-ω-2 epitopes); and the γ-gliadin DQ2.5-glia-γ-1 epitope [31–34]. Of note, many of the gluten T-cell stimulatory sequences have been identified thanks to the availability of stable T-cell lines and T-cell clones raised from intestinal mucosa tissues. However, the intestinal T-cell cultures have several technical restrictions mainly due to: (i) the limited numbers of cells that can be obtained from intestinal biopsies, (ii) long time necessary to establish growing T-cell cultures. Because of that, there is the need to find new tools that allow to investigate the gluten-specific CD4+ T-cell response in CD.

3. Current and Emerging Therapies

To date, the only valid treatment for celiac patients is the GFD [35], based on the strict avoidance of wheat, rye, barley, and all related cereals, including spelt (a wheat variant). After a strict GFD, the intestine recovers a normal morphology and function, and concomitantly, all symptoms and serological disease markers disappear. If from one side the GFD allows the restoration of the intestinal physiological function, from the other side it is expensive and provides several social restrictions, and compliance to GFD is not optimal, particularly in adolescence [36,37]. Nutritional properties of gluten free foods, as for example the high glycemic index and caloric power, increase the risk of treated celiacs to develop nutritional alterations, obesity, or metabolic syndromes [38,39]. In addition, there is a minority of patients that suffers from a refractory condition, in which the diet is not efficacious, and requires a pharmacological, anti-inflammatory treatment [40,41]. A deeper knowledge of CD pathophysiology has opened to the investigation of several therapeutic drug-based approaches in the last decade, some of them currently on clinical trial phase II to assess their efficacy [42]. This promising scenario strongly demands the availability of a rapid, safe, and reproducible *in vivo* assay to assess the efficacy of emerging novel therapies to treat CD [43].

4. Gluten Oral Challenge as Tool to Monitor Intestinal Gluten-Reactive T-Cells

The gluten challenge is a clinical approach widely used in the last decades to have a diagnosis of celiac disease. It consists in the introduction of gluten containing foods in subjects previously on a gluten free diet, for a time frame necessary to provoke a clinical response (from two weeks up to four months). About 75% of adults received a clear diagnosis in at least two weeks [44], however the response rates and the onset of symptoms were highly variable among different patients [45,46]. Either histological, serological, and symptomatic changes are evaluated, to monitor the efficacy of gluten challenge. However, the extensive gluten challenge has some limitations, such as the risk of the overt disease induction (especially in younger patients), and the invasive endoscopy as final exam. Altogether, these findings have raised the need of alternative, less invasive, procedures to investigate the role of gluten-specific T-cells in the pathogenesis of CD.

4.1. Interferon-γ ELISPOT Assay on Peripheral Blood Cells after a Three Day Gluten Challenge

For long time, all the efforts to isolate gliadin-specific memory T-cells from peripheral blood samples of CD patients gave poor results, due to the low frequency in the blood of gluten-primed intestinal CD4+ T-cells, and to a substantial functional differences (in particular a diverse HLA restriction) that has been reported between gliadin-specific T-cell clones raised from the gut or blood [26,47,48]. As consequence, peripheral blood samples have, for a long time, been considered not optimal tissue material to study the anti-gluten T-cell immunity. At the beginning of this century, Anderson and co-workers published a study describing a new *in vivo* approach to analyze T-cell response to gluten in peripheral blood, overcoming in this way all the technical problems related to the use of intestinal T-cells [6]. This procedure requires the oral administration of bread slices (approximately 200 g/day) for three days to CD patients on a strict GFD, and blood samples obtained at different time points during the gluten challenge. The gluten-reactive T-cells are monitored in peripheral blood mononuclear cells (PBMCs) by detecting those releasing IFN-γ, the prominent mediator of the inflammatory cascade in celiac mucosa, by ELISPOT assay. The ELISPOT is a sensitive technique able to catch single cell secreting cytokine, or other immune mediators, upon specific stimuli. In this pilot study, Anderson and co-workers found that the SGC rarely causes problems, as only few volunteers, out of 16 adult CD patients enrolled, showed clinical symptoms of disease (usually mild), or had histological signs of intestinal mucosa inflammation. The classical serological markers of CD, as the anti-endomysium and anti-tTG2 antibodies, remained negative after the SGC. The gluten challenge induced in celiac patients a transient IFN-γ response to tTG-treated chymotrypsin-digested gliadin that was maximum six days after the volunteers began eating bread slices. A 660% increment of IFN-γ spot-forming cells (IFN-γ-SFC) was reported at day six compared to responses before the challenge, whilst only a 37% of IFN-γ-SFC increment was detected in DQ2+ control group. In addition, the gut origin of these circulating T lymphocytes, mobilized in response to the gluten challenge, was supported by the expression of the α4β7 integrin [7,8], a classical marker of gut homing [49,50]. Similarly, the restriction of gluten response by HLA class II DQ2 molecules, associated to CD risk, was also demonstrated.

A subsequent study from our group performed in adolescent CD patients has reported that the SGC is a reproducible assay. To further demonstrate that the SGC is a valid instrument to investigate the gluten induced immune response, 14 young celiac patients on GFD underwent two separate gluten consumptions, with the same procedure described by Anderson *et al.* After three to five months of gluten wash-out, the celiac cohort underwent a second cycle of wheat-containing food challenge. We found that the IFN-γ responses significantly increased in peripheral blood sampled six days after the second challenge, and interestingly, gliadin reactive cells were more frequent compared to the first challenge, most likely due to the increased frequency of memory T-cells activated upon the first gluten exposure [8].

4.2. Interferon-γ ELISA Assay and Multiparametric Masscytometry to Monitor the Anti-Gluten T-Cells Response after a Three Day Gluten Challenge

Other studies have reported *in vitro* read-outs different from ELISPOT assay to assess the specific immune response elicited by gluten challenge. Ontiveros *et al.* have developed a whole blood assay to detect gluten-specific T-cells by dosing IFN-γ in the serum by ELISA after stimulation of blood with gluten/peptides [51]. The same research group has also analyzed the peripheral blood cell response to gluten upon the three days of wheat consumption by measuring the cell proliferation and found results consistent with the IFN-γ ELISPOT findings [6].

Despite the central role given by HLA class II in CD, being the main genetic risk factor and the key restriction molecules of pathogenic CD4+ T-cells, studies from our group have demonstrated that gliadin contain peptides able to stimulate cytotoxic CD8+ T-cells in an antigen restricted manner when presented on surface of antigen presenting cells (APC), such as B- or enterocytes by HLA class I molecules [52]. Of note, a more recent study from Mark Davis and co-workers using the potent multiparametric CyTOF technology approach, that allows to monitor simultaneously more than 50 different T-cell markers, showed that the three days gluten challenge induced in peripheral blood of CD patients a remarkable increased of either TCRαβ- and TCRγδ- bearing CD8+ T lymphocytes, other than the CD4+ T-cells [53]. These lymphocytes, expressed the gut homing markers, such as CD103 (intestinal epithelial-homing markers αE) and β7-integrins, thus demonstrating their origin from intestinal mucosa. The percentage of each cell subset mobilized by gluten intake varies among single patients, but ranged from 1% up to 10% of total peripheral CD8+ cells. This keynote study has demonstrated that memory CD8+ T-cells are activated by the oral gluten challenge and circulate from the target intestinal tissue to peripheral blood. However, further studies are necessary to assess the gluten specificity of these CD8+ T cells mobilized by the SGC.

4.3. HLA-DQ2-Tetramers as Probe to Detect Gliadin-Specific Cells in Peripheral Blood

In the recent years, much attention has been paid to the use of tetramers technology to dissect specific T-cell responses to a variety of antigenic sources [20]. Tetramers are composed by four major histocompatibility complex (MHC) molecules each of them loaded with a single antigenic peptide, labelled with fluoresceinated biotin-streptavidin complex. The MHC-peptide construct binds to a single T-cell receptor on the surface membrane of cognate T-cells. When the tetramer is bound, the cells can be visualized by flow cytometry analysis [54]. This sensitive assay allows to quantify the cell frequency, to assess their phenotype, or to separate the cell subset that specifically reacts to a single antigen. Tetramer complexes have been widely and successfully used to study MHC class I-restricted CD8+ T lymphocytes specific for infectious diseases or tumor antigens [55].

DQ2-gliadin-tetramer tests were first used by Raki and co-workers to monitor CD4+ T lymphocyte specific for two immunodominant gluten epitopes, DQ2.5-glia-α1a and DQ2.5-glia-α2, in PBMCs of celiac patients underwent the SGC [10]. The response rate of such test (approximately 85% sensitive and 100% specific evaluated in HLA-DQ2.5+ celiac patients *vs.* HLA-matched controls) is comparable to that found in IFN-γ ELISPOT assay [10]. Frequencies of positive cells identified after gluten challenge is similar between the two approaches (number of IFN-γ secreting cells found by ELISPOT ranging from 1 to 5000 in comparison to DQ2.5-glia-α1a tetramer positive cells ranging 1:1000 and DQ2.5-glia-α2 tetramer positive cells 1:5000). Similarly to the IFN-γ ELISPOT findings, no tetramer positive cells were detected in DQ2+ healthy controls, either before or after the brief gluten exposure. Interestingly, in subjects with a diagnosis of CD, 5%–8% of total CD4+ cells were stained with tetramer specific for both DQ2.5 α epitopes [10]. More recently, other studies from the same group have monitored gluten-specific T-cells in peripheral blood of celiac patients by tetramer technology without the gluten oral challenge [20]. More specifically, gliadin-tetramer positive cells have been detected in peripheral blood of both treated and untreated DQ2-positive subjects with CD.

In addition, a single cell-TCR sequence analysis performed on DQ2-gliadin-tetramer specific T-cells, mobilized upon the gluten challenge, has demonstrated how highly focused the TCR repertoire is of CD4+ T-cells specific for the immunodominant gluten epitopes [53,56–58]. Collectively, all these studies demonstrated the great potentiality of the tetramer technology as a tool to investigate the anti-gluten T-cell responses. However, tetramer assay has both pros and cons. The main advantage is that it allows to quantify the antigen-specific cells independently by their immune function or activation state. More specifically, this technology can also monitor cells not releasing a specific cytokine [9]. However, despite the high sensitivity, tetramers allow the identification of only cells specific for a single peptide, whereas ELISPOT assay allows simultaneous monitoring for T cells reacting to a wider repertoire of gluten epitopes. Tetramer production, furthermore, is challenging, being laborious, expensive, and time consuming all factors that render this technology difficult in application, especially in a clinical practice context. Notwithstanding the above advantages or disadvantages, it is evident that larger cohort of patients and healthy controls are needed to validate the sensitivity of tetramer technology to diagnose CD, independently of the gluten challenge.

5. Translational Applications of the Short Gluten Oral Challenge

5.1. Identification of Gluten Immunogenic Peptides

Since the first description, the short oral gluten challenge has become an attractive tool for all researchers interested in the identification of the complete repertoire of gluten (and of other prolamin) toxic sequences [32,59] (Table 1). Tye-Din and co-workers found a high degree of T-cell peptide cross reactivity in adult celiacs underwent the SGC by screening a large library (almost 3000) of 20-mer peptides derived from gluten, hordein, and secalin [32]. Interestingly, though many peptides were immunogenic, only the T-cell clones specific for three peptides containing five epitopes (DQ2.5-glia-α1a/DQ2.5-glia-α2; DQ2.5-glia-ω-1/DQ2.5-glia-ω-2; DQ2.5-Hor-1) were found responsible for the great majority of responses in adult CD, thus demonstrating a high T-cell stimulatory peptide redundancy.

A recent study from Hardy and co-workers [60] has expanded such peptide repertoire analysis to a pediatric cohort of CD patients. A comparable pattern of peptide recognition was found between children and adult with CD. These similarities in the nature of the T-cells induced by the *in vivo* SGC between pediatric and adult CD can have a great potentiality for the applications also in celiac children of the peptide-based therapy designed for adults.

5.2. Validation of Therapeutic Drugs

Many studies aimed to identify new strategies to detoxify wheat gluten, and several of these are based on enzymatic technologies that degrade fragments or mask gluten immune-stimulatory sequences [34] (Table 1). The high content in proline and glutamine-rich peptides make gluten resistant to proteolysis by gastric, pancreatic, and intestinal brush border membrane enzymes. Partially digested gluten fragments stimulate the immune system and became toxic for celiac disease patients [11]. The identification of a combination of enzymes that can break proline and glutamine bounds is a fascinating goal for celiac researchers, and it represents an interesting future perspective for pharmaceutical sector that aims to produce oral drugs. To this specific purpose, several gluten-specific proteases, called glutenases, have been isolated from bacteria, fungi, and cereals and are currently under clinical trial investigation. ALV003 is a promising mixture of two glutenases which cleaves gluten fragments at site enriched in proline and glutamine: a cysteine-endoprotease derived from germinated barley seeds (EP-B2), able to breaks gluten protein, and a prolyl endopeptidase (PEP) from S. capsulate (SC-PEP) that cleaves proline residues. When combined in 1:1 ratio these two glutenases maximized the enzymatic activity [61]. In a clinical trial, 20 patients with celiac disease on GFD were randomized to eat either gluten (16 g/day for three days) pre-treated with ALV003, or gluten pre-treated with placebo. Patients who received ALV003 gluten had significantly lower peripheral T-cell IFN-γ response to the immunodominant α-gliadin 33-mer multi-epitope peptide, or whole gliadin, compared to the group that received the placebo [62]. The relevance of the SGC to monitor drug efficacy has been demonstrated in a follow-up study, where a double blind, placebo-controlled trial was performed on 41 adults CD patients randomized to assume ALV003, or the placebo, along with a gluten daily intake (2 g/day) for six weeks [63]. In this second study, the main clinical read-out was the evaluation of the small intestinal mucosa damage that appeared. Signs of lymphocytes activation, and intraepithelial infiltration of CD3+ lymphocytes, both TCRα/β and TCRγ/δ, were found significantly increased only in the placebo-treated patients, while these markers remained almost unchanged in ALV003 treated group. Though very promising, this drug shows an interesting expectative for its future application, further investigations are necessary to monitor the long term effects.

Other strategies have been developed to directly detoxify wheat flour, as the extensive hydrolysis during the sourdough fermentation with a mixture of acid bacteria proteases [64], or the transamidation with methyl-lysine of specific glutamines that are target of the tTG [65] (Table 1). The demonstration of the immuno-stimulatory properties of fermented or transamidated wheat after a short challenge may provide rapid and preliminary information about the safety and efficacy of these novel and promising strategies to produce wheat-based gluten free food for celiac disease.

5.3. Diagnostic Relevance

In recent times, a great attention has been paid to develop clinical practices less invasive than endoscopy to diagnose celiac disease (Table 1). Moreover, the increased attention paid by the general public to food related problems, as well as the improved distribution of gluten free foods, has spread the belief that gluten free diet coincides with a healthy life style; as a consequence more and more people voluntary exclude gluten from their diet without a clear diagnosis of celiac disease [66]. This makes difficult for clinicians to formulate a definitive diagnosis of celiac disease in unclear cases, as both serological and histological tests revert to the normal value on GFD. Even the HLA genotyping of such individuals complaining gluten related disorders, and on arbitrary GFD, does not help to make a definitive diagnosis of CD in DQ2 or DQ8 positive subjects, having this test only a negative prediction value. To date, the only instrument to practice a correct diagnosis in such doubtful cases consists in the evaluation of histological lesions after a long-term gluten challenge. A recent study conducted in adults has shown that at least two weeks of gluten consumption allow a clear diagnosis of celiac disease in over 75% of CD population [44]. However, the time frame of the gluten challenge is variable, as indicated by several studies, and may be longer than two weeks. In fact it is clear that sensitivity to gluten exposure varies greatly between coeliac patients and some may take much longer before showing signs of relapse [4,46]. This long-term gluten challenge makes this diagnostic procedure difficult to practice. Moreover a long-term challenge is not suggested in children younger than five years old and during a pubertal growth spurt. The short-time (only three days) of the gluten challenge and the sensitivity of immunological tests offer an interesting perspective for using the SGC as a diagnostic tool. Pilot studies of gluten challenge as diagnostic tool for subjects coming to the observation when they are already on gluten free diet came from Brottveit *et al.* [10]. The authors enrolled 35 subjects with uncertain diagnosis and on GFD for at least four weeks and 13 patients with treated CD. All the enrolled subjects underwent the SGC and endoscopy for biopsy sampling at day 0 and day 4 of the gluten challenge. By the positive detection of tetramers the authors have observed gliadin-specific T-cells in 11/13 CD patients, and in only 2/35 with uncertain CD, thus identifying a group of subjects clinically gluten-sensitive and yet negative to this test.

In order to validate the SGC as a procedure to support diagnosis of celiac disease in uncertain cases, it is mandatory the assessment of its sensitivity and specificity. Regarding the sensitivity, there is a large variability in the cut-off applied to define subject responders to the gluten challenge among the different studies. In our recent experience of brief gluten challenge performed on a cohort of 36 DQ2+ CD adolescent celiacs [8,60], each single patient was considered responsive to oral challenge when showed levels of INF-γ secreting cells in response to whole gliadin, and/or dominant gliadin peptides, that exceeded two-fold the INF-γ responses at day 0 (Fold Increase-FI $\geq$ 2) and a difference of SFC/well (ΔSFC) of at least 10 between day 6 and day 0. Based on these criteria, we found that almost 73% of our 36 patients are responsive (Figure 1). Other studies reporting a higher frequency of DQ2+ CD responders (by ELISPOT) ranging from 85% to 92% of responder cases [6–8,51]. These un-matched results, obtained in different celiac cohorts, highlighted how it is important to identify common and unique criteria to validate unequivocally the subjects that positively respond to gluten challenge (responders), and to distinguish from the non-responder ones. It is evident that further work is necessary to validate the SGC as diagnostic tool for celiac disease; it is particularly fundamental to expand such an analysis to HLA DQ2+ non celiac healthy control to assess its specificity, which is to date poorly investigated. Indeed the classical diagnostic approach characterized by the long gluten challenge, and monitored by serology and histology, is more stable and reliable than the brief challenge, despite that there is the need to have a shorter and less invasive test to apply to the clinical practice. As stated above, the tetramers are promising diagnostic tools, however several technological limits still remain to be solved for their use large-scale.

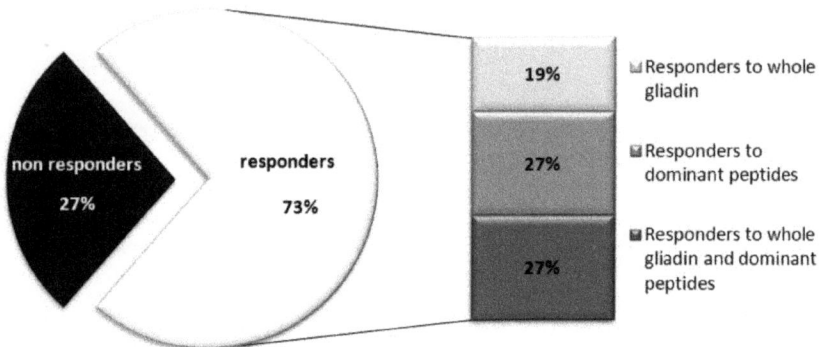

Figure 1. Percentage of subject responders to the short gluten challenge. A cohort of 36 Italian DQ2-positive young celiac patients [8,60] consumed 3–4 wheat bread slices (corresponding to 9–12 g of gluten/die) for three days. Immunoreactivity was evaluated in peripheral blood at day 0 and day 6 by INF-γ-ELISPOT assay, in response to either whole gliadin or immunodominant α-gliadin peptides.

Table 1. Possible translational applications of brief gluten challenge.

Application	Clinical/Research Purpose	References
Diagnosis	Confirmation of diagnosis in uncertain celiac disease cases	[10,67]
Therapies	Validation of new therapeutic drugs	[62]
Therapies	Validation of biochemical or enzymatic strategies to detoxify gluten.	[64,65]
Therapies	Searching of wheat cultivars with reduced immunotoxic gluten sequences	[68]
Pathogenesis	Identification of immunogenic gluten epitopes	[32,60]
Pathogenesis	Phenotypic analysis of cell population involved in celiac disease	[53]

6. Conclusions

The short (three days) gluten challenge is a validated tool for the evaluation and monitoring in peripheral blood of gluten-specific T-cell response that are elicited in the gut after gluten exposure. Since its first demonstration in early 2000 [6], this *in vivo* procedure, less invasive than the endoscopy, has allowed the screening of large peptide library and provided a great help for the characterization of a repertoire of immunostimulatory gluten sequences, a fundamental step to constructing a peptide-base immunotherapy for the treatment of CD [29,32]. Furthermore, the short oral challenge has been a powered instrument to demonstrate that gluten mobilizes intestinal CD8+ T-cells, corroborating their role in CD pathogenesis. The SGC is a promising tool to assess the efficacy of novel treatments aimed to reduce the load of toxic gluten or of immunomodulatory drugs.

Finally, thanks to several sensitive assays to measure anti-gluten T response in blood cells, as IFN-γ ELISPOT/ELISA or tetramers-flow cytometry technologies, it is thinkable to apply this innovative approach to clinical practice, in order to help specialists in making a correct and definitive diagnosis of celiac disease in those cases in which subjects are arbitrarily on gluten free diet, or can help the diagnosis in case of potential celiac disease. To make this technique adapt to clinical practice, several parameters still have to be addressed. Further work is necessary to reach a high sensitivity, to keep lowest number of false negative subjects. So far, the main limitations playing against the wide use of oral challenge for clinical practice are less sensitivity and specificity compared to available serology tests, and the high cost of ELISPOT and tetramers immune assays. Notwithstanding, these limitations do not lessen the value of the oral challenge, as a rapid tool to assess the efficacy of several alternative therapies currently under investigation.

Acknowledgments: This work has been supported by funding from CNR-DSB Progetto Bandiera "InterOmics" (MIUR PNR 2011-2013).

Conflicts of Interest: The authors declare no conflict of interest.

References

1. Lundin, K.E.A.; Qiao, S.-W.; Snir, O.; Sollid, L.M. Coeliac disease—From genetic and immunological studies to clinical applications. *Scand. J. Gastroenterol.* **2015**, *50*, 708–717. [CrossRef] [PubMed]

2. Korponay-Szabó, I.R.; Troncone, R.; Discepolo, V. Adaptive diagnosis of coeliac disease. *Best Pract. Res. Clin. Gastroenterol.* **2015**, *29*, 381–398. [CrossRef] [PubMed]

3. Walker-Smith, J.A.; Guandalini, S.; Schmitz, J.; Shmerling, D.H.; Visakorpi, J.K. Revised criteria for diagnosis of coeliac disease. *Arch. Dis. Child.* **1990**, *65*, 909–911.

4. Husby, S.; Koletzko, S.; Korponay-Szabó, I.R.; Mearin, M.L.; Phillips, A.; Shamir, R.; Troncone, R.; Giersiepen, K.; Branski, D.; Catassi, C.; *et al.* European Society for Pediatric Gastroenterology, Hepatology, and Nutrition Guidelines for the Diagnosis of Coeliac Disease. *J. Pediatr. Gastroenterol. Nutr.* **2012**, *54*, 136–160. [CrossRef] [PubMed]

5. Currier, J.R.; Kuta, E.G.; Turk, E.; Earhart, L.B.; Loomis-Price, L.; Janetzki, S.; Ferrari, G.; Birx, D.L.; Cox, J.H. A panel of MHC class I restricted viral peptides for use as a quality control for vaccine trial ELISPOT assays. *J. Immunol. Methods* **2002**, *260*, 157–172. [CrossRef]

6. Anderson, R.P.; Degano, P.; Godkin, A.J.; Jewell, D.P.; Hill, A.V. *In vivo* antigen challenge in celiac disease identifies a single transglutaminase-modified peptide as the dominant A-gliadin T-cell epitope. *Nat. Med.* **2000**, *6*, 337–342. [CrossRef] [PubMed]

7. Anderson, R.P.; van Heel, D.A.; Tye-Din, J.A.; Barnardo, M.; Salio, M.; Jewell, D.P.; Hill, A.V.S. T cells in peripheral blood after gluten challenge in coeliac disease. *Gut* **2005**, *54*, 1217–1223. [CrossRef] [PubMed]

8. Camarca, A.; Radano, G.; di Mase, R.; Terrone, G.; Maurano, F.; Auricchio, S.; Troncone, R.; Greco, L.; Gianfrani, C. Short wheat challenge is a reproducible *in vivo* assay to detect immune response to gluten. *Clin. Exp. Immunol.* **2012**, *169*, 129–136. [CrossRef] [PubMed]

9. Ráki, M.; Fallang, L.-E.; Brottveit, M.; Bergseng, E.; Quarsten, H.; Lundin, K.E.A.; Sollid, L.M. Tetramer visualization of gut-homing gluten-specific T cells in the peripheral blood of celiac disease patients. *Proc. Natl. Acad. Sci. USA* **2007**, *104*, 2831–2836. [CrossRef] [PubMed]

10. Brottveit, M.; Ráki, M.; Bergseng, E.; Fallang, L.-E.; Simonsen, B.; Løvik, A.; Larsen, S.; Løberg, E.M.; Jahnsen, F.L.; Sollid, L.M.; Lundin, K.E.A. Assessing possible celiac disease by an HLA-DQ2-gliadin Tetramer Test. *Am. J. Gastroenterol.* **2011**, *106*, 1318–1324. [CrossRef] [PubMed]

11. Abadie, V.; Sollid, L.M.; Barreiro, L.B.; Jabri, B. Integration of genetic and immunological insights into a model of celiac disease pathogenesis. *Annu. Rev. Immunol.* **2011**, *29*, 493–525. [CrossRef] [PubMed]

12. Van Heel, D.A.; Hunt, K.; Greco, L.; Wijmenga, C. Genetics in coeliac disease. *Best Pract. Res. Clin. Gastroenterol.* **2005**, *19*, 323–339. [CrossRef] [PubMed]

13. Sollid, L.M.; Thorsby, E. HLA susceptibility genes in celiac disease: Genetic mapping and role in pathogenesis. *Gastroenterology* **1993**, *105*, 910–922. [PubMed]

14. Karell, K.; Louka, A.S.; Moodie, S.J.; Ascher, H.; Clot, F.; Greco, L.; Ciclitira, P.J.; Sollid, L.M.; Partanen, J. HLA types in celiac disease patients not carrying the DQA1*05-DQB1*02 (DQ2) heterodimer: Results from the European Genetics Cluster on Celiac Disease. *Hum. Immunol.* **2003**, *64*, 469–477. [CrossRef]

15. Kumar, V.; Gutierrez-Achury, J.; Kanduri, K.; Almeida, R.; Hrdlickova, B.; Zhernakova, D.V.; Westra, H.J.; Karjalainen, J.; Ricaño-Ponce, I.; Li, Y.; *et al.* Systematic annotation of celiac disease loci refines pathological pathways and suggests a genetic explanation for increased interferon-gamma levels. *Hum. Mol. Genet.* **2015**, *24*, 397–409. [CrossRef] [PubMed]

16. Bodd, M.; Ráki, M.; Bergseng, E.; Jahnsen, J.; Lundin, K.E.A.; Sollid, L.M. Direct cloning and tetramer staining to measure the frequency of intestinal gluten-reactive T cells in celiac disease. *Eur. J. Immunol.* **2013**, *43*, 2605–2612. [CrossRef] [PubMed]

17. Oberhuber, G.; Granditsch, G.; Vogelsang, H. The histopathology of coeliac disease: Time for a standardized report scheme for pathologists. *Eur. J. Gastroenterol. Hepatol.* **1999**, *11*, 1185–1194. [CrossRef] [PubMed]

18. Ludvigsson, J.F.; Leffler, D.A.; Bai, J.C.; Biagi, F.; Fasano, A.; Green, P.H.R.; Hadjivassiliou, M.; Kaukinen, K.; Kelly, C.P.; Leonard, J.N.; *et al.* The Oslo definitions for coeliac disease and related terms. *Gut* **2013**, *62*, 43–52. [CrossRef] [PubMed]

19. Auricchio, R.; Tosco, A.; Piccolo, E.; Galatola, M.; Izzo, V.; Maglio, M.; Paparo, F.; Troncone, R.; Greco, L. Potential celiac children: 9-year follow-up on a gluten-containing diet. *Am. J. Gastroenterol.* **2014**, *109*, 913–921. [CrossRef] [PubMed]

20. Christophersen, A.; Ráki, M.; Bergseng, E.; Lundin, K.E.; Jahnsen, J.; Sollid, L.M.; Qiao, S.-W. Tetramer-visualized gluten-specific CD4+ T cells in blood as a potential diagnostic marker for coeliac disease without oral gluten challenge. *United Eur. Gastroenterol. J.* **2014**, *2*, 268–278. [CrossRef] [PubMed]

21. Gianfrani, C.; Auricchio, S.; Troncone, R. Adaptive and innate immune responses in celiac disease. *Immunol. Lett.* **2005**, *99*, 141–145. [CrossRef] [PubMed]

22. Matysiak-Budnik, T.; Moura, I.C.; Arcos-Fajardo, M.; Lebreton, C.; Ménard, S.; Candalh, C.; ben-Khalifa, K.; Dugave, C.; Tamouza, H.; van Niel, G.; *et al.* Secretory IgA mediates retrotranscytosis of intact gliadin peptides via the transferrin receptor in celiac disease. *J. Exp. Med.* **2008**, *205*, 143–154. [CrossRef] [PubMed]

23. Tripathi, A.; Lammers, K.M.; Goldblum, S.; Shea-Donohue, T.; Netzel-Arnett, S.; Buzza, M.S.; Antalis, T.M.; Vogel, S.N.; Zhao, A.; Yang, S.; *et al.* Identification of human zonulin, a physiological modulator of tight junctions, as prehaptoglobin-2. *Proc. Natl. Acad. Sci. USA* **2009**, *106*, 16799–16804. [CrossRef] [PubMed]

24. Lammers, K.M.; Lu, R.; Brownley, J.; Lu, B.; Gerard, C.; Thomas, K.; Rallabhandi, P.; Shea-Donohue, T.; Tamiz, A.; Alkan, S.; *et al.* Gliadin induces an increase in intestinal permeability and zonulin release by binding to the chemokine receptor CXCR3. *Gastroenterology* **2008**, *135*, 194–204. [CrossRef] [PubMed]

25. Fasano, A.; Not, T.; Wang, W.; Uzzau, S.; Berti, I.; Tommasini, A.; Goldblum, S.E. Zonulin, a newly discovered modulator of intestinal permeability, and its expression in coeliac disease. *Lancet* **2000**, *355*, 1518–1519. [CrossRef]

26. Molberg, O.; Mcadam, S.N.; Körner, R.; Quarsten, H.; Kristiansen, C.; Madsen, L.; Fugger, L.; Scott, H.; Norén, O.; Roepstorff, P.; *et al.* Tissue transglutaminase selectively modifies gliadin peptides that are recognized by gut-derived T cells in celiac disease. *Nat. Med.* **1998**, *4*, 713–717. [CrossRef] [PubMed]

27. Pinkas, D.M.; Strop, P.; Brunger, A.T.; Khosla, C. Transglutaminase 2 undergoes a large conformational change upon activation. *PLoS Biol.* **2007**. [CrossRef] [PubMed]

28. Sollid, L.M.; Jabri, B. Celiac disease and transglutaminase 2: A model for posttranslational modification of antigens and HLA association in the pathogenesis of autoimmune disorders. *Curr. Opin. Immunol.* **2011**, *23*, 732–873. [CrossRef] [PubMed]

29. Camarca, A.; del Mastro, A.; Gianfrani, C. Repertoire of gluten peptides active in celiac disease patients: Perspectives for translational therapeutic applications. *Endocr. Metab. Immune Disord. Drug Targets* **2012**, *12*, 207–219. [CrossRef] [PubMed]

30. Wieser, H. Chemistry of gluten proteins. *Food Microbiol.* **2007**, *24*, 115–119. [CrossRef] [PubMed]

31. Shan, L.; Molberg, Ø.; Parrot, I.; Hausch, F.; Filiz, F.; Gray, G.M.; Sollid, L.M.; Khosla, C. Structural basis for gluten intolerance in celiac sprue. *Science* **2002**, *297*, 2275–2279. [CrossRef] [PubMed]

32. Tye-Din, J.A.; Stewart, J.A.; Dromey, J.A.; Beissbarth, T.; van Heel, D.A.; Tatham, A.; Henderson, K.; Mannering, S.I.; Gianfrani, C.; Jewell, D.P.; *et al.* Comprehensive, quantitative mapping of T cell epitopes in gluten in celiac disease. *Sci. Transl. Med.* **2010**. [CrossRef] [PubMed]

33. Camarca, A.; Anderson, R.P.; Mamone, G.; Fierro, O.; Facchiano, A.; Costantini, S.; Zanzi, D.; Sidney, J.; Auricchio, S.; Sette, A.; *et al.* Intestinal T cell responses to gluten peptides are largely heterogeneous: Implications for a peptide-based therapy in celiac disease. *J. Immunol.* **2009**, *182*, 4158–4166. [CrossRef] [PubMed]

34. Sollid, L.M.; Qiao, S.-W.; Anderson, R.P.; Gianfrani, C.; Koning, F. Nomenclature and listing of celiac disease relevant gluten T-cell epitopes restricted by HLA-DQ molecules. *Immunogenetics* **2012**, *64*, 455–460. [CrossRef] [PubMed]

35. Sollid, L.M.; Lundin, K.E.A. Diagnosis and treatment of celiac disease. *Mucosal Immunol.* **2009**, *2*, 3–7. [CrossRef] [PubMed]

36. Greco, L.; Mayer, M.; Ciccarelli, G.; Troncone, R.; Auricchio, S. Compliance to a gluten-free diet in adolescents, or "what do 300 coeliac adolescents eat every day?". *Ital. J. Gastroenterol. Hepatol.* **1997**, *29*, 305–310. [PubMed]

37. Errichiello, S.; Esposito, O.; di Mase, R.; Camarca, M.E.; Natale, C.; Limongelli, M.G.; Marano, C.; Coruzzo, A.; Lombardo, M.; Strisciuglio, P.; *et al.* Celiac disease: Predictors of compliance with a gluten-free diet in adolescents and young adults. *J. Pediatr. Gastroenterol. Nutr.* **2010**, *50*, 54–60. [CrossRef] [PubMed]

38. Lamacchia, C.; Camarca, A.; Picascia, S.; Di Luccia, A.; Gianfrani, C. Cereal-based gluten-free food: How to reconcile nutritional and technological properties of wheat proteins with safety for celiac disease patients. *Nutrients* **2014**, *6*, 575–590. [CrossRef] [PubMed]

39. Diamanti, A.; Capriati, T.; Basso, M.S.; Panetta, F.; di Ciommo Laurora, V.M.; Bellucci, F.; Cristofori, F.; Francavilla, R. Celiac disease and overweight in children: An update. *Nutrients* **2014**, *6*, 207–220. [CrossRef] [PubMed]

40. Ryan, B.M.; Kelleher, D. Refractory celiac disease. *Gastroenterology* **2000**, *119*, 243–251. [CrossRef] [PubMed]

41. Malamut, G.; Cellier, C. Complications of coeliac disease. *Best Pract. Res. Clin. Gastroenterol.* **2015**, *29*, 451–458. [CrossRef] [PubMed]

42. Kaukinen, K.; Lindfors, K.; Mäki, M. Advances in the treatment of coeliac disease: An immunopathogenic perspective. *Nat. Rev. Gastroenterol. Hepatol.* **2014**, *11*, 36–44. [CrossRef] [PubMed]

43. Ludvigsson, J.F.; Card, T.; Ciclitira, P.J.; Swift, G.L.; Nasr, I.; Sanders, D.S.; Ciacci, C. Support for patients with celiac disease: A literature review. *United Eur. Gastroenterol. J.* **2015**, *3*, 146–159. [CrossRef] [PubMed]

44. Leffler, D.; Schuppan, D.; Pallav, K.; Najarian, R.; Goldsmith, J.D.; Hansen, J.; Kabbani, T.; Dennis, M.; Kelly, C.P. Kinetics of the histological, serological and symptomatic responses to gluten challenge in adults with coeliac disease. *Gut* **2013**, *62*, 996–1004. [CrossRef] [PubMed]

45. Tack, G.J.; van de Water, J.M.W.; Bruins, M.J.; Kooy-Winkelaar, E.M.C.; van Bergen, J.; Bonnet, P.; Vreugdenhil, A.C.E.; Korponay-Szabo, I.; Edens, L.; von Blomberg, B.M.E.; *et al.* Consumption of gluten with gluten-degrading enzyme by celiac patients: A pilot-study. *World J. Gastroenterol.* **2013**, *19*, 5837–5847. [CrossRef] [PubMed]

46. Mayer, M.; Greco, L.; Troncone, R.; Grimaldi, M.; Pansa, G. Early prediction of relapse during gluten challenge in childhood celiac disease. *J. Pediatr. Gastroenterol. Nutr.* **1989**, *8*, 474–479. [CrossRef] [PubMed]

47. Gjertsen, H.A.; Sollid, L.M.; Ek, J.; Thorsby, E.; Lundin, K.E. T cells from the peripheral blood of coeliac disease patients recognize gluten antigens when presented by HLA-DR, -DQ, or -DP molecules. *Scand. J. Immunol.* **1994**, *39*, 567–574. [CrossRef] [PubMed]

48. Jensen, K.; Sollid, L.M.; Scott, H.; Paulsen, G.; Kett, K.; Thorsby, E.; Lundin, K.E. Gliadin-specific T cell responses in peripheral blood of healthy individuals involve T cells restricted by the coeliac disease associated DQ2 heterodimer. *Scand. J. Immunol.* **1995**, *42*, 166–170. [CrossRef] [PubMed]

49. Quiding-Järbrink, M.; Ahlstedt, I.; Lindholm, C.; Johansson, E.L.; Lönroth, H. Homing commitment of lymphocytes activated in the human gastric and intestinal mucosa. *Gut* **2001**, *49*, 519–525. [CrossRef] [PubMed]

50. Berlin, C.; Berg, E.L.; Briskin, M.J.; Andrew, D.P.; Kilshaw, P.J.; Holzmann, B.; Weissman, I.L.; Hamann, A.; Butcher, E.C. Alpha 4 beta 7 integrin mediates lymphocyte binding to the mucosal vascular addressin MAdCAM-1. *Cell* **1993**, *74*, 185–195. [CrossRef]

51. Ontiveros, N.; Tye-Din, J.A.; Hardy, M.Y.; Anderson, R.P. *Ex-vivo* whole blood secretion of interferon (IFN)-γ and IFN-γ-inducible protein-10 measured by enzyme-linked immunosorbent assay are as sensitive as IFN-γ enzyme-linked immunospot for the detection of gluten-reactive T cells in human leucocyte antigen (HLA)-DQ2·5(+) -associated coeliac disease. *Clin. Exp. Immunol.* **2014**, *175*, 305–315. [PubMed]

52. Mazzarella, G.; Stefanile, R.; Camarca, A.; Giliberti, P.; Cosentini, E.; Marano, C.; Iaquinto, G.; Giardullo, N.; Auricchio, S.; Sette, A.; *et al.* Gliadin activates HLA class I-restricted CD8+ T cells in celiac disease intestinal mucosa and induces the enterocyte apoptosis. *Gastroenterology* **2008**, *134*, 1017–1027. [CrossRef] [PubMed]

53. Han, A.; Newell, E.W.; Glanville, J.; Fernandez-Becker, N.; Khosla, C.; Chien, Y.-H.; Davis, M.M. Dietary gluten triggers concomitant activation of CD4+ and CD8+ αβ T cells and γδ T cells in celiac disease. *Proc. Natl. Acad. Sci. USA* **2013**, *110*, 13073–13078. [CrossRef] [PubMed]

54. Altman, J.D.; Moss, P.A.; Goulder, P.J.; Barouch, D.H.; McHeyzer-Williams, M.G.; Bell, J.I.; McMichael, A.J.; Davis, M.M. Phenotypic analysis of antigen-specific T lymphocytes. *Science* **1996**, *274*, 94–96. [CrossRef] [PubMed]

55. Klenerman, P.; Cerundolo, V.; Dunbar, P.R. Tracking T cells with tetramers: New tales from new tools. *Nat. Rev. Immunol.* **2002**, *2*, 263–272. [CrossRef] [PubMed]

56. Qiao, S.-W.; Ráki, M.; Gunnarsen, K.S.; Løset, G.-Å.; Lundin, K.E.A.; Sandlie, I.; Sollid, L.M. Posttranslational modification of gluten shapes TCR usage in celiac disease. *J. Immunol.* **2011**, *187*, 3064–3071. [CrossRef] [PubMed]

57. Qiao, S.-W.; Christophersen, A.; Lundin, K.E.A.; Sollid, L.M. Biased usage and preferred pairing of α- and β-chains of TCRs specific for an immunodominant gluten epitope in coeliac disease. *Int. Immunol.* **2014**, *26*, 13–19. [CrossRef] [PubMed]

58. Broughton, S.E.; Petersen, J.; Theodossis, A.; Scally, S.W.; Loh, K.L.; Thompson, A.; van Bergen, J.; Kooy-Winkelaar, Y.; Henderson, K.N.; Beddoe, T.; *et al.* Biased T-cell receptor usage directed against human leukocyte antigen DQ8-restricted gliadin peptides is associated with celiac disease. *Immunity* **2012**, *37*, 611–621. [CrossRef] [PubMed]

59. Tanner, G.J.; Howitt, C.A.; Forrester, R.I.; Campbell, P.M.; Tye-Din, J.A.; Anderson, R.P. Dissecting the T-cell response to hordeins in coeliac disease can develop barley with reduced immunotoxicity. *Aliment. Pharmacol. Ther.* **2010**, *32*, 1184–1191. [CrossRef] [PubMed]

60. Hardy, M.Y.; Girardin, A.; Pizzey, C.; Cameron, D.J.; Watson, K.A.; Picascia, S.; Auricchio, R.; Greco, L.; Gianfrani, C.; La Gruta, N.L.; *et al.* Consistency in Polyclonal T-cell Responses to Gluten Between Children and Adults with Celiac Disease. *Gastroenterology* **2015**, *6*, 1541–1552. [CrossRef] [PubMed]

61. Freeman, H.J. Emerging drugs for celiac disease. *Expert Opin. Emerg. Drugs* **2015**, *20*, 129–135. [CrossRef] [PubMed]

62. Tye-Din, J.A.; Anderson, R.P.; Ffrench, R.A.; Brown, G.J.; Hodsman, P.; Siegel, M.; Botwick, W.; Shreeniwas, R. The effects of ALV003 pre-digestion of gluten on immune response and symptoms in celiac disease *in vivo*. *Clin. Immunol.* **2010**, *134*, 289–295. [CrossRef] [PubMed]

63. Lähdeaho, M.-L.; Kaukinen, K.; Laurila, K.; Vuotikka, P.; Koivurova, O.-P.; Kärjä-Lahdensuu, T.; Marcantonio, A.; Adelman, D.C.; Mäki, M. Glutenase ALV003 attenuates gluten-induced mucosal injury in patients with celiac disease. *Gastroenterology* **2014**, *146*, 1649–1658. [CrossRef] [PubMed]

64. Greco, L.; Gobbetti, M.; Auricchio, R.; di Mase, R.; Landolfo, F.; Paparo, F.; di Cagno, R.; de Angelis, M.; Rizzello, C.G.; Cassone, A.; *et al.* Safety for patients with celiac disease of baked goods made of wheat flour hydrolyzed during food processing. *Clin. Gastroenterol. Hepatol.* **2011**, *9*, 24–29. [CrossRef] [PubMed]

65. Gianfrani, C.; Siciliano, R.A.; Facchiano, A.M.; Camarca, A.; Mazzeo, M.F.; Costantini, S.; Salvati, V.M.; Maurano, F.; Mazzarella, G.; Iaquinto, G.; *et al.* Transamidation of wheat flour inhibits the response to gliadin of intestinal T cells in celiac disease. *Gastroenterology* **2007**, *133*, 780–789. [CrossRef] [PubMed]

66. NPD Group. *Dieting Monitor: Eating Patterns in America*; NPD Group: Port Washington, NY, USA, 2013.

67. Brottveit, M.; Beitnes, A.C.; Tollefsen, S.; Bratlie, J.E.; Jahnsen, F.L.; Johansen, F.E.; Sollid, L.M.; Lundin, K.E.A. Mucosal Cytokine Response After Short-Term Gluten Challenge in Celiac Disease and Non-Celiac Gluten Sensitivity. *Am. J. Gastroenterol.* **2013**, *108*, 842–850. [CrossRef] [PubMed]

68. Gianfrani, C.; Camarca, A.; Mazzarella, G.; di Stasio, L.; Giardullo, N.; Ferranti, P.; Picariello, G.; Rotondi Aufiero, V.; Picascia, S.; Troncone, R.; *et al.* Extensive *in vitro* gastrointestinal digestion markedly reduces the immune-toxicity of Triticum monococcum wheat: Implication for celiac disease. *Mol. Nutr. Food Res.* **2015**. [CrossRef] [PubMed]

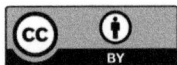

Section 2:
Clinical Aspects

nutrients

MDPI

Review

DQ2, DQ7 and DQ8 Distribution and Clinical Manifestations in Celiac Cases and Their First-Degree Relatives

Magdalena Araya [1,*], Amaya Oyarzun [1], Yalda Lucero [2], Nelly Espinosa [3] and Francisco Pérez-Bravo [4]

[1] Human Nutrition, Institute of Nutrition and Food Technology (INTA), University of Chile, Santiago, Chile; amaya.oyarzun@gmail.com
[2] Department of Pediatrics, Faculty of Medicine, University of Chile, Santiago, Chile; ylucero@gmail.com
[3] Hospital Militar, Santiago, Chile; nespinosap@yahoo.es
[4] Nutrition Department, Faculty of Medicine, University of Chile, Santiago, Chile; fperez@med.uchile.cl
* Author to whom correspondence should be addressed; maraya@inta.uchile.cl; Tel.: +56-2-29781411; Fax: +56-2-22140230.

Received: 20 April 2015; Accepted: 5 June 2015; Published: 18 June 2015

Abstract: HLA-linked genes are relevant to celiac disease (CD); the potential genetic differences present worldwide are not fully understood. Previous results suggest that the distribution of HLA-DQ2/DQ7/DQ8 in Chile may differ from that in Europe and North America. In celiac patients and their first-degree relatives (FDRS), we assessed their clinical, serological and histological characteristics, determined HLA-DQ2, HLA-DQ7 and HLA-DQ8 alleles and genotypes, and evaluated the relations between them. A total of 222 individuals were assessed (56 cases, 166 FDRs). 16.9% of FDRs were tTG positive; 53.6% of them showed overweight/obesity and 3% undernourishment; they spontaneously declared being asymptomatic, but detailed questioning revealed that 60.7% experienced symptoms, which had not been investigated. DQ2 was present in 53.9% and 43.9.0% of cases and FDRs ($p < 0.05$). The most frequent genotype distribution was DQ2/DQ7 (fr 0.392 (cases) and 0.248 (FDRs), respectively, $p < 0.02$). The next most common genotypes were HLA-DQ2/DQ8 (fr 0.236 in FDRs and 0.176 in cases, $p < 0.05$). 3.92% cases were not HLA-DQ2/DQ8 carriers. Among tTG positive FDRs, 57.4%, 22.3% and 20.2% carried DQ2, DQ7 and DQ8, respectively. In cases, 72.7% of the biopsies classified Marsh ≥ 3 carried at least one DQ2; 91.7% of DQ2/DQ2 and 88.3% of DQ2/DQ7 were Marsh ≥ 3. Thus, DQ2 frequency is lower than reported; the higher frequency found for DQ8 and DQ7 concur with recent publications from Argentine and Brazil. These results suggest that although CD may manifest clinically in ways similar to those described in other populations, some genetic peculiarities in this region deserve further study.

Keywords: celiac disease; first degree relatives; HLA- DQ2; HLA-DQ7; HLA-DQ8

1. Introduction

Celiac disease (CD) is a heritable, frequent, chronic disorder that involves small intestinal inflammation and autoimmune manifestations in response to dietary gluten. The condition results from the interplay of genetic and environmental factors (mainly dietary gluten) [1–3]; the host immune system and microbiota are also involved in the development of CD [2,4–7]. Although knowledge has progressed greatly in the last decades, several aspects of the condition remain unclear. Until the 90s, CD was thought to occur mainly among white Europeans [8,9] and there was no clear explanation as to why countries with rather large white populations of European origin reported low incidence of the disease [10]. The significant geographical differences reported [9] refer mainly to prevalence of CD [11–13] while genetic characteristics in some areas of the globe are still insufficient and not fully understood. It is well-agreed that a significant proportion of the genetic predisposition for CD comes from human leukocyte antigen (HLA)-linked genes, estimated to account for up to 40% of the genetic load [14]. The southern cone of South America is one of the areas where available evidence is incomplete and still unclear. The estimated prevalence of CD in Chile [15] and in Argentine [16] is 0.6%; in both countries and HLA-DQ8 frequencies seem to be higher than described elsewhere [17,18]. Also, there is data suggesting that the frequency of cases not carrying HLA-DQ2 or DQ8 may be higher than reported in other areas [19,20]. It has been speculated that these features might be related to common native genetic (Mapuche) background; in Chile, there is evidence that diabetes mellitus (DMT1) would be infrequent in the Mapuche native group [21]. The first objective in this protocol was to assess the frequency and distribution of HLA-DQ2, HLA-DQ8 and HLA-DQ7 in a family study of celiac patients and their first-degree relatives (FDRs).

Better diagnostic tools and recognition of the extra intestinal and autoimmune manifestations have proved that CD is frequent in most countries that actively search for it. Recognition of atypical, incomplete or non-classical forms of CD and the application of active search in risk groups has yielded good evidence for an increased prevalence of CD among FDRs of celiac patients [17,22–26]. However, evidence about the global frequency of the disease in this group and their clinical and genetic characteristics is largely insufficient. In an effort to contribute to expand our knowledge on these issues, we set as a second objective the determination of serologically positive FDRs of known celiac cases (susceptible group) and their clinical characterization.

Thus, in this study we measured HLA-DQ2, HLA-DQ8 and HLA-DQ7 in celiac cases and their FDRs and characterized their symptoms, nutritional status, serological and histologic data. Then we calculated the percentage of serologically positive FDRs, analyzed their characteristics and compared serologically positive FDRs with cases and serologically negative FDRs. Finally, we related the genetic findings to clinical and serological characteristics of cases and FDRs.

2. Experimental Section

2.1. Patients and First-Degree Relatives (FDRs)

Patients consulting for CD at the outpatient clinic of INTA during 2012–2014 were evaluated as potential candidates for the study. Following current diagnostic criteria [3,22,27] the 57 biopsy-proven celiac patients and their 171 FDRs were invited to participate in the study. Participants gave their written informed consent prior to incorporation to the protocol. INTA's Institutional Review Board approved the study. Cases and their families participated in an interview where the medical history of each family member was registered, including previous consultations and diagnoses; the presence of clinical symptoms was asked for in the form of "do you have it", "did you have it at the time of diagnosis" and "have you ever had it".

Clinical presentations were defined on the basis of symptoms present at diagnosis—classical when initial diagnosis was led to by digestive symptoms, non-classical when non-digestive symptoms (extra-intestinal and/or autoimmune manifestations and/or being a FDR) led to the initial investigation. At the end of the interview, weight and height were registered and nutritional status was classified following the World Health Organization (body mass index (BMI) for adolescents and adults and Z score weight/height for children under 5 years) [28]. A blood sample was obtained from the antecubital vein for serological and genetic analyses.

2.2. Laboratory testing

Serum IgA was measured using an ELISA commercial kit (Alpco®, Salem, NH, USA). IgA-anti-endomysial antibodies (EMA) were determined by indirect immunofluorescence using slides with monkey esophagus sections as substrate (IMMCO Diagnostics®, Buffalo, NY. USA), IgA anti-tTG2 antibodies (tTG) were measured using a commercial ELISA kit (AESKU®, Wendelsheim, Germany), expressing the results as suggested by the manufacturer: negative ≤ 12 U, borderline = 12–18 U and positive $\geq$ 18 U. When IgA-tTG was negative and total serum IgA was below the cut off for age, IgA/IgG tTG was measured using Celicheck (a kit that measures IgA- and IgG- transglutaminase antibodies, (AESKU®, Wendelsheim, Germany), expressing the results as negative $\leq$ 16 U, borderline = 16–24 U and positive $\geq$ 24 U. Mucosal lesions in the small intestinal biopsies were graded according to Marsh classification [29]: M1 = more than 25 IELs/100 enterocytes in the epithelium (lymphocytic enteritis); M2 = with crypt hyperplasia; M3a = with moderate villous atrophy, M3b = with subtotal villous atrophy; M3c = total villous atrophy. Genetic studies were performed using the commercial kit DQ-CD Typing plus (BioDiagene®, Palermo, Italy). After blood lysis, DNA was amplified by polymerase chain reaction (PCR) (12 per sample) and identification of alleles was carried out by agarose gel electrophoresis. HLA- DQ typing for celiac susceptibility included the single sequence specific primer-PCR home based method to detect the presence of the HLA heterodimer DQA1*0501 - DQB1*0201 [30,31]. Then we used a sequence specific oligonucleotide-PCR based method to type the HLA DQB1*locus (Dynal Biotech Ltd, Bromborough, UK) to confirm the presence/absence of the DQB1*02 allele or to verify the presence of the other DQB1*03 risk allele. Finally, the sequence-specific primer-PCR technique (Dynal Biotech Ltd, Bromborough, UK) was used to resolve the DQB1*03 locus, showing the presence/absence of the DQB1*0302 allele. HLA DR typing HLA-DRB1 typing was performed by a sequence specific oligonucleotide-PCR-based method (Dynal Biotech LTD, Bromborough, UK) that determined the phased DR-DQ genotypes of all individuals. Results are expressed nominating DQ2 = DQA1*0501, DQB1*0201. DQ7 = DQB1*0301/04. DQ8 = DQA1*03, DQB1*0302.

2.3. Statistical Analysis

Analysis of general data included descriptive statistics for variables with normal or non-normal distribution. Allele and genotype frequencies were computed as sample proportions. Comparison of such frequencies in cases and FDRs was statistically assessed by a chi-square test corrected by multiple comparisons [26].

3. Results

3.1. Clinical Data

A total of 56 out of 57 celiac cases agreed to participate, providing 166 FDRs (48 fathers, 50 mothers, 8 sons/daughters and 60 siblings). Their sex distribution, mean age and nutritional status are shown in Table 1. Women were more frequent among patients with classical presentations and in symptomatic FDRs. Only three (non-classical) cases were under 8 years of age at diagnosis; they were investigated because of anemia (n = 1) or failure to thrive (n = 2). Overweight/obesity was present in 21.4% and 53.6% of cases and FDRs, respectively. There was no morbid obesity in cases or FDRs; 10.7% of cases and 3% of FDRs were undernourished.

Twenty cases (35.7%) initially presenting classical digestive features required hospitalization at diagnosis. Among celiac cases, both in those initially investigated for classical digestive symptoms or other reasons, abdominal distension, abdominal pain, weight loss/undernutrition and diarrhea were the most frequent findings (Table 2). Many FDRs declared they were asymptomatic, but detailed and directed questioning revealed that they experienced a variety of symptoms (Table 2), abdominal pain and constipation being the most frequent ones. In 23.2% of cases and in 12% of FDRs an autoimmune condition was already diagnosed at the time of this study, Hashimoto's thyroiditis being the most frequent diagnosis. Since appearance of symptoms, children and adult patients' first consultation occurred after 0.1 and 5.9 years and diagnosis was reached after 0.9 and 6 years, respectively. No differences were detected between genders in time to first consultation or to reach diagnosis. Cases with non-classical courses consulted and reached diagnosis in shorter times in comparison to patients with classical symptoms; comparing the periods 2000–2009 and 2010–2014, mean time to reach diagnosis among adult patients decreased from 108 months to 62 months.

Table 1. Sex, age and nutritional status in celiac cases and their first degree relatives.

	Cases (*n* = 56)		First Degree Relatives (*n* = 166)		Total (*n* = 222)
	Classical	Non-Classical	Symptomatics	Subclinical	
Females *n* (%)	32 (68.1)	4 (44.4)	57 (66.3)	33 (41.3)	126 (100)
Age y (mean)					
0–8	19 (4.2 y)	3 (4.5 y)	9 (4.5 y)	8 (4.0 y)	39 (100)
8–12	5 (9.7 y)	4 (9.4 y)	2 (10.1 y)	7 (10.2 y)	18 (100)
12–18	6 (14.9 y)	2 (12.7 y)	7 (14.3 y)	4 (14.6 y)	19 (100)
>18	17 (31.1 y)	0	68 (42.9 y)	61 (44.1 y)	146 (100)
Nutritional status					
Undernourished	4 (8.5)	2 (22.2)	3 (3.5)	2 (2.5)	11 (100)
Well nourished	31 (66)	7 (77.8)	39 (45.3)	33 (41.3)	110 (100)
Overweight	11 (23.4)	0	29 (33.7)	33 (41.3)	73 (100)
Obesity type I	1 (2.1)	0	12 (14)	11 (13.8)	24 (100)
Obesity type II	0	0	3 (3.5)	1 (1.3)	4 (100)
Total	47 (100)	9 (100)	86 (100)	80 (100)	222

Table 2. Symptoms, autoimmune diseases and other diagnoses detected in celiac cases and their first-degree relatives.

	Cases (*n* = 56)			First Degree Relatives (*n* = 166)		
	Total *n* (%)	Classical *n* (%)	Non-Classical *n* (%)	Total *n* (%)	Symptomatic *n* (%)	Subclinical *n* (%)
Symptoms						
Abdominal distension	49 (87.5)	44 (78.6)	5 (8.9)	2 (1.2)	2 (1.2)	0 -
Abdominal pain	41 (73.2)	37 (66.1)	4 (7.1)	48 (28.9)	48 (28.9)	0 -
Weight loss	41 (73.2)	36 (64.3)	5 (8.9)	1 (0.6)	1 (0.6)	0 -
Diarrhea	40 (71.4)	39 (69.6)	1 (1.8)	3 (1.8)	3 (1.8)	0 -
Malaise	33 (58.9)	32 (57.1)	1 (1.8)	1 (0.6)	1 (0.6)	0 -
Constipation	27 (48.2)	24 (42.9)	3 (5.4)	30 (18.1)	30 (18.1)	0 -
Steatorrhea	22 (39.3)	22 (39.3)	0 -	2 (1.2)	2 (1.2)	0 -
Vomiting	23 (41.1)	21 (37.5)	2 (3.6)	0 -	0 -	0 -
Malnutrition	20 (35.7)	16 (28.6)	4 (7.1)	2 (1.2)	2 (1.2)	0 -
Anorexia	14 (25.0)	13 (23.2)	1 (1.8)	0 -	0 -	0 -
Edema	8 (14.3)	8 (14.3)	0 -	1 (0.6)	1 (0.6)	0 -
Autoimmune disease						
Autoimmune thyroiditis	9 (16.1)	9 (16.1)	0 (0)	17 (10.2)	13 (7.8)	4 (2.4)
DM type 1	2 (3.6)	1 (1.8)	1 (1.8)	2 (1.2)	2 (1.2)	0 -
Down Syndrome	1 (1.8)	1 (1.8)	0 -	0 -	0 -	0 -
Autoimmune hepatitis	1 (1.8)	1 (1.8)	0 -	1 (0.6)	1 (0.6)	0 -

About half of cases showed positive serologic studies at the time of current assessment; in only 5 out of 25 tTG positive cases, EMA was also positive. Among FDRs, 28 out of 166 (16.9%) were tTG positive, of which 5 were also EMA positive (Table 3). All 28 positive FDRs were advised a small intestinal biopsy but only 10 (35.7%) underwent the procedure; of these 4 (2 adult women and 2 adult men) were diagnosed CD; two were eutrophic and two overweight, three had digestive symptoms and one was asymptomatic. In all, diagnosis was reached after the intestinal biopsy showed lesions Marsh ≥ 2 and clinical improvement after gluten free diet was demonstrated.

Biopsy records of cases were available in 44 of 56 cases (Table 4). Of these, 35 of 44 (79.5%) showed mucosal lesions classified as Marsh 3 or more; no differences were observed in the proportion of Marsh 3 lesions between classical and non-classical cases.

Table 3. Antiendomysial antibodies and antitransglutaminases in celiac cases and first-degree relatives.

	Cases (*n* = 56)		First Degree Relatives (*n* = 166)	
	Classical *n* = 47	Non-Classical *n* = 9	Symptomatic *n* = 83	Subclinical *n* = 84
EMA * (+)	5 (10.6%)	0 -	3 (3.6%)	2 (2.4%)
tTG ** (+)	25 (53.2%)	4 (44.4%)	19 (22.9%)	9 (10.7%)

* = Antiendomysial antibodies. ** = transglutaminase antibodies.

Table 4. Small intestinal biopsy lesions and genotypes in 44 cases of celiac disease.

		Genotypes							
		DQ2/DQ2	DQ2/DQ7	DQ2/DQ8	DQ7/DQ7	DQ7/DQ8	DQ8/DQ8	DQ8/ND	Total
Marsh	*n* (%)								
2–3	9 (20.5)	1 (2.3)	2 (4.5)	2 (4.5)	1 (2.3)	0	3 (6.8)	0	9 (100)
≥3	35 (79.5)	11 (25)	15 (34.1)	6 (13.6)	1 (2.3)	0	1 (2.3)	1 (2.3)	35 (100)
Total	44 (100)	12 (27.3)	17 (38.6)	8 (18.2)	2 (4.5)	0	4 (9.1)	1 (2.3)	44 (100)

ND = Not Detected (represents an allele not detected by the techniques used).

3.2. Genetic Data

Distribution of genotypes found and biopsy lesions observed in cases also appear in Table 4. In relation to duodenal lesion and DQ assessment, 91.4% of biopsies classified Marsh ≥ 3 carried at least one DQ2; 91.7% of DQ2/DQ2 was Marsh ≥ 3 and 88.2% were DQ2/DQ7 (Table 4).

Table 5 shows the DQ2, DQ7, DQ8 allele and genotypic distribution in cases and FDRs. Contribution of DQ2 in celiac cases and FDRs was 53.9% and 43.9% ($p < 0.05$), respectively, with no differences detected for DQ7 or DQ8 distribution between CD cases and FDRs.

Table 5. Alleles and genotype frequencies in 51 celiac cases and 157 tTG first-degree relatives (FDRs).

	Cases (*n* = 51) N (fr)	FDRs (*n* = 157) N (fr)	*p* value
Alleles			
DQ2	55 0.539	138 0.439	<0.05
DQ7	24 0.235	82 0.261	NS
DQ8	22 0.215	82 0.261	NS
Others	1 0.011	12 0.039	-
Genotypes			
DQ2/DQ2	13 0.255	27 0.172	NS
DQ2/DQ7	20 0.392	39 0.248	<0.02
DQ2/DQ8	9 0.176	37 0.236	NS
DQ2/ND	0	7 0.045	-
DQ7/DQ7	2 0.039	14 0.089	NS
DQ7/DQ8	0 0.000	15 0.096	-
DQ8/DQ8	6 0.118	14 0.089	NS
DQ8/DQ2	0	1 0.006	-
DQ8/ND	1 0.020	1 0.006	-
ND/ND	0	2 0.013	-

ND = allele not detected.

Among celiac cases, DQ2, DQ7 and DQ8 frequency in genotypes was 55, 24 and 22, respectively. Two cases (3.92%) were not HLA-DQ2/DQ8 carriers. As for FDRs, DQ8 was more frequent than among cases, with DQ2, DQ7 and DQ8 frequencies contributing 138, 82 and 82, respectively. Table 5 also shows that the most frequent genotype distribution was DQ2/DQ7 (fr 0.392 and 0.248 in cases and FDRs, respectively, $p < 0.02$). The second-most common genotype was DQ2/DQ8 (fr 0.236 in FDRs and 0.176 in cases, *p* < 0.05). DQ2/DQ2 was third in frequency, without differences between cases or FDRs. 3/48 cases.

Among tTG positive FDRs, 57.4% carried DQ2 while 22.3% and 20.2% carried DQ7 and DQ8, respectively. This distribution was not different among tTG-negative FDRs. As for the four FDRs diagnosed CD, 2 carried DQ2/DQ2, 1 DQ2/DQ8 and 1 DQ2/DQ7.

4. Discussion

4.1. Clinical Aspects

Results show that active search yielded 16.9% of tTG-positive FDRs, a figure that is in the higher range of values reported [22,32,33]. Overweight/obesity among FDRs was close to 50%, not different from the range currently described in our country's general population, with no differences between symptomatic and subclinical individuals [15]; as expected, overweight/obesity was more frequent among tTG negative (57.2%) than tTG positive (35.7%, *p* < 0.01) FDRs; at the same time, under-nutrition was marginally present in all FDRs (Table 1). All this emphasizes the new scenario of CD. As described by other authors, symptoms in FDRs were less frequent (Table 2), mainly abdominal pain (28.9%) and constipation (18.1%) [22,27]. However, results showed some rather unexpected findings in this group; it was surprising that the majority of FDRs spontaneously declared they were asymptomatic, but the more detailed questioning revealed that 60.7% did experience some kind of symptoms; these were similar to those observed in celiac cases, and their frequency among tTG-positive FDRs was not different from that of tTG-negative FDRs (54.3%). It was not possible to clarify to what extent lower intensity of symptoms could be responsible for the lack of awareness of disease. It was unfortunate that only a few of the serologically positive FDRs accepted an endoscopic biopsy; this represents the main limitation to this study; reluctance to accept being investigated seems to be common among these individuals and has also been reported by other authors [34]; in the four newly diagnosed FDRs, DQ2 was present in all them.

Among celiac cases, at time of diagnosis, 35.7% of them required hospitalization, which we interpret as suggesting late consultation and/or diagnosis. This clearly draws attention to a public health problem, the need for promoting active search; at present, the large group of professionals responsible for public health systems does not apply it in several countries. As expected, the frequency of autoimmune disorders was found to be higher than in the general population [35,36]. Other conditions and diagnoses, such as anemia and short stature, were present both in celiac cases and FDRs. Time to consult since the appearance of symptoms was clearly longer among adult patients (data not shown), as also was the time to reach diagnosis; although the study was not designed to assess this issue, chart analysis suggested that at present, although diagnosis is indeed delayed, people in the community seem to be more aware of non-classical presentations of CD and spontaneously look for help earlier. The fact that about half of cases showed positive serologic studies at the time of our current assessment reveals poor adherence to treatment; unfortunately, this finding is not different from what we have found in previous evaluations [17].

4.2. Genetic Data

The results obtained in the celiac cases confirmed that DQ2 is the main allele associated with CD [14] and with more intense damage to the intestinal mucosa [37,38]. Although DQ2 exhibits the highest frequency in this study, it is clearly lower than reported (Tables 4 and 5) [22]. DQ8 appears to be less frequent than in our own previous studies, sharing the second frequency with DQ7, a relevant finding considering similar recent publications in the South American region [18,20]. In relation to DQ8 findings, our present results agree with what we found in 2010 [19] and differ from older data obtained in 1999, which showed that DQ8 was more prevalent [17]. There is no clear explanation for the differences observed; the three groups assessed 15 years ago represented an unselected local population receiving medical care in the public health systems of Santiago. However, the protocols applied had different designs; the results of this study cannot clarify whether this may be responsible for the different results obtained. It is also worth mentioning that in the present study the frequency of cases not carrying HLA-DQ2 or HLA-DQ8 was 3.92%, a figure still higher than that reported in Europe, but somewhat lower than our own previous results that showed 7% [18].

In summary, results of this study contribute to improving global knowledge of CD, in this case in Chile as part of the southern cone of South America. tTG-positive FDRs were found at 16.9%, a figure in the higher range of those previously described, which contributes to characterizing this group; about half of FDRs were overweight/obese, emphasizing the new scenario of CD; and 60.7% reported symptoms which had not been investigated. This finding among FDRs, the long time elapsed between initiation of symptoms and diagnosis and the high percentage of cases meant to be treated but tTG-positive at the time of this study strongly stress the need for improving public health management of CD. Genetic analyses showed that HLA-DQ2 alleles were first in frequency (53.9%), but the figure found is lower than those reported elsewhere, with HLA-DQ7 and DQ8 making significant contributions, both as alleles and genotypes. These findings agree with recent communications originating from the same geographical region and suggest that, although CD may manifest clinically in ways similar to those described in other areas (mainly Europe and North America) in this region, it seems to have some genetic peculiarities that deserve further study.

Acknowledgments: This project was funded by the Institute of Nutrition and Food Technology and the University of Chile. We thank the patients and their families for their valuable participation. The authors acknowledge BioDiagene and Grifols for supplying kits to analyze alleles and genotypes.

Author Contributions: MA is responsible for the work; she conceived and designed the study, participated in analysis and interpretation of data and wrote the manuscript. AO participated in study design, acquisition, analysis and interpretation of data and manuscript critical review. YL participated in designing the protocol, and in acquisition and critical review of the manuscript. NE participated in acquisition and critical review of the manuscript and FP-B conceived and designed the study and participated in analysis, interpretation of data and critical revision of the manuscript.

Conflicts of Interest: The authors declare no conflict of interest.

References

1. McNeish, A.S.; Anderson, C.M. Coeliac disease. The disorder in childhood. *Clin. Gastroenterol.* **1974**, *3*, 127–144. [PubMed]
2. Kupfer, S.S.; Jabri, B. Pathophysiology of celiac disease. *Gastrointest. Endosc. Clin. N. Am.* **2012**, *22*, 639–660. [CrossRef] [PubMed]
3. Ludvigsson, J.F.; Leffler, D.A.; Bai, J.C.; Biagi, F.; Fasano, A.; Green, P.H.; Hadjivassiliou, M.; Kaukinen, K.; Kelly, C.P.; Leonard, J.N.; *et al.* The Oslo definitions for coeliac disease and related terms. *Gut* **2013**, *62*, 43–52. [CrossRef] [PubMed]
4. Olivares, M.; Neef, A.; Castillejo, G.; Palma, G.D.; Varea, V.; Capilla, A.; Palau, F.; Nova, E.; Marcos, A.; Polanco, I.; *et al.* The HLA-DQ2 genotype selects for early intestinal microbiota composition in infants at high risk of developing coeliac disease. *Gut* **2015**, *64*, 406–417. [CrossRef] [PubMed]
5. Wacklin, P.; Laurikka, P.; Lindfors, K.; Collin, P.; Salmi, T.; Lahdeaho, M.L.; Saavalainen, P.; Maki, M.; Matto, J.; Kurppa, K.; *et al.* Altered duodenal microbiota composition in celiac disease patients suffering from persistent symptoms on a long-term gluten-free diet. *Am. J. Gastroenterol.* **2014**, *109*, 1933–1941. [CrossRef] [PubMed]
6. Sanchez, E.; de Palma, G.; Capilla, A.; Nova, E.; Pozo, T.; Castillejo, G.; Varea, V.; Marcos, A.; Garrote, J.A.; Polanco, I.; *et al.* Influence of environmental and genetic factors linked to celiac disease risk on infant gut colonization by Bacteroides species. *Appl. Environ. Microbiol.* **2011**, *77*, 5316–5323. [CrossRef] [PubMed]
7. Peng, J.; Narasimhan, S.; Marchesi, J.R.; Benson, A.; Wong, F.S.; Wen, L. Long term effect of gut microbiota transfer on diabetes development. *J. Autoimmun.* **2014**, *53*, 85–94. [CrossRef] [PubMed]
8. Gardiner, A.J.; Mutton, K.J.; Walker-Smith, J.A. A family study of coeliac disease. *Aust. Paediatr. J.* **1973**, *9*, 18–24. [CrossRef] [PubMed]

9. Kang, J.Y.; Kang, A.H.; Green, A.; Gwee, K.A.; Ho, K.Y. Systematic review: Worldwide variation in the frequency of coeliac disease and changes over time. *Aliment. Pharmacol. Ther.* **2013**, *38*, 226–245. [CrossRef] [PubMed]

10. Fasano, A. Where have all the American celiacs gone? *Acta Paediatr. Suppl.* **1996**, *412*, 20–24. [CrossRef] [PubMed]

11. Cummins, A.G.; Roberts-Thomson, I.C. Prevalence of celiac disease in the Asia-Pacific region. *J. Gastroenterol. Hepatol.* **2009**, *24*, 1347–1351. [CrossRef] [PubMed]

12. Wang, X.Q.; Liu, W.; Xu, C.D.; Mei, H.; Gao, Y.; Peng, H.M.; Yuan, L.; Xu, J.J. Celiac disease in children with diarrhea in 4 cities in China. *J. Pediatr. Gastroenterol. Nutr.* **2011**, *53*, 368–370. [PubMed]

13. Akbari, M.R.; Mohammadkhani, A.; Fakheri, H.; Javad Zahedi, M.; Shahbazkhani, B.; Nouraie, M.; Sotoudeh, M.; Shakeri, R.; Malekzadeh, R. Screening of the adult population in Iran for coeliac disease: Comparison of the tissue-transglutaminase antibody and anti-endomysial antibody tests. *Eur. J. Gastroenterol. Hepatol.* **2006**, *18*, 1181–1186. [CrossRef] [PubMed]

14. Bevan, S.; Popat, S.; Braegger, C.P.; Busch, A.; O'Donoghue, D.; Falth-Magnusson, K.; Ferguson, A.; Godkin, A.; Hogberg, L.; Holmes, G.; *et al.* Contribution of the MHC region to the familial risk of coeliac disease. *J. Med. Genet.* **1999**, *36*, 687–690. [PubMed]

15. Chile, M.D.S.D. Encuesta Nacional de Salud 2009–2010 (National health Survey). Avaialable online: http://www.minsal.gob.cl/portal/docs/page/minsalcl/g_home/ (accessed on 27 March 2015).

16. Gomez, J.C.; Selvaggio, G.S.; Viola, M.; Pizarro, B.; la Motta, G.; de Barrio, S.; Castelletto, R.; Echeverria, R.; Sugai, E.; Vazquez, H.; Maurino, E.; Bai, J.C. Prevalence of celiac disease in Argentina: Screening of an adult population in the La Plata area. *Am. J. Gastroenterol.* **2001**, *96*, 2700–2704. [CrossRef] [PubMed]

17. Araya, M.; Mondragon, A.; Perez-Bravo, F.; Roessler, J.L.; Alarcon, T.; Rios, G.; Bergenfreid, C. Celiac disease in a Chilean population carrying Amerindian traits. *J. Pediatr. Gastroenterol. Nutr.* **2000**, *31*, 381–386. [CrossRef] [PubMed]

18. Motta, P.M.; López, M.; Marinic, K.; Picón, S.O.; Stafuza, M.G.; Habegger de Sorrentino, A. Alta frecuencia de DQ8 en la población celíaca de la provincia del Chaco, Argentina. *Acta Gastroenterol. Latinoam.* **2014**, *44*, 16–21. [PubMed]

19. Parada, A.; Araya, M.; Perez-Bravo, F.; Mendez, M.; Mimbacas, A.; Motta, P.; Martin, G.; Botero, J.; Espinosa, N.; Alarcon, T.; Canales, P. Amerindian mtDNA haplogroups and celiac disease risk HLA haplotypes in mixed-blood Latin American patients. *J. Pediatr. Gastroenterol. Nutr.* **2011**, *53*, 429–434. [CrossRef] [PubMed]

20. Kotze, L.M.; Nisihara, R.; Utiyama, S.R.; Kotze, L.R. Absence of HLA-DQ2 and HLA-DQ8 does not exclude celiac disease in Brazilian patients. *Rev. Esp. Enferm. Dig.* **2014**, *106*, 561–562. [PubMed]

21. Perez-Bravo, F.; Carrasco, E.; Santos, J.L.; Calvillan, M.; Larenas, G.; Albala, C. Prevalence of type 2 diabetes and obesity in rural Mapuche population from Chile. *Nutrition* **2001**, *17*, 236–238. [CrossRef]

22. Husby, S.; Koletzko, S.; Korponay-Szabo, I.R.; Mearin, M.L.; Phillips, A.; Shamir, R.; Troncone, R.; Giersiepen, K.; Branski, D.; Catassi, C.; *et al.* European Society for Pediatric Gastroenterology, Hepatology, and Nutrition guidelines for the diagnosis of coeliac disease. *J. Pediatr. Gastroenterol. Nutr.* **2012**, *54*, 136–160. [CrossRef] [PubMed]

23. Murch, S.; Jenkins, H.; Auth, M.; Bremner, R.; Butt, A.; France, S.; Furman, M.; Gillett, P.; Kiparissi, F.; Lawson, M.; *et al.* Joint BSPGHAN and Coeliac UK guidelines for the diagnosis and management of coeliac disease in children. *Arch. Dis. Child.* **2013**, *98*, 806–811. [CrossRef] [PubMed]

24. Book, L.; Zone, J.J.; Neuhausen, S.L. Prevalence of celiac disease among relatives of sib pairs with celiac disease in U.S. families. *Am. J. Gastroenterol.* **2003**, *98*, 377–381. [CrossRef] [PubMed]

25. Uenishi, R.H.; Gandolfi, L.; Almeida, L.M.; Fritsch, P.M.; Almeida, F.C.; Nobrega, Y.K.; Pratesi, R. Screening for celiac disease in 1st degree relatives: A 10-year follow-up study. *BMC Gastroenterol.* **2014**, *14*, 36. [CrossRef] [PubMed]

26. Vitoria, J.C.; Arrieta, A.; Astigarraga, I.; Garcia-Masdevall, D.; Rodriguez-Soriano, J. Use of serological markers as a screening test in family members of patients with celiac disease. *J. Pediatr. Gastroenterol. Nutr.* **1994**, *19*, 304–309. [CrossRef] [PubMed]

27. Rubio-Tapia, A.; Hill, I.D.; Kelly, C.P.; Calderwood, A.H.; Murray, J.A. ACG clinical guidelines: Diagnosis and management of celiac disease. *Am. J. Gastroenterol.* **2013**, *108*, 656–676. [CrossRef] [PubMed]

28. De Onis, M.; Lobstein, T. Defining obesity risk status in the general childhood population: Which cut-offs should we use? *Int. J. Pediatr. Obes.* **2010**, *5*, 458–460. [CrossRef] [PubMed]

29. Marsh, M.N. The immunopathology of the small intestinal reaction in gluten-sensitivity. *Immunol. Investig.* **1989**, *18*, 509–531. [CrossRef]

30. Sacchetti, L.; Tinto, N.; Calcagno, G.; Improta, P.; Salvatore, F. Multiplex PCR typing of the three most frequent HLA alleles in celiac disease. *Clin. Chim. Acta* **2001**, *310*, 205–207. [CrossRef] [PubMed]

31. Bourgey, M.; Calcagno, G.; Tinto, N.; Gennarelli, D.; Margaritte-Jeannin, P.; Greco, L.; Limongelli, M.G.; Esposito, O.; Marano, C.; Troncone, R.; *et al.* HLA related genetic risk for coeliac disease. *Gut* **2007**, *56*, 1054–1059. [CrossRef] [PubMed]

32. Evans, K.E.; Hadjivassiliou, M.; Sanders, D.S. Is it time to screen for adult coeliac disease? *Eur. J. Gastroenterol. Hepatol.* **2011**, *23*, 833–838. [CrossRef] [PubMed]

33. Freeman, H.J. Risk factors in familial forms of celiac disease. *World J. Gastroenterol.* **2010**, *16*, 1828–1831. [CrossRef] [PubMed]

34. Bonamico, M.; Ferri, M.; Mariani, P.; Nenna, R.; Thanasi, E.; Luparia, R.P.; Picarelli, A.; Magliocca, F.M.; Mora, B.; Bardella, M.T.; *et al.* Serologic and genetic markers of celiac disease: A sequential study in the screening of first degree relatives. *J. Pediatr. Gastroenterol. Nutr.* **2006**, *42*, 150–154. [CrossRef] [PubMed]

35. Barton, S.H.; Murray, J.A. Celiac disease and autoimmunity in the gut and elsewhere. *Gastroenterol. Clin. N. Am.* **2008**, *37*, 411–428. [CrossRef] [PubMed]

36. Catassi, C.; Kryszak, D.; Bhatti, B.; Sturgeon, C.; Helzlsouer, K.; Clipp, S.L.; Gelfond, D.; Puppa, E.; Sferruzza, A.; Fasano, A. Natural history of celiac disease autoimmunity in a USA cohort followed since 1974. *Ann. Med.* **2010**, *42*, 530–538. [CrossRef] [PubMed]

37. Al-Toma, A.; Al-Toma, A.; Goerres, M.S.; Meijer, J.W.; Pena, A.S.; Crusius, J.B.; Mulder, C.J. Human leukocyte antigen-DQ2 homozygosity and the development of refractory celiac disease and enteropathy-associated T-cell lymphoma. *Clin. Gastroenterol. Hepatol.* **2006**, *4*, 315–319. [CrossRef] [PubMed]

38. Congia, M.; Cucca, F.; Frau, F.; Lampis, R.; Melis, L.; Clemente, M.G.; Cao, A.; de Virgiliis, S. A gene dosage effect of the DQA1 * 0501/DQB1 * 0201 allelic combination influences the clinical heterogeneity of celiac disease. *Hum. Immunol.* **1994**, *40*, 138–142. [CrossRef]

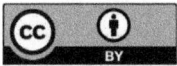

nutrients

Review

The Spectrum of Differences between Childhood and Adulthood Celiac Disease

Rachele Ciccocioppo [1,*], Peter Kruzliak [2], Giuseppina C. Cangemi [1], Miroslav Pohanka [3,4], Elena Betti [1], Eugenia Lauret [5] and Luis Rodrigo [5]

[1] Rachele Ciccocioppo, Center for the Study and Cure of Celiac Disease, Clinica Medica I, Department of Internal Medicine, IRCCS Policlinico San Matteo Foundation, University of Pavia, 19–27100 Pavia, Italy; cangemi.giusy@gmail.com (G.C.C.); elena.betti19@gmail.com (E.B.)

[2] International Clinical Research Center, St. Anne's University Hospital and Masaryk University, 65691 Brno, Czech Republic; peter.kruzliak@savba.sk

[3] Faculty of Military Health Sciences, University of Defence, Trebešská 1575-500 01 Hradec Kralove, Czech Republic; miroslav.pohanka@gmail.com

[4] Department of Geology and Pedology, Faculty of Forestry and Wood Technology, Mendel University in Brno, 61300 Brno, Czech Republic

[5] Gastroenterology Unit, Hospital Universitario Central de Asturias, 33000 Oviedo, Spain; meugelb@hotmail.com (E.L.); lrodrigosaez@gmail.com (L.R.)

* Correspondence: rachele.ciccocioppo@unipv.it; Tel.: +39-382-502-786; Fax: +39-382-502-618

Received: 1 August 2015; Accepted: 12 October 2015; Published: 22 October 2015

Abstract: An old saying states that "children are not little adults" and this certainly holds true for celiac disease, as there are many peculiar aspects regarding its epidemiology, diagnosis, clinical presentations, associated diseases, and response to treatment in pediatric compared to adult populations, to such an extent that it merits a description of its own. In fact, contrary to the past when it was thought that celiac disease was a disorder predominantly affecting childhood and characterized by a malabsorption syndrome, nowadays it is well recognized that it affects also adult and elderly people with an impressive variability of clinical presentation. In general, the clinical guidelines for diagnosis recommend starting with specific serologic testing in all suspected subjects, including those suffering from extraintestinal related conditions, and performing upper endoscopy with appropriate biopsy sampling of duodenal mucosa in case of positivity. The latter may be omitted in young patients showing high titers of anti-transglutaminase antibodies. The subsequent management of a celiac patient differs substantially depending on the age at diagnosis and should be based on the important consideration that this is a lifelong condition.

Keywords: adulthood; associated diseases; childhood; complications

1. Introduction

Celiac disease (CD) is a chronic, immune-mediated enteropathy caused by the ingestion of gluten-containing cereals (wheat, rye, and barley) in genetically predisposed individuals [1,2]. Left untreated, CD may cause malabsorption [3], reduced quality of life [4], iron deficiency [5], osteoporosis [6,7], and an increased risk of lymphoma [8,9]. CD patients may complain of not only gastrointestinal symptoms, but also extraintestinal symptoms and, most importantly, they may often be asymptomatic [10]. Moreover, CD is associated with several autoimmune diseases [11], mostly diabetes mellitus type 1 [12] and thyroiditis [13]. The ubiquitous transglutaminase type 2 (TG2) enzyme plays a crucial role in CD pathogenesis, not only because it is the main autoantigen and the target of the specific auto-antibodies (TG2A), but also for the ordered and precise deamidation of gliadins that generates epitopes which bind more efficiently to histocompatibility locus antigen (HLA)-DQ2/DQ8 molecules [14]. Mucosal CD4$^+$ T lymphocytes, in turn, become activated by these immunodominat epitopes, thus resulting in the development of an immune reaction where interleukin (IL)-15 [14,15] and interferon-α are involved [16]. The TG2A are produced by B-cells localized in the intestinal mucosa, and detected in patients' serum. Moreover, TG2 activity may lead to unmasking of further auto-antigens thus causing additional autoimmune conditions [17]. The activation of these complex pathogenic mechanisms leads to various degrees of alteration of small intestine architecture eventually resulting in malfunction of the intestine [18]. Currently, the only effective treatment available is a strict life-long gluten-free diet (GFD), which improves symptoms, nutritional status [19,20], serological and histological changes [19], and possibly body composition in most patients [19–21].

2. Epidemiology and Genetics

It is estimated that CD affects approximately 1% of the whole world population [22]. Recent epidemiological research based on serological studies of the general population in Europe and in the United States of America has also shown that both the incidence and prevalence has grown in recent years not only thanks to increased awareness and better diagnostic tests, but also due to a real spread of the disease [22]. Scandinavian, Irish and United Kingdom populations tended to show a higher prevalence of CD compared to the rest of Europe [23]. On the other hand, there are regions with very low or no incidence of CD North, Sub-and Saharan Africa, India, China, Japan, and the Caribbean [24,25]. The low incidence is probably due in part to eating habits, but genetic disposition may also play a role. Unavailability of proper diagnostic facilities can be another reason why incidence appears to be so low in these regions [25]. With regard to gender, there is an increased prevalence of CD amongst women compared to men with a male: female ratio of 1:2.8 [26]. However, a gap has emerged between the prevalence rate obtained through serological screening and that resulting from clinical studies. This is due to the fact that oligo-a-symptomatic patients or those with atypical forms too often remain unrevealed [24]. In fact, the ratio between diagnosed and undiagnosed cases was as high as 1 to 7 (the "celiac iceberg") [27]; for instance, the Danish National Patient Registry records about 50 cases of patients per 100,000 persons [28].

As far as genetic predisposition is concerned, it is estimated that almost all CD patients carry the HLA-DQ2 or HLA-DQ8 haplotype (with HLA-DQ2 prevalence being >90% and HLA-DQ8 approximately 5%) [29]. The molecules encoded by these genes play a key role in the pathogenesis of the disease since they form a heterodimer expressed on the surface of antigen-presenting cells which displays high affinity to gliadin peptides, thus triggering and sustaining the abnormal adaptive immune response to these epitopes [30]. Nevertheless, HLA-DQ2 and HLA-DQ8 occur in about 30% of the Caucasian population, thus HLA genotyping did not increase the diagnostic accuracy of the serological tests, since a positive result has low specificity [31]. On the other hand, it has a strong negative predictive value, since the absence of HLA-DQ2 and HLA-DQ8 can most likely exclude CD. Thus, HLA-DQ2/8 genotyping can be used as complementary analysis in some specific situations, e.g., in patients with a discrepancy between serology and histology, and where complications are suspected [32]. Further genetic *loci* have been shown to be related to CD susceptibility and possibly also to its pathogenesis [33]. The most important ones are the following: CELIAC1 on chromosome 6, CELIAC2 on chromosome 5q31-33 [34], CELIAC3 on chromosome 2q33 [35], and CELIAC4 on chromosome 19p13.1 [36].

3. Serologic and Histologic Differences between CD in Children and Adults

The diagnosis of CD has traditionally depended upon the results of several (four to six) intestinal biopsies, currently considered to be the gold standard, and has been extended to include also an array of serological markers.

The Guidelines of the North American Societies for Gastroenterology usually require at least a duodenal biopsy for diagnosis [37,38]. Recently, the European Society for Pediatric Gastroenterology, Hepatology, and Nutrition (ESPGHAN) published new guidelines allowing the diagnosis of CD without a biopsy in some situations, mainly related to presence of high titers of TG2A, higher than

100 IU/L [39]. CD is usually diagnosed when the duodenal or jejunal mucosa displays changes including not only a different degree of villous atrophy but also crypt hyperplasia, and an increase in intraepithelial lymphocytes (IELs) [40].

However, other diseases unrelated to gluten-dependent enteropathy can induce a flat mucosa, thus mimicking CD (see below), whilst CD may exist even in the presence of a normal small bowel mucosal architecture [41]. In addition, often the lack of technical proficiency in using biopsy forceps and/or of orientation of the mucosal specimens are the cause of perplexing interpretations of the original histologic preparations, indeed they have been shown to be sufficient for CD diagnosis in only 90% of cases [42].

Furthermore, CD may be overlooked during histological examinations, owing to differences in pathologists' assessments. Because of this, and also due to the inconvenience and the cost associated with jejunal biopsy and the high prevalence of CD in the general population, less-invasive tests are required. Over the last 20 years, several new serological tests have been used for the diagnosis of CD, leading to a significant improvement in accuracy. For practical and ethical reasons, patients with negative serology sometimes do not undergo a biopsy unless clinical indications of CD are evident (IgA deficiency). This procedure causes a verification bias because the gold standard (histology of the mucosa) is not always available for negative tests [43]

A positive correlation between serum levels of TG2A and duodenal histopathology has been previously described, both for pediatric and adult CD populations [44,45]. In a prospective clinical study, when comparing the findings of TG2A in these two populations, a positive correlation between the TG2A titers and the mucosal lesions according to Marsh grades was consistently observed in the pediatric population [46].

Although TG2A levels correlated with duodenal histopathology both in the adult [47] and pediatric populations [46], the higher percentage of Marsh type 3 lesions observed in children [48] makes a high antibody titer especially interesting for CD prediction in this group. The choice of an upper cut-off limit of 30 U/mL TG2A yielded the highest area under the receiver operating characteristic curve (0.854). Based on the predictive value of this cut-off point, up to 95% of children and only 53% of adults would be correctly diagnosed without biopsy. Thus, the authors conclude that duodenal biopsy may be avoided when high TG2A titers are present, generally over 100 IU/mL [46].

Several additional studies in extensive series of celiac patients have clearly shown that TG2A sensitivity varies depending on the severity of duodenal damage, and reaches almost 100% in the presence of complete villous atrophy (more common in children under three years), 70% for subtotal atrophy, and up to 30% when only an increase in IELs is present [49]. However, TG2A titers and histologic lesion degree exhibit an inverse correlation with age [50]. Thus, as the age of diagnosis increases, the antibody titers decrease and histological damage is less marked. It is common to find adults without villous atrophy, showing only an inflammatory pattern in the duodenal mucosa biopsies, *i.e.*, increased number of IELs (Marsh I) with/without crypt hyperplasia (Marsh II) (Figure 1) [50].

However, a note of caution should be inserted when diagnosing CD in children younger than two years of age, since the biopsies before and after the gluten challenge may be omitted only in the presence of anti-endomysial antibodies (EMA) positivity and Marsh IIIc lesions at histology [48].

4. Associated Diseases

The number of conditions possibly associated with CD is extensive enough to justify active screening for most of them, with an estimated prevalence of 30.1% in adulthood and 20.7% in childhood [51]. The most frequent are the autoimmune disorders, both systemic and organ-specific, which tend to occur more frequently as the age at diagnosis increases, which can be taken as an index of the duration of gluten exposure [52]. In this regard, the protective role of the GFD was highlighted in a study where those strictly adherent to a GFD were found to acquire fewer autoimmune diseases than those not compliant with the strict dietetic regimen [53]. However, there is significant controversy surrounding the notion that early detection and treatment of CD may result in a decreased risk of developing further autoimmune diseases [54,55]. It is conceivable that, similarly to inflammatory bowel disease [56], the onset and activity of some of them are connected to the full-blown status and duration of the intestinal disease, whilst others are completely unrelated. The exact nature of this association is still not fully understood [57]. Predominant and not mutually exclusive hypotheses include the presence of a linkage disequilibrium of genes that generally predispose to autoimmune diseases [58], the loss of intestinal barrier integrity [59], an altered microbiome [60], and posttranslational modifications of immunogenic peptides [61], with a conceivable high relevance of genetics in childhood and immunity in adulthood (Figure 2). From a clinical point of view, the relevance of this association regards either the detrimental effect that an autoimmune disease may have on CD (and *vice versa*), or the possibility of diagnosing those CD patients presenting only or apparently with symptoms of secondary autoimmunity. In fact, in a substantial number of cases, both in adults and children, the disease remains clinically silent and the only manifestation is the associated disease/s [62,63] for which they are referred to specialists other than gastroenterologists, *i.e.*, endocrinologists, rheumatologists, orthopedists *etc.*, who need to be aware of this association [64]. Here below, we review the spectrum of associated diseases in CD and discuss their possible pathophysiologic mechanisms (Figure 2).

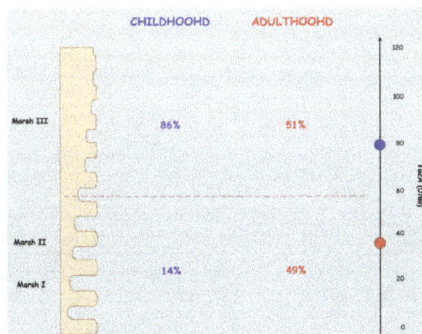

Figure 1. Serologic and histologic findings in childhood and adulthood celiac disease. The prevalence of major and minor intestinal lesions, as defined according to Marsh's classification, in terms of percentages in both childhood and adult celiac disease is shown. Moreover, the mean values of anti-tissue transglutaminase antibodies (TG2A) is given on the right hand side, with the blue spot indicating childhood age and the red one adult age. The data are presented according to [50].

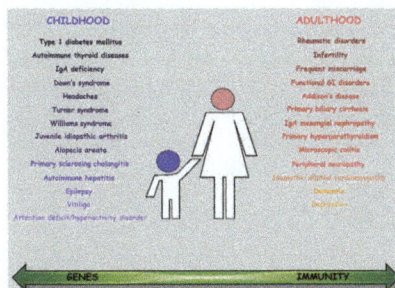

Figure 2. Associated diseases. The most common associated diseases listed in descending order of frequency for childhood (**left**) and adulthood (**right**) celiac disease. The green arrow shows the prevalent role played by genes or immunity in the pathogenesis of these conditions. Abbreviations: GI: gastrointestinal; Ig: immunoglobulin.

4.1. Type 1 Diabetes Mellitus

Surely, diabetes mellitus type I is the most frequent autoimmune disease associated with CD [65], with a prevalence of CD in type 1 diabetes that is higher in children (6.2%) than in adults (2.7%) [66]. In the former, the risk of having both the diseases is three times higher in those diagnosed with type 1 diabetes aged <4 years than in those diagnosed aged >9 years [67]. Moreover, type 1 diabetes is only seldom found in individuals already diagnosed with CD, mostly within five years of CD diagnosis and before 20 years of age [68], while in the vast majority of cases, CD is detected via screening antibodies at the time of or after the diagnosis of diabetes [69]. The need for CD screening is also justified by the evidence of potential improvement in symptoms (if present) [70], body composition [70–72], diabetic control [71,72], and reduction in hypoglycemia episodes after diagnosis of CD and implementation of a GFD [73], despite the higher glycemic index and fat content of gluten-free foods compared to their gluten-containing counterparts [74]. As regards the pathogenic mechanisms, other than a shared genetic background, namely the HLA genotype DR3-DQ2, gluten seems to be involved in both the diseases [75]. In fact, non-obese diabetic (NOD) mice fed with a GFD showed a lower incidence of diabetes, possibly also related to changes in the gut microbiome [76], and children with diabetes display a deranged immune response to gliadin [77], and the presence of TG2A deposits in the small intestinal mucosa [78]. This association represents a unique example of how our understanding of one disease improves knowledge and management of the other and *vice versa*.

4.2. Autoimmune Thyroid Disease

An increased prevalence of autoimmune thyroid diseases, namely Hashimoto's and Graves' diseases, has been described in adults and to a greater extent in children with CD, although the rate varies amongst studies [79–82]. In fact, when screening 90 children and adolescents with autoimmune thyroid diseases by using EMA, a rate of 7.7% of positivity was found [80], whilst when using the TG2A-IgA in a mixed population, a rate of 4.6% was observed, with only 2.3% of them having biopsy confirmed CD [82]. The decreased specificity of TG2A in this subset of patients compared to the general population was attributed to co-morbidities including type 1 diabetes and Down's syndrome [82], even though the possibility that a considerable number of them suffer from potential CD cannot be ruled out. However, although CD seems to be more common in children with autoimmune thyroid diseases, the reverse is not necessarily true. A prospective study including 545 children and adolescents with CD on a GFD showed that autoimmune thyroid disease was no more common in these patients than in controls, and that patients who had been on a GFD longer were less likely to suffer from thyroid disorders [81]. Consequently, the authors suggest that screening CD children for autoimmune thyroid disorders should be performed only in those who are symptomatic or suspected of having this condition [81]. By contrast, when screening adolescents with CD for autoantibodies against thyroid peroxidase, a prevalence of 7.2% was observed in comparison with 2.8% found in controls [83]. On the other hand, the institution of a GFD did not prevent the progression of established autoimmune thyroid disease [84] or the appearance of anti-thyroid antibodies [85] after the diagnosis of CD. As in type 1 diabetes, a close overlap in the risk haplotypes between these conditions has been shown, with a frequent presence of HLA DQA1*0301 (linked to DR4), DQB1*0301 (linked to DR5), and DQB1*0201 (linked to DR3) [86].

4.3. Other Immune-Mediated Disorders

Other than type 1 diabetes and thyroid autoimmune diseases, further endocrine conditions, such as Addison's disease [87] and primary hyperparathyroidism [88], together with a substantial number of additional immune-mediated disorders [89] have been reported in association with CD. These include rheumatic and connective tissue diseases, *i.e.*, Sjögren's syndrome [90], systemic lupus erythematosus [91], and juvenile idiopathic arthritis [92], skin disorders [93], hepatic diseases [94], neurological abnormalities [95], cardiological illnesses, including autoimmune myocarditis [96] and idiopathic dilated cardiomyopathy [97], although a recent nationwide study found only a moderately but not statistically significantly increased risk of this latter condition in patients with biopsy-verified CD [98]. Similarly, the previously reported association with immunoglobulin (Ig)A mesangial nephropathy [99], has been recently contested [100]. Here below, we summarize the most frequent conditions associated with CD, while referring readers to the cited references for the others.

4.4. Rheumatic Disorders

Sjogren's syndrome is an autoimmune exocrinopathy characterized by dry eyes, dry mouth, and circulating antibodies against intracellular proteins. The association between Sjogren's syndrome and CD was first described in 1965 [101]. Since then, two further series reported prevalence rates of CD amongst adult Sjogren's patients as high as 12% [102] and 14.4% [103]. With these values, Sjogren's syndrome can be considered the most common rheumatic disorder associated with CD. In this regard, it should be emphasized that 56% of Sjogren's adult patients carry the HLA-DQ2 haplotype [103]. The second most frequent rheumatic disorder associated with CD is antiphospholipid syndrome, with a prevalence of 14% in adults diagnosed with this condition [104]. The prevalence of CD amongst patients with chronic arthritis ranged from 1.5% to 2.5% [102,105,106], whilst its occurrence in patients with systemic lupus erythematosus is under debate, since despite reported findings of an increased rate [91,102], no case of CD was found in a large series of 103 systemic lupus erythematosus patients [107].

4.5. Selective IgA Deficiency

Selective IgA deficiency is one of the most frequent immunologic disorders associated with CD, with a reported frequency of 1:39 in populations of both adult and childhood CD [108], compared to an estimated frequency of 1:600 in the general population [109]. The reverse is also true, as there is an increased prevalence of CD found in children with IgA deficiency [110]. This close association may be largely due to a higher prevalence of the HLA-DQ2 genotype in the IgA deficient population too [111]. While IgA deficiency does not seem to affect CD presentation, it significantly impacts the diagnostic process since celiac antibodies utilized for the serological screening are primarily of the IgA subtype.

4.6. Neuro-Psychiatric Conditions

Other than gluten ataxia, a wide range of neurological and psychiatric disorders, such as peripheral neuropathy, epilepsy, headaches, dementia, depression, autism, and schizophrenia has been reported in association with CD, both in childhood and adulthood, although the risk seems higher in adulthood [95]. In particular, the syndrome of epilepsy with occipital calcifications was reported in childhood CD [112], although the strength of this association has recently been questioned, following evidence that only seven out 2893 epileptic children (0.2%) screened for CD presented with cerebral calcifications, possibly because cerebral calcifications might develop later in life [113]. Moreover, when considering the different types of epilepsy overall, the reported prevalence in CD is in line with that found in the general population [113]. The other neurological disorder of early childhood that has been associated with gluten ingestion, rather than with actual CD, is autism [114], stemming from the reported benefit of a gluten-free/casein-free diet in these patients [115]. Nevertheless, the association between autism and CD has not yet been conclusively proved [116]. Instead, there is some evidence of an increased prevalence of milder neurologic disorders in childhood CD, such as chronic headaches, hypotonia, attention deficit/hyperactivity disorder, and developmental delay [117]. Specifically, pediatric CD carries a three-fold increased relative risk of chronic headache, as compared to controls, a situation that improves dramatically after the implementation of a GFD [113].

4.7. Skin and Annexes

The relationship between dermatomyositis and CD has been suggested, both in young adult and adults [118,119], with some evidence of amelioration following a GFD [120]. Again, close association with DQA1*0501 heterodimer has been reported [121]. A similar benefit of GFD was shown also in a child with vitiligo [122], and in a few cases of alopecia areata associated with CD [123–125]. However, the scarcity of the cases described and the lack of systematic studies, do not allow for definite conclusions in skin disorders [93].

4.8. Liver

Possible conditions associated with CD, mainly in childhood, include elevated serum aminotransferases, without any specific histological changes that promptly reverse after a course of GFD, now known as "celiac hepatitis" [94], as well as autoimmune hepatitis, and primary sclerosing cholangitis. Primary biliary cirrhosis, whose diagnosis often precedes that of CD, has been found only in adults, while natural history is totally independent from the establishment of a GFD [94,126,127].

4.9. Reproduction

Obviously, this problem affects only CD in adulthood, where the association of infertility in both women and men [128] is recognized to such an extent that screening for CD is part of the routine diagnostic workup of infertile couples [129], also because the possibility of successful reproduction and pregnancy improves after diagnosis of CD and the start of a GFD [130]. Furthermore, celiac women also experience delayed menarche and early menopause more frequently than controls, thus leading to a shorter fertile life span [131]. Apparently, this finding was not confirmed in a recent study, showing that celiac women do not have a greater likelihood of clinically recorded fertility problems than non-celiac women do, even though this was not true in those diagnosed with CD between 25–39 years of age [132].

4.10. Genetic Disorders

Following the established association with some genetic disorders, namely Down's, Turner, and Williams syndrome, CD screening is highly recommended for these conditions. The prevalence of CD in Down's syndrome patients, indeed, ranges from 4% to 18%, according to several studies performed in both the USA and Europe [133–135], with a higher rate in adults than in children [136]. Whether it depends on a real increased prevalence with age or a missed diagnosis during childhood is unknown. CD has also been found to be associated with Turner syndrome, with reported prevalence ranging from 4.5% to 8.1% [137,138]. Finally, the association with Williams syndrome has been well documented, with an estimated prevalence of CD as high as 9.3% in a representative cohort of 63 patients, in an Italian multicenter study [139]. This relationship between genetic syndromes and CD does not seem to be dependent on a larger percentage of patients carrying the HLA-DQ2 or HLA-DQ8 haplotypes compared to the general population, but to a propensity to develop autoimmune associated diseases, including CD. For instance, a relationship with the pro-inflammatory cytokine interferon-α, which plays a key role in eliciting the intestinal immune response in celiac disease [16], has been suggested, since its receptor is encoded on chromosome 21 [140].

5. Response to GFD and Prognosis

Pending a better understanding of its pathogenesis [1,2], the treatment of CD is still based on the GFD, as originally proposed by the Dutch Pediatrician, Doctor Willem-Karel Dicke [141], which requires the complete elimination from the diet of all types of foods containing or prepared with wheat, rye, barley grains, and their derivatives. Although this treatment guarantees the recovery from both clinical symptoms and intestinal damage in almost all cases, it seriously affects the patient's quality of life, since its stringency and lifelong duration cause chronic distress and it segregates patients in a sort of "social apartheid" [142]. This is the reason why compliance is very often suboptimal, ranging from 52% to 95% in the pediatric population [143], with adolescents having serious difficulties with permanent adherence to the GFD [144]. In general, factors that improve chances of compliance are early age diagnosis [145], the presence of symptoms after gluten ingestion [146], a good awareness in the family [147], and frequent follow-ups by both a physician and a meticulous nutritionist [148]. Similarly, in adults the adherence to a GFD improves by having regular follow-ups, even by telephone, within the setting of a dedicated adult celiac unit [149]. Therefore, patients' education, close supervision with scheduled nutritional counselling, and maintenance of dietary adherence when travelling or dining out, are all crucial factors needed to achieve full compliance [150]. This treatment carries the additional burden of a wide range of minor side effects, such as constipation, intestinal bloating, changes in body composition, modification of dietary intake, and poor vitamin status [151,152]. In fact, in a substantial proportion of adults, the presence of several nutritional problems has been found after a long-term course of GFD: calorie/protein imbalance, fiber, folate, niacin, vitamin B12, and riboflavin deficiencies [21]. In this regard, the nutritional adequacy of the GFD is particularly important in childhood, when maximum energy is required for growth, development and activity. In recent years, attention has been focused on the nutritional quality of the gluten-free products (GFPs) available on the market, and it has emerged that these are of lower quality and poorer nutritional value than their gluten-containing counterparts [74]. A further emerging problem is represented by excess weight and obesity [153,154], since 81% of patients on a GFD had gained weight after two years, including 82% of those who were initially overweight patients, in both adults and children [151]. Reasons for the weight gain are related to the improved intestinal absorption and the hypercaloric content of commercial or natural gluten-free food due to its high lipid and protein content, thus attentive follow-ups with an experienced dietitian is strongly recommended. Finally, in the last few years, a gap has emerged between the clinical and mucosal recovery, mainly in the adult population, since when re-biopsing treated CD patients only half of them had healed mucosa, despite the negativity of serologic markers [155,156]. This makes the follow-up of CD patients extremely difficult. In this regard, it has been recently shown that measuring the circulating levels of intestinal-fatty acid binding protein may provide a useful tool for monitoring compliance with a GFD [157]. Following the exclusion of gluten from the diet, the clinical symptoms and mucosal architecture usually improve very quickly in children [158], whilst in a mixed population, the histological response requires more time, reaching a complete recovery in 95% of cases within two years [159]. In fact, mostly in adulthood, the establishment of a strict GFD has intrinsic difficulties, from both a practical and psychological point of view. Moreover, both the clinical and mucosal recovery may be slower than expected in this age group, with as many as 60% of patients showing persistent villous atrophy after the same time course of two years on a GFD [160,161]. This is why a second biopsy is not required in childhood [39], whilst in adulthood it is the only tool that can detect an unsatisfactory histological response [162]. This indication arises also from the evidence that the persistence of intestinal damage carries an increased risk development of a malignant T-cell lymphoma [156,163], albeit not of overall mortality [164] and that the GFD does not fully protect patients from developing complications [156,163]. Since the latter are very rare conditions [163], the persistence or recurrence of symptoms should first prompt the clinicians to revise the accuracy of the original diagnosis and, if necessary, to perform a course of gluten challenge followed by new mucosal sampling [165]. Afterwards, it is advisable to carry out systematic evaluation for alternative and associated diseases, possibly responsible for the apparent refractoriness to GFD [166,167]. In this regard, false refractoriness may be divided on the basis of the mucosal architecture, in those conditions with a normal duodenal mucosa, and those causing complete or partial alteration of mucosal architecture which firstly include poor compliance to GFD, then a number of conditions, as shown in Figure 3.

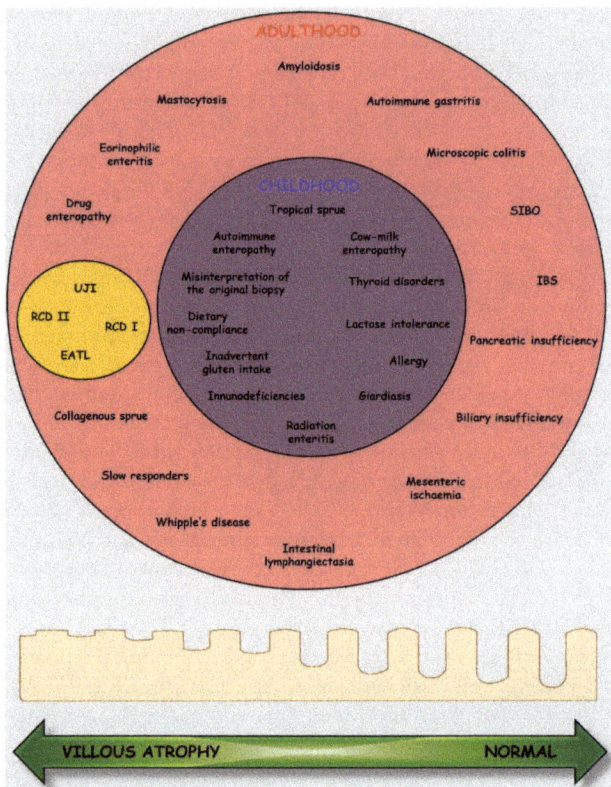

Figure 3. Possible causes of refractoriness to a gluten-free diet. A series of conditions responsible for refractoriness to gluten-free diet is presented according to their "true" (inside the yellow circle) or "false" relationship (all the others) with celiac disease, and to their prevalence in adulthood (**red circle**) or childhood (**blue circle**). At the bottom, a schematic representation of the duodenal mucosa architecture is given as a continuum (**green arrow**) from villus atrophy to a normal appearance, going from left to right, thus the place where each pathological condition is inserted in the circles depends on the status of the small intestinal mucosa. Abbreviations: EATL: enteropathy-type-associated T cell lymphoma; IBS: irritable bowel syndrome; RCD: refractory celiac disease; SIBO: small intestinal bacterial overgrowth; UJI: ulcerative jejunoileitis.

5.1. Complicated Celiac Disease

The term complicated CD encompasses a spectrum of different conditions, namely refractory CD (RCD), ulcerative jejunoileitis (UJI), and enteropathy-type-associated T cell lymphoma (EATL), which represent a biological continuum and are estimated to affect only a few cases in the adult CD population [2,3,163]. The only two exceptions are an eight-year-old boy suffering from refractory CD, who was successfully treated with azathioprine [168], and a 13-year-old girl with CD and evidence of ulcerative lesions in the jejunum, who responded to a GFD [169]. However, in our opinion, the latter cannot be considered a true refractory case, firstly because of the response to a GFD and secondly for the absence of both a monoclonal re-arrangement of the T-cell receptor and an aberrant population of intraepithelial lymphocytes (IELs), which are the hallmarks of CD-associated UJI. Further causes capable of inducing ulcerative lesions in the small intestine should have been actively ruled out. On the other hand, since a systematic study with wireless capsule endoscopy or enteroscopy has not yet been carried out in the pediatric CD population, we cannot exclude the possibility that a number of erosions/ulcers may be present in pediatric active CD patients, devoid of the biological significance of a complication. In fact, the diagnostic criteria for the presence of refractoriness are very strictly defined as the persistence or recurrence of both malabsorption syndrome and intestinal villous atrophy after 6–12 months of a controlled GFD [32]. Over the last decade, two distinct conditions have been identified on the basis of the amount of aberrant IELs, named type I and type II [170]. The latter has a poor prognosis, largely due to the frequent development of an overt lymphoma [171]. By contrast, in type I RCD, intestinal lymphocytes have an almost normal phenotype, symptoms are usually mild and sometimes difficult to differentiate from uncomplicated celiac disease, except for the resistance to a GFD. Ulcerative jejunoileitis is characterized by the presence of several ulcerations possibly involving all layers of the intestinal wall, which may evolve in strictures, bleeding or perforation and often results in a life-threatening condition [172]. As a consequence, the main clinical features are colicky central abdominal pain, distension, fever, diarrhea, and weight loss. The current management of these conditions relies on a combination of nutritional support, immunosuppressive or biological therapies (steroids, azathioprine, cladribine, anti-CD52 or anti-CD30 monoclonal antibodies), and autologous hematopoietic stem cell transplantation whose choice is based on non-controlled studies in small cohorts of patients and personal experience [173]. However, their prognosis remains bleak.

In conclusion, despite previous evidence that adult CD carries a twofold increase in all-cause mortality, and 60-fold increase in non-Hodgkin lymphoma compared with the general population [174], a recent competing risk analysis showed that overall, people with CD have no major excess risk of cancer, related digestive disease or respiratory disease or cardiovascular mortality compared with the general population, although an excess risk for non-Hodgkin lymphoma was confirmed [156,175]. Although these findings reassure both CD patients and clinicians involved in managing their care, it should be emphasised that the increased mortality risk is actually restricted to those diagnosed with CD after 40 years of age, where more vigorous follow-up is then recommended [176].

6. Conclusions

Taken together, these findings highlight how different CD in children appears compared to CD in adults. First, the disease seems more common in children than in adults [177,178] probably because of the frequent presence of malabsorption symptoms mainly in the early pediatric age. Secondly, coexisting autoimmune diseases are more common in adulthood, thus making the diagnosis in this age group more difficult. Thirdly, the CD-related complications, including the malignant forms, are almost exclusively found in adults. Finally, considering that this illness is a permanent intolerance to gluten, the relevance and intrinsic difficulty of the transition phase between these two periods of life deserves our utmost attention, since it represents a cornerstone in the modern management of chronic diseases. Transition, indeed, is recognised as not just a simple "transfer" of patients from the pediatric service to adult health care [179], but relies on a complex and scheduled process, aimed at ensuring continuity, coordination, flexibility and sensitivity in a multi-disciplinary context [180].

Author Contributions: Rachele Ciccocioppo reviewed the literature and wrote the abstract and Sections 4–6, and planned the figures. Luis Rodrigo and Eugenia Lauret reviewed the literature and wrote Sections 2 and 3. Giuseppina C. Cangemi and Elena Betti drafted the figures and gave substantial technical contributions. Peter Kruzliak and Miroslav Pohanka reviewed the literature and wrote Sections 1 and 2.

Conflicts of Interest: The authors have no conflict of interest to declare.

References

1. Green, P.H.; Cellier, C. Celiac disease. *N. Engl. J. Med.* **2007**, *357*, 1731–1743. [CrossRef] [PubMed]
2. Di Sabatino, A.; Corazza, G.R. Coeliac disease. *Lancet* **2009**, *373*, 1480–1493. [CrossRef]
3. Wright, D.H. The major complications of coeliac disease. *Baillieres Clin. Gastroenterol.* **1995**, *9*, 351–369. [CrossRef]

4.   Sainsbury, K.; Mullan, B.; Sharpe, L. Reduced quality of life in coeliac disease is more strongly associated with depression than gastrointestinal symptoms. *J. Psychosom. Res.* **2013**, *75*, 135–141. [PubMed]

5.   Wierdsma, N.J.; van Bokhorst-de van der Schueren, M.A.; Berkenpas, M.; Mulder, C.J.; van Bodegraven, A.A. Vitamin and mineral deficiencies are highly prevalent in newly diagnosed celiac disease patients. *Nutrients* **2013**, *5*, 3975–3992. [CrossRef] [PubMed]

6.   Mazure, R.; Vazquez, H.; Gonzalez, D.; Mautalen, C.; Pedreira, S.; Boerr, L.; Bai, J.C. Bone mineral affection in asymptomatic adult patients with celiac disease. *Am. J. Gastroenterol.* **1994**, *89*, 2130–2134. [PubMed]

7.   Stein, E.M.; Rogers, H.; Leib, A.; McMahon, D.J.; Young, P.; Nishiyama, K.; Guo, X.E.; Lewis, S.; Green, P.H.; Shane, E. Abnormal skeletal strength and microarchitecture in women with celiac disease. *J. Clin. Endocrinol. Metable* **2015**, *100*, 2347–2353. [CrossRef] [PubMed]

8.   Spencer, J.; MacDonald, T.T.; Diss, T.C.; Walker-Smith, J.A.; Ciclitira, P.J.; Isaacson, P.G. Changes in intraepithelial lymphocyte subpopulations in coeliac disease and enteropathy associated T cell lymphoma (malignant histiocytosis of the intestine). *Gut* **1989**, *30*, 339–346. [CrossRef] [PubMed]

9.   Grigg-Gutierrez, N.M.; Estremera-Marcial, R.; Caceres, W.W.; Toro, D.H. Primary enteropathy-associated t-cell lymphoma type 2: An emerging entity? *Cancer Control.* **2015**, *22*, 242–247. [PubMed]

10.   Hernandez, L.; Green, P.H. Extraintestinal manifestations of celiac disease. *Curr. Gastroenterol. Rep.* **2006**, *8*, 383–389. [CrossRef] [PubMed]

11.   Trigoni, E.; Tsirogianni, A.; Pipi, E.; Mantzaris, G.; Papasteriades, C. Celiac disease in adult patients: Specific autoantibodies in the diagnosis, monitoring, and screening. *Autoimmun. Dis.* **2014**, *2014*, 623514. [CrossRef] [PubMed]

12.   Kakleas, K.; Soldatou, A.; Karachaliou, F.; Karavanaki, K. Associated autoimmune diseases in children and adolescents with type 1 diabetes mellitus (T1DM). *Autoimmun. Rev.* **2015**, *14*, 781–797. [CrossRef] [PubMed]

13.   Berti, I.; Trevisiol, C.; Tommasini, A.; Città, A.; Neri, E.; Geatti, O.; Giammarini, A.; Ventura, A.; Not, T. Usefulness of screening program for celiac disease in autoimmune thyroiditis. *Dig. Dis. Sci.* **2000**, *45*, 403–406. [CrossRef] [PubMed]

14.   Molberg, O.; Mcadam, S.N.; Körner, R.; Quarsten, H.; Kristiansen, C.; Madsen, L.; Fugger, L.; Scott, H.; Norén, O.; Roepstorff, P.; *et al.* Tissue transglutaminase selectively modifies gliadin peptides that are recognized by gut-derived T cells in celiac disease. *Nat. Med.* **1998**, *4*, 713–717. [CrossRef] [PubMed]

15.   Di Sabatino, A.; Ciccocioppo, R.; Cupelli, F.; Cinque, B.; Millimaggi, D.; Clarkson, M.M.; Paulli, M.; Cifone, M.G.; Corazza, G.R. Epithelium derived interleukin 15 regulates intraepithelial lymphocyte Th1 cytokine production, cytotoxicity, and survival in coeliac disease. *Gut* **2006**, *55*, 469–477. [CrossRef] [PubMed]

16.   Monteleone, G.; Pender, S.L.; Alstead, E.; Hauer, A.C.; Lionetti, P.; McKenzie, C.; MacDonald, T.T. Role of interferon alpha in promoting T helper cell type 1 responses in the small intestine in coeliac disease. *Gut* **2001**, *48*, 425–429. [CrossRef] [PubMed]

17.   Fasano, A.; Catassi, C. Current approaches to diagnosis and treatment of celiac disease: An evolving spectrum. *Gastroenterology* **2001**, *120*, 636–651. [CrossRef] [PubMed]

18.   Du Pre, M.F.; Sollid, L.M. T-cell and B-cell immunity in celiac disease. *Best Pract. Res. Clin. Gastroenterol.* **2015**, *29*, 413–423. [CrossRef] [PubMed]

19.   Haines, M.L.; Anderson, R.P.; Gibson, P.R. Systematic review: The evidence base for long-term management of coeliac disease. *Aliment. Pharmacol. Ther.* **2008**, *28*, 1042–1066. [CrossRef] [PubMed]

20.   Smecuol, E.; Gonzalez, D.; Mautalen, C.; Siccardi, A.; Cataldi, M.; Niveloni, S.; Mazure, R.; Vazquez, H.; Pedreira, S.; Soifer, G.; *et al.* Longitudinal study on the effect of treatment on body composition and anthropometry of celiac disease patients. *Am. J. Gastroenterol.* **1997**, *92*, 639–643. [PubMed]

21.   Bardella, M.T.; Fredella, C.; Prampolini, L.; Molteni, N.; Giunta, A.M.; Bianchi, P.A. Body composition and dietary intakes in adult celiac disease patients consuming a strict gluten-free diet. *Am. J. Clin. Nutr.* **2000**, *72*, 937–939. [PubMed]

22.   Kang, J.Y.; Kang, A.H.Y.; Green, A.; Gwee, K.A.; Ho, K.Y. Systematic review: Worldwide variation in the frequency of coeliac disease and changes over time. *Aliment. Pharmacol. Ther.* **2013**, *38*, 226–245. [CrossRef] [PubMed]

23.   Elson, C.O.; Ballew, M.; Banard, J.A. NIH Consensus Development Conference on Celiac Disease. *NIH Consens. State Sci. Statements* **2004**, *21*, 1–23.

24.   Lionetti, E.; Gatti, S.; Pulvirenti, A.; Catassi, C. Celiac disease from a global perspective. *Best Pract. Res. Clin. Gastroenterol.* **2015**, *29*, 365–379. [CrossRef] [PubMed]

25. Catassi, C.; Gatti, S.; Lionetti, E. World perspective and celiac disease epidemiology. *Dig. Dis.* **2015**, *33*, 141–146. [CrossRef] [PubMed]

26. Thomas, H.J.; Ahmad, T.; Rajaguru, C.; Barnardo, M.; Warren, B.F.; Jewell, D.P. Contribution of histological, serological, and genetic factors to the clinical heterogeneity of adult-onset coeliac disease. *Scand. J. Gastroenterol.* **2009**, *44*, 1076–1083. [CrossRef] [PubMed]

27. Catassi, C.; Fabiani, E.; Ratsch, I.M.; Coppa, G.V.; Giorgi, P.L.; Pierdomenico, R.; Alessandrini, S.; Iwanejko, G.; Domenici, R.; Mei, E.; *et al.* The coeliac iceberg in Italy. A multicentre antigliadin antibodies screening for coeliac disease in school-age subjects. *Acta Paediatr. Suppl.* **1996**, *412*, 29–35. [CrossRef] [PubMed]

28. Horwitz, A.; Skaaby, T.; Kårhus, L.L.; Schwarz, P.; Jørgensen, T.; Rumessen, J.J.; Linneberg, A. Screening for celiac disease in Danish adults. *Scand. J. Gastroenterol.* **2015**, *50*, 824–831. [CrossRef] [PubMed]

29. Sollid, L.M.; Markussen, G.; Ek, J.; Gjerde, H.; Vartdal, F.; Thorsby, E. Evidence for a primary association of celiac disease to a particular HLA-DQ alpha/beta heterodimer. *J. Exp. Med.* **1989**, *169*, 345–350. [CrossRef] [PubMed]

30. Tjon, J.M.; van Bergen, J.; Koning, F. Celiac disease: How complicated can it get? *Immunogenetics* **2010**, *62*, 641–651. [CrossRef] [PubMed]

31. Hadithi, M.; von Blomberg, B.M.; Crusius, J.B.; Bloemena, E.; Kostense, P.J.; Meijer, J.W.; Mulder, C.J.; Stehouwer, C.D.; Peña, A.S. Accuracy of serologic tests and HLA-DQ typing for diagnosing celiac disease. *Ann. Intern. Med.* **2007**, *147*, 294–302. [CrossRef] [PubMed]

32. Malamut, G.; Meresse, B.; Cellier, C.; Cerf-Bensussan, N. Refractory celiac disease: From bench to bedside. *Semin. Immunopathol.* **2012**, *34*, 601–613. [CrossRef] [PubMed]

33. Polvi, A.; Eland, C.; Koskimies, S.; Mäki, M.; Partanen, J. HLA DQ and DP in Finnish families with celiac disease. *Eur. J. Immunogenet.* **1996**, *23*, 221–234. [CrossRef]

34. Koskinen, L.L.; Einarsdottir, E.; Korponay-Szabo, I.R.; Kurppa, K.; Kaukinen, K.; Sistonen, P.; Pocsai, Z.; Széles, G.; Adány, R.; Mäki, M.; *et al.* Fine mapping of the CELIAC2 locus on chromosome 5q31-q33 in the Finnish and Hungarian populations. *Tissue Antigens* **2009**, *74*, 408–416. [CrossRef] [PubMed]

35. Holopainen, P.; Naluai, A.T.; Moodie, S.; Percopo, S.; Coto, I.; Clot, F.; Ascher, H.; Sollid, L.; Ciclitira, P.; Greco, L.; *et al.* Candidate gene region 2q33 in European families with coeliac disease. *Tissue Antigens* **2004**, *63*, 212–222. [CrossRef] [PubMed]

36. Van Belzen, M.J.; Meijer, J.W.; Sandkuijl, L.A.; Bardoel, A.F.; Mulder, C.J.; Pearson, P.L.; Houwen, R.H.; Wijmenga, C. A major non-HLA locus in celiac disease maps to chromosome 19. *Gastroenterology* **2003**, *125*, 1032–1041. [CrossRef]

37. Hill, I.D.; Dirks, M.H.; Liptak, G.D.; Colletti, R.B.; Fasano, A.; Guandalini, S.; Hoffenberg, E.J.; Horvath, K.; Murray, J.A.; Pivor, M.; *et al.* Guideline for the diagnosis and treatment of celiac disease in children: Recommendations of the North American Society for Pediatric Gastroenterology Hepatology and Nutrition. *J. Pediatr. Gastroenterol. Nutr.* **2005**, *40*, 1–19. [CrossRef] [PubMed]

38. James, S.P. National Institutes of Health Consensus Development Conference Statement on Celiac Disease. *Gastroenterology* **2005**, *128*, 1–9. [CrossRef]

39. Husby, S.; Koletzko, S.; Korponay-Szabo, I.R.; Mearin, M.L.; Phillips, A.; Shami, R.; Troncone, R.; Giersiepen, K.; Branski, D.; Catassi, C.; *et al.* European Society for Pediatric Gastroenterology, Hepatology and Nutrition Guidelines for the diagnosis of Coeliac disease. *JPGN* **2012**, *54*, 136–160. [CrossRef] [PubMed]

40. Dickson, B.C.; Streutker, C.J.; Chetty, R. Coeliac disease: An update for pathologists. *Rev. J. Clin. Path.* **2006**, *59*, 1008–1016. [CrossRef] [PubMed]

41. Mohamed, B.M.; Feighery, C.; Coates, C.; O'Shea, U.; Delaney, D.; O'Briain, S.; Kelly, J.; Abuzakouk, M. The absence of a mucosal lesion on standard histological examination does not exclude diagnosis of celiac disease. *Dig. Dis. Sci.* **2008**, *53*, 52–61. [CrossRef] [PubMed]

42. Kaukinen, K.; Collin, P.; Mäki, M. Latent coeliac disease or coeliac disease beyond villous atrophy? *Gut* **2007**, *56*, 1339–1340. [CrossRef] [PubMed]

43. Mubarak, A.; Nikkels, P.; Houwen, R.; Kate, F.T. Reproducibility of the histological diagnosis of celiac disease. *Scand. J. Gastroenterol.* **2011**, *46*, 1065–1073. [CrossRef] [PubMed]

44. Barker, C.C.; Mitton, C.; Jevon, G.; Mock, T. Can tissue transglutaminase antibody titers replace small-bowel biopsy to diagnose celiac disease in select pediatric populations? *Pediatrics* **2005**, *115*, 1341–1346. [CrossRef] [PubMed]

45. Donaldson, M.R.; Book, L.S.; Leiferman, K.M.; Zone, J.J.; Neuhausen, S.L. Strongly positive tissue transglutaminaseantibodies are associated with Marsh 3 histopathology in adult and pediatric celiac disease. *J. Clin. Gastroenterol.* **2008**, *42*, 256–260. [PubMed]

46. Vivas, S.; de Morales, J.G.R.; Riestra, S.; Arias, L.; Fuentes, D.; Alvarez, N.; Calleja, S.; Hernando, M.; Herrero, B.; Casqueiro, J.; *et al.* Duodenal biopsy may be avoided when high transglutaminase antibody titers are present. *World J. Gastroenterol.* **2009**, *15*, 4775–4780. [CrossRef] [PubMed]

47. Tortora, R.; Imperatore, N.; Capone, P.; de Palma, G.D.; de Stefano, G.; Gerbino, N.; Caporaso, N.; Rispo, A. The presence of anti-endomysial antibodies and the level of anti-tissue transglutainase can be used to diagnose adult coeliac disease without duodenal biopsy. *Aliment. Pharmacol. Ther.* **2014**, *40*, 1223–1229. [CrossRef] [PubMed]

48. Misak, Z.; Hojsak, I.; Jadresin, O.; Kekez, A.J.; Abdovic, S.; Kolacek, S. Diagnosis of coeliac disease in children younger than 2 years. *J. Pediatr. Gastroenterol. Nutr.* **2013**, *56*, 201–205. [CrossRef] [PubMed]

49. Vermeersch, P.; Geboes, K.; Marien, G.; Hoffman, I.; Hiele, M.; Bossuyt, X. Serological diagnosis of celiac disease: Comparative analysis of different strategies. *Clin. Chimic. Acta* **2012**, *413*, 1761–1767. [CrossRef] [PubMed]

50. Bürgin-Wolff, A.; Mauro, B.; Faruk, H. Intestinal biopsy is not always required to diagnose celiac disease: A retrospective analysis of combined antibody tests. *BMC Gastroenterol.* **2013**, *13*, 19. [CrossRef] [PubMed]

51. Bottaro, G.; Cataldo, F.; Rotolo, N.; Spina, M.; Corazza, G.R. The clinical pattern of subclinical/silent celiac disease: An analysis on 1026 consecutive cases. *Am. J. Gastroenterol.* **1999**, *94*, 691–696. [PubMed]

52. Ventura, A.; Magazzu, G.; Greco, L. Duration of exposure to gluten and risk for autoimmune disorders in patients with celiac disease. *Gastroenterology* **1999**, *117*, 297–303. [CrossRef] [PubMed]

53. Cosnes, J.; Cellier, C.; Viola, S.; Colombel, J.F.; Michaud, L.; Sarles, J.; Hugot, J.P.; Ginies, J.L.; Dabadie, A.; Mouterde, O.; *et al.* Nion-Larmurier IIncidence of autoimmune diseases in celiacdisease: Protective effect of the gluten-free diet. *Clin. Gastroenterol. Hepatol.* **2008**, *6*, 53–58. [CrossRef] [PubMed]

54. Sategna-Guidetti, C.; Solerio, E.; Scaglione, N.; Aimo, G.; Mengozzi, G. Duration of gluten exposure in adult coeliac disease does not correlate with the risk for autoimmune disorders. *Gut* **2001**, *49*, 502–505. [CrossRef] [PubMed]

55. Viljamaa, M.; Kaukinen, K.; Huhtala, H.; Kyrönpalo, S.; Rasmussen, M.; Collin, P. Coeliac disease, autoimmune diseases and gluten exposure. *Scand. J. Gastroenterol.* **2005**, *40*, 437–443. [CrossRef] [PubMed]

56. Ott, C.; Schölmerich, J. Extraintestinal manifestations and complications in IBD. *Nat. Rev. Gastroenterol. Hepatol.* **2013**, *10*, 585–595. [CrossRef] [PubMed]

57. Denham, J.M.; Hill, D. Celiac disease and autoimmunity: Review and controversies. *Curr. Allergy Asthma Rep.* **2013**, *13*, 347–353. [CrossRef] [PubMed]

58. Gutierrez-Achury, J.; de Almeida, R.C.; Wijmenga, C. Shared genetics in coeliac disease and other immune-mediated diseases. *J. Intern. Med.* **2011**, *269*, 591–603. [CrossRef] [PubMed]

59. Lammers, K.M.; Lu, R.; Brownley, J.; Lu, B.; Gerard, C.; Thomas, K.; Rallabhandi, P.; Shea-Donohue, T.; Tamiz, A.; Alkan, S.; *et al.* Gliadin induces an increase in intestinal permeability and zonulin release by binding to the chemokine receptor CXCR3. *Gastroenterology* **2008**, *135*, 194–204. [CrossRef] [PubMed]

60. McLean, M.H.; Dieguez, D., Jr.; Miller, L.M.; Young, H.A. Does the microbiota play a role in the pathogenesis of autoimmune diseases? *Gut* **2015**, *64*, 332–341. [CrossRef] [PubMed]

61. Koning, F.; Thomas, R.; Rossjohn, J.; Toes, R.E. Coeliac disease and rheumatoid arthritis: Similar mechanisms, different antigens. *Nat. Rev. Rheumatol.* **2015**. [CrossRef] [PubMed]

62. Guandalini, S.; Assiri, A. Celiac disease: A review. *JAMA Pediatr.* **2014**, *168*, 272–278. [CrossRef] [PubMed]

63. Volta, U.; Caio, G.; Stanghellini, V.; de Giorgio, R. The changing clinical profile of celiac disease: A 15-year experience (1998–2012) in an Italian referral center. *BMC Gastroenterol.* **2014**, *14*, 194. [CrossRef] [PubMed]

64. Sharma, M.; Singh, P.; Agnihotri, A.; Das, P.; Mishra, A; Verma, A.K.; Ahuja, A.; Sreenivas, V.; Khadgawat, R.; Gupta, S.D.; *et al.* Celiac disease: A disease with varied manifestations in adults and adolescents. *J. Dig. Dis.* **2013**, *14*, 518–525. [CrossRef] [PubMed]

65. Holmes, G.K. Coeliac disease and type 1 diabetes mellitus: An important association. *J. Diab. Nurs.* **2015**, *19*, 111–116.

66. Elfström, P.; Sundström, J.; Ludvigsson, J.F. Systematic review with meta-analysis: Associations between coeliac disease and type 1 diabetes. *Alim. Pharmacol. Ther.* **2014**, 1123–1132. [CrossRef] [PubMed]

67. Cerutti, F.; Bruno, G.; Chiarelli, F.; Lorini, R.; Meschi, F.; Sacchetti, C. Younger age at onset and sex predict celiac disease in children and adolescents with type 1diabetes: An Italian multicenter study. *Diabetes Care* **2004**, *27*, 1294–1298. [CrossRef] [PubMed]

68. Ludvigsson, J.F.; Ludvigsson, J.; Ekbom, A.; Montgomery, S.M. Celiac disease and risk of subsequent type 1 diabetes: A general population cohort study of children and adolescents. *Diabetes Care* **2006**, *29*, 2483–2488. [CrossRef] [PubMed]

69. Pocecco, M.; Ventura, A. Coeliac disease and insulin-dependent diabetes mellitus: A causal association? *Acta. Paediatr.* **1995**, *84*, 1432–1433. [CrossRef] [PubMed]

70. Hansen, D.; Brock-Jacobsen, B.; Lund, E.; Bjorn, C.; Hansen, L.P.; Nielsen, C.; Fenger, C.; Lillevang, S.T.; Husby, S. Clinical benefit of a gluten-free diet in type 1 diabetic children with screening-detected celiac disease: A population-based screening study with 2 years' follow-up. *Diabetes Care* **2006**, *29*, 2452–2456. [CrossRef] [PubMed]

71. Amin, R.; Murphy, N.; Edge, J.; Ahmed, M.L.; Acerini, C.L.; Dunger, D.B. A longitudinal study of the effects of a gluten-free diet on glycemic control and weight gain in subjects with type 1 diabetes and celiac disease. *Diabetes Care* **2002**, *25*, 1117–1122. [CrossRef] [PubMed]

72. Sanchez-Albisua, I.; Wolf, J.; Neu, A.; Geiger, H.; Wascher, I.; Stern, M. Coeliac disease in children with type 1 diabetes mellitus: The effect of the gluten-free diet. *Diabet. Med.* **2005**, *22*, 1079–1082. [CrossRef] [PubMed]

73. Mohn, A.; Cerruto, M.; Iafusco, D.; Prisco, F.; Tumini, S.; Stoppoloni, O.; Chiarelli, F. Celiac disease in children and adolescents with type I diabetes: Importance of hypoglycemia. *J. Pediatr. Gastroenterol. Nutr.* **2001**, *32*, 37–40. [CrossRef] [PubMed]

74. Penagini, F.; Dilillo, D.; Meneghin, F.; Mameli, C.; Fabiano, V.; Zuccotti, G.V. Gluten-free diet in children: an approach to a nutritionally adequate and balanced diet. *Nutrients* **2013**, *5*, 4553–4565. [CrossRef] [PubMed]

75. Troncone, R.; Discepolo, V. Celiac disease and autoimmunity. *J. Pediatr. Gastroenterol. Nutr.* **2014**, *59*, S9–S11. [CrossRef] [PubMed]

76. Marietta, E.V.; Gomez, A.M.; Yeoman, C.; Tilahun, A.Y.; Clark, C.R.; Luckey, D.H.; Murray, J.A.; White, B.A.; Kudva, Y.C.; Rajagopalan, G. Low incidence of spontaneous type 1 diabetes in non-obese diabetic mice raised on gluten-free diets is associated with changes in the intestinal microbiome. *PLoS ONE* **2013**, *8*, e78687. [CrossRef] [PubMed]

77. Auricchio, R.; Paparo, F.; Maglio, M.; Franzese, A.; Lombardi, F.; Valerio, G.; Nardone, G.; Percopo, S.; Greco, L.; Troncone, R. *In vitro*-deranged intestinal immune response to gliadin in type 1 diabetes. *Diabetes* **2004**, *53*, 1680–1683. [CrossRef] [PubMed]

78. Maglio, M.; Florian, F.; Vecchiet, M.; Auricchio, R.; Paparo, F.; Spadaro, R.; Zanzi, D.; Rapacciuolo, L; Franzese, A.; Sblattero, D.; *et al.* Majority of children with type 1 diabetes produce and deposit anti-tissue transglutaminase antibodies in the small intestine. *Diabetes* **2009**, *58*, 1578–1584. [CrossRef] [PubMed]

79. Sategna-Guidetti, C.; Volta, U.; Ciacci, C.; Usai, P.; Carlino, A.; de Franceschi, L.; Camera, A.; Pelli, A.; Brossa, C. Prevalence of thyroid disorders in untreated adult celiac disease patients and effect of gluten withdrawal: An Italian multicenter study. *Am. J. Gastroenterol.* **2001**, *96*, 751–757. [CrossRef] [PubMed]

80. Larizza, D.; Calcaterra, V.; de Giacomo, C.; de Silvestri, A.; Asti, M.; Badulli, C.; Autelli, M.; Coslovich, E.; Martinetti, M. Celiac disease in children with autoimmune thyroid disease. *J. Pediatr.* **2001**, *139*, 738–740. [CrossRef] [PubMed]

81. Diamanti, A.; Ferretti, F.; Guglielmi, R.; Panetta, F.; Colistro, F.; Cappa, M.; Daniele, A.; Sole Basso, M.; Noto, C.; Crisogianni, M.; *et al.* Thyroid autoimmunity in children with coeliac disease: A prospective survey. *Arch. Dis. Child.* **2011**, *96*, 1038–1041. [CrossRef] [PubMed]

82. Sattar, N.; Lazare, F.; Kacer, M.; Aguayo-Figueroa, L.; Desikan, V.; Garcia, M.; Lane, A.; Chawla, A.; Wilson, T. Celiac disease in children, adolescents, and young adults with autoimmune thyroid disease. *J. Pediatr.* **2011**, *158*, 272–275. [CrossRef] [PubMed]

83. Van der Pals, M.; Ivarsson, A.; Norström, F.; Högberg, L.; Svensson, J.; Carlsson, A. Prevalence of thyroid autoimmunity in children with celiac disease compared to healthy 12-year olds. *Autoimmun. Dis.* **2014**. [CrossRef] [PubMed]

84. Metso, S.; Hyytia-Ilmonen, H.; Kaukinen, K.; Huhtala, H.; Jaatinen, P.; Salmi, J.; Taurio, J.; Collin, P. Gluten-free diet and autoimmune thyroiditis in patients with celiac disease. A prospective controlled study. *Scand. J. Gastroenterol.* **2012**, *47*, 43–48. [CrossRef] [PubMed]

85. Kalyoncu, D.; Urganci, N. Antithyroid antibodies and thyroid function in pediatric patients with celiac disease. *Inter. J. Endocrinol.* **2015**. [CrossRef] [PubMed]

86. Ergür, A.T.; Öçal, G.; Berberoglu, M.; Adıyaman, P.; Sıklar, Z.; Aycan, Z.; Evliyaoğlu, O.; Kansu, A.; Girgin, N.; Ensari, A. Celiac disease and autoimmune thyroid disease in children with type 1 diabetes mellitus: Clinical and HLA-genotyping results. *J. Clin. Res. Ped. Endocrinol.* **2010**, *2*, 151–154. [CrossRef] [PubMed]

87. Biagi, F.; Campanella, J.; Soriani, A.; Vailati, A.; Corazza, G.R. Prevalence of coeliac disease in Italian patients affected by Addison's disease. *Scand. J. Gastroenterol.* **2006**, *41*, 302–305. [CrossRef] [PubMed]

88. Ludvigsson, J.F.; Kämpe, O.; Lebwohl, B.; Green, P.H.; Silverberg, S.J.; Ekbom, A. Primary hyperparathyroidism and celiac disease: A population-based cohort study. *J. Clin. Endocrinol. Metable* **2012**, *97*, 897–904. [CrossRef] [PubMed]

89. Lauret, E.; Rodrigo, L. Celiac disease and autoimmune-associated conditions. *Biol. Med. Res. Int.* **2013**. [CrossRef] [PubMed]

90. Roblin, X.; Helluwaert, F.; Bonaz, B. Celiac disease must be evaluated in patients with Sjögren syndrome. *Arch. Intern. Med.* **2004**, *164*, 2387. [CrossRef] [PubMed]

91. Ludvigsson, J.F.; Rubio-Tapia, A.; Chowdhary, V.; Murray, J.A.; Simard, J.F. Increased risk of systemic lupus erythematosus in 29,000 patients with biopsy-verified celiac disease. *J. Rheumatol.* **2012**, *39*, 1964–1970. [CrossRef] [PubMed]

92. De Maddi, F.; Pellegrini, F.; Raffaele, C.G.; Tarantino, G.; Rigante, D. Celiac disease and juvenile idiopathic arthritis: A still enigmatic crossover. *Scand. J. Gastroenterol.* **2013**, *48*, 511–512. [CrossRef] [PubMed]

93. Abenaoli, L.; Proietti, I.; Leggio, L.; Ferrulli, A.; Vonghia, L.; Capizzi, R.; Rotoli, M.; Amerio, P.L.; Gasbarrini, G.; Addolorato, G. Cutaneous manifestations in celiac disease. *World J. Gastroenterol.* **2006**, *12*, 843–852.

94. Rubio-Tapia, A.; Murray, J.A. The liver in celiac disease. *Hepatology* **2007**, *46*, 1650–1658. [CrossRef] [PubMed]

95. Grossman, G. Neurological complications of coeliac disease: What is the evidence? *Pract. Neurol.* **2008**, *8*, 77–89. [CrossRef] [PubMed]

96. Frustaci, A.; Cuoco, L.; Chimenti, C.; Pieroni, M.; Fioravanti, G.; Gentiloni, N.; Maseri, A.; Gasbarrini, G. Celiac disease associated with autoimmune myocarditis. *Circulation* **2002**, *105*, 2611–2618. [CrossRef] [PubMed]

97. Curione, M.; Barbato, M.; de Biase, L.; Viola, F.; lo Russo, L.; Cardi, E. Prevalence of coeliac disease in idiopathic dilated cardiomyopathy. *Lancet* **1999**, *354*, 222–223. [CrossRef]

98. Emilsson, L.; Andersson, B.; Elfström, P.; Green, P.H.R.; Ludvigsson, J.F. Risk of idiopathic dilated cardiomyopathy in 29,000 patients with celiac disease. *J. Am. Heart Assoc.* **2012**, *1*, e001594. [CrossRef] [PubMed]

99. Welander, A.; Sundelin, B.; Fored, M.; Ludvigsson, J.F. Increased risk of IgA nephropathy among individuals with celiac disease. *J. Clin. Gastroenterol.* **2013**, *47*, 678–683. [CrossRef] [PubMed]

100. Moeller, S.; Canetta, P.A.; Taylor, A.K.; Arguelles-Grande, C.; Snyder, H.; Green, P.H.; Kiryluk, K.; Alaedini, A. Lack of serologic evidence to link IgA nephropathy with celiac disease or immune reactivity to gluten. *PLoS ONE* **2014**, *9*, e94677. [CrossRef] [PubMed]

101. Pittman, F.E.; Holub, D.A. Sjoegren's syndrome and adult celiac disease. *Gastroenterology* **1965**, *48*, 869–876. [PubMed]

102. Luft, L.M.; Barr, S.G.; Martin, L.O.; Chan, E.K.; Fritzler, M.J. Autoantibodies to tissue transglutaminase in Sjogren's syndrome and related rheumatic diseases. *J. Rheumatol.* **2003**, *30*, 2613–2619. [PubMed]

103. Iltanen, S.; Collin, P.; Korpela, M.; Holm, K.; Partanen, J.; Polvi, A.; Mäki, M. Celiac disease and markers of celiac disease latency in patients with primary Sjogren's syndrome. *Am. J. Gastroenterol.* **1999**, *94*, 1042–1046. [PubMed]

104. Shamir, R.; Shoenfeld, Y.; Blank, M.; Eliakim, R.; Lahat, N.; Sobel, E.; Shinar, E.; Lerner, A. The prevalence of coeliac disease antibodies in patients with the antiphospholipid syndrome. *Lupus* **2003**, *12*, 394–399. [CrossRef] [PubMed]

105. George, E.K.; Hertzberger-ten Cate, R.; van Suijlekom-Smit, L.W.; von Blomberg, B.M.; Stapel, S.O.; van Elburg, R.M.; Mearin, M.L. Juvenile chronic arthritis and coeliac disease in The Netherlands. *Clin. Exp. Rheumatol.* **1996**, *14*, 571–575. [PubMed]

106. Lepore, L.; Martelossi, S.; Pennesi, M.; Falcini, F.; Ermini, M.L.; Ferrari, R.; Perticarari, S.; Presani, G.; Lucchesi, A.; Lapini, M.; *et al.* Prevalence of celiac disease in patients with juvenile chronic arthritis. *J. Pediatr.* **1996**, *129*, 311–313. [CrossRef]

107. Rensch, M.J.; Szyjkowski, R.; Shaffer, R.T.; Fink, S.; Kopecky, C.; Grissmer, L.; Enzenhauer, R.; Kadakia, S. The prevalence of celiac disease autoantibodies in patients with systemic lupus erythematosus. *Am. J. Gastroenterol.* **2001**, *96*, 1113–1115. [CrossRef] [PubMed]

108. Wang, N.; Shen, N.; Vyse, T.J.; Anand, V.; Gunnarson, I.; Sturfelt, G.; Rantapaa-Dahlqvist, S.; Elvin, K.; Truedsson, L.; Andersson, B.A.; *et al.* Selective IgA deficiency in autoimmune diseases. *Mol. Med.* **2011**, *17*, 1383–1396. [PubMed]

109. Pan-Hammarstrom, Q.; Hammarstrom, L. Antibody deficiency diseases. *Eur. J. Immunol.* **2008**, *38*, 327–333. [CrossRef] [PubMed]

110. Meini, A.; Pillan, N.M.; Villanacci, V.; Monafo, V.; Ugazio, A.G.; Plebani, A. Prevalence and diagnosis of celiac disease in IgA-deficient children. *Ann. Allergy Asthma Immunol.* **1996**, *77*, 333–336. [CrossRef]

111. Fiore, M.; Pera, C.; Delfino, L.; Scotese, I.; Ferrara, G.B.; Pignata, C. DNA typing of DQ and DR alleles in IgA-deficient subjects. *Eur. J. Immunogenet.* **1995**, *22*, 403–411. [CrossRef] [PubMed]

112. Arroyo, H.A.; de Rosa, S.; Ruggieri, V.; de Davila, M.T.; Fejerman, N. Epilepsy, occipital calcifications, and oligosymptomatic celiac disease in childhood. *J. Child. Neurol.* **2002**, *17*, 800–806. [CrossRef] [PubMed]

113. Lionetti, E.; Francavilla, R.; Pavone, P.; Pavone, L.; Francavilla, T.; Pulvirenti, A.; Giugno, R.; Ruggieri, M. The neurology of coeliac disease in childhood: What is the evidence? A systematic review and meta-analysis. *Dev. Med. Child. Neurol.* **2010**, *52*, 700–707. [CrossRef] [PubMed]

114. Buie, T. The relationship of autism and gluten. *Clin. Ther.* **2013**, *35*, 579–583. [CrossRef] [PubMed]

115. Millward, C.; Ferriter, M.; Calver, S.; Connell-Jones, G. Gluten- and casein-free diets for autistic spectrum disorder. *Cochrane Database Syst. Rev.* **2004**. [CrossRef]

116. Batista, I.C.; Gandolfi, L.; Nobrega, Y.K.; Almeida, R.C.; Almeida, L.M.; Campos Junior, D.; Pratesi, R. Autism spectrum disorder and celiac disease: No evidence for a link. *Arq. Neuropsiquiatr.* **2012**, *70*, 28–33. [CrossRef] [PubMed]

117. Zelnik, N.; Pacht, A.; Obeid, R.; Lerner, A. Range of neurologic disorders in patients with celiac disease. *Pediatrics* **2004**, *113*, 1672–1676. [CrossRef] [PubMed]

118. Falcini, F.; Porfirio, B.; Lionetti, P. Juvenile dermatomyositis and celiac disease. *J. Rheumatol.* **1999**, *26*, 1419–1420. [PubMed]

119. Marie, I.; Lecomte, F.; Hachulla, E.; Antonietti, M.; François, A.; Levesque, H.; Courtois, H. An uncommon association: Celiac disease and dermatomyositis in adults. *Clin. Exper. Rheumatol.* **2001**, *19*, 201–203.

120. Song, M.S.; Farber, D.; Bitton, A.; Jass, J.; Singer, M.; Karpati, G. Dermatomyositis associated with celiac disease: Response to a gluten-free diet. *Canadian J. Gastroenterol.* **2006**, *20*, 433–435.

121. Reed, A.M.; Pachman, L.; Ober, C. Molecular genetic studies of major histocompatibility complex genes in children with juvenile dermatomyositis: Increased risk associated with HLADQA1*0501. *Hum. Immunol.* **1991**, *32*, 235–240. [CrossRef]

122. Rodríguez-García, C.; González-Hernández, S.; Pérez-Robayna, N.; Guimerá, F.; Fagundo, E.; Sánchez, R. Repigmentation of vitiligo lesions in a child with celiac disease after a gluten-free diet. *Pediatr. Dermatol.* **2011**, *28*, 209–210. [CrossRef] [PubMed]

123. Corazza, G.R.; Andreani, M.L.; Venturo, N.; Bernardi, M.; Tosti, A.; Gasbarrini, G. Celiac disease and alopecia areata: Report of a new association. *Gastroenterology* **1995**, *109*, 1333–1337. [CrossRef]

124. Bardella, M.T.; Marino, R.; Barbareschi, M.; Bianchi, F.; Faglia, G.; Bianchi, P. Alopecia areata and coeliac disease: No effect of a gluten-free diet on hair growth. *Dermatology* **2000**, *200*, 108–110. [CrossRef] [PubMed]

125. Fessatou, S.; Kostaki, M.; Karpathios, T. Coeliac disease and alopecia areata in childhood. *J. Paediatr. Child. Health* **2003**, *39*, 152–154. [CrossRef] [PubMed]

126. Caprai, S.; Vajro, P.; Ventura, A.; Sciveres, M.; Maggiore, G.; SIGENP Study Group for Autoimmune Liver Disorders in Celiac Disease. Autoimmune liver disease associated with celiac disease in childhood: A multicenter study. *Clin. Gastroenterol. Hepatol.* **2008**, *6*, 803–806. [CrossRef] [PubMed]

127. Van Gerven, N.M.; Bakker, S.F.; de Boer, Y.S.; Witte, B.I.; Bontkes, H.; van Nieuwkerk, C.M.; Mulder, C.J.; Bouma, G.; Dutch AIH working group. Seroprevalence of celiac disease in patients with autoimmune hepatitis. *Eur. J. Gastroenterol. Hepatol.* **2014**, *26*, 1104–1107. [CrossRef] [PubMed]

128. Rostami, K.; Steegers, E.A.; Wong, W.Y.; Braat, D.D.; Steegers-Theunissen, R.P. Coeliac disease and reproductive disorders: A neglected association. *Eur. J. Obstet. Gynecol. Reprod. Biol.* **2001**, *96*, 146–149. [CrossRef]

129. Choi, J.M.; Lebwohl, B.; Wang, J.; Lee, S.K.; Murray, J.A.; Sauer, M.V.; Green, P.H. Increased prevalence of celiac disease in patients with unexplained infertility in the United States. *J. Reprod. Med.* **2011**, *56*, 199–203. [PubMed]

130. Zugna, D.; Richiardi, L.; Akre, O.; Stephansson, O.; Ludvigsson, J.F. A nationwide population-based study to determine whether coeliac disease is associated with infertility. *Gut* **2010**, *59*, 1471–1475. [CrossRef] [PubMed]

131. Santonicola, A.; Iovino, P.; Cappello, C.; Capone, P.; Andreozzi, P.; Ciacci, C. From menarche to menopause: The fertile life span of celiac women. *Menopause* **2011**, *18*, 1125–1130. [CrossRef] [PubMed]

132. Dhalwani, N.N.; West, J.; Sultan, A.A.; Ban, L.; Tata, L.J. Women with celiac disease present with fertility problems no more often than women in the general population. *Gastroenterology* **2014**, *147*, 1267–1274. [CrossRef] [PubMed]

133. Gale, L.; Wimalaratna, H.; Brotodiharjo, A.; Duggan, J.M. Down's syndrome is strongly associated with coeliac disease. *Gut* **1997**, *40*, 492–496. [CrossRef] [PubMed]

134. Zachor, D.A.; Mroczek-Musulman, E.; Brown, P. Prevalence of celiac disease in Down syndrome in the United States. *J. Pediatr. Gastroenterol. Nutr.* **2000**, *31*, 275–279. [CrossRef] [PubMed]

135. Bonamico, M.; Mariani, P.; Danesi, H.M.; Crisogianni, M.; Failla, P.; Gemme, G.; Quartino, A.R.; Giannotti, A.; Castro, M.; Balli, F.; *et al.* Prevalence and clinical picture of celiac disease in Italian Down syndrome patients: A multicenter study. *J. Pediatr. Gastroenterol. Nutr.* **2001**, *33*, 139–143. [CrossRef] [PubMed]

136. Henderson, A.; Lynch, S.A.; Wilkinson, S.; Hunter, M. Adults with Down's syndrome: The prevalence of complications and health care in the community. *Br. J. Gen. Pract.* **2007**, *57*, 50–55. [PubMed]

137. Ivarsson, S.A.; Carlsson, A.; Bredberg, A.; Alm, J.; Aronsson, S.; Gustafsson, J.; Hagenas, L.; Hager, A.; Kristrom, B.; Marcus, C.; *et al.* Prevalence of coeliac disease in Turner syndrome. *Acta. Paediatr.* **1999**, *88*, 933–936. [CrossRef] [PubMed]

138. Bonamico, M.; Pasquino, A.M.; Mariani, P.; Danesi, H.M.; Culasso, F.; Mazzanti, L.; Petri, A.; Bona, G. Prevalence and clinical picture of celiac disease in Turner syndrome. *J. Clin. Endocrinol. MeTable* **2002**, *87*, 5495–5498. [CrossRef] [PubMed]

139. Giannotti, A.; Tiberio, G.; Castro, M.; Virgili, F.; Colistro, F.; Ferretti, F.; Digilio, M.C.; Gambarara, M.; Dallapiccola, B. Coeliac disease in Williams syndrome. *J. Med. Genet.* **2001**, *38*, 767–768. [CrossRef] [PubMed]

140. Abadie, V.; Sollid, L.M.; Barreiro, L.B.; Jabri, B. Integration of genetic and immunological insights into a model of celiac disease pathogenesis. *Annu. Rev. Immunol.* **2011**, *29*, 493–525. [CrossRef] [PubMed]

141. Van de Kamer, J.; Weijers, H.; Dicke, W. Coeliac disease. Some experiments on the cause of the harmful effect of wheat gliadin. *Acta. Paediatr. Scand.* **1953**, *42*, 223–231.

142. Lee, A.R.; Ng, D.L.; Diamond, B.; Ciaccio, E.J.; Green, P.H. Living with coeliac disease: Survey results from the USA. *J. Hum. Nutr. Diet* **2012**, *25*, 233–238. [CrossRef] [PubMed]

143. Rashid, M.; Cranney, A.; Zarkadas, M.; Graham, I.D.; Switzer, C.; Case, S.; Molloy, M.; Warren, R.E.; Burrows, V.; Butzner, J.D. Celiac disease: Evaluation of the diagnosis and dietary compliance in Canadian children. *Pediatrics* **2005**, *116*, e754–e759. [CrossRef] [PubMed]

144. Panzer, R.M.; Dennis, M.; Kelly, C.P.; Weir, D.; Leichtner, A.; Leffler, D.A. Navigating the gluten-free diet in college. *J. Pediatr. Gastroenterol. Nutr.* **2012**, *55*, 740–744. [CrossRef] [PubMed]

145. Wagner, G.; Berger, G.; Sinnreich, U.; Grylli, V.; Schober, E.; Huber, W.D.; Karwautz, A. Quality of life in adolescents with treated coeliac disease: Influence of compliance and age at diagnosis. *J. Pediatr. Gastroenterol. Nutr.* **2008**, *47*, 555–561. [CrossRef] [PubMed]

146. Fabiani, E.; Taccari, L.M.; Ratsch, I.M.; di Giuseppe, S.; Coppa, G.V.; Catassi, C. Compliance with gluten-free diet in adolescents with screening-detected celiac disease: A 5-year follow-up study. *J. Pediatr.* **2000**, *136*, 841–843. [CrossRef]

147. Anson, O.; Weizman, Z.; Zeevi, N. Celiac disease: Parental knowledge and attitudes of dietary compliance. *Pediatrics* **1990**, *85*, 98–103. [PubMed]

148. Jadresin, O.; Misak, Z.; Sanja, K.; Sonicki, Z.; Zizic, V. Compliance with gluten-free diet in children with coeliac disease. *J. Pediatr. Gastroenterol. Nutr.* **2008**, *47*, 344–348. [CrossRef] [PubMed]

149. Mulder, C.J.; Wierdsma, N.J.; Berkenpas, M.; Jacobs, M.A.; Bouma, G. Preventing complications in celiac disease: Our experience with managing adult celiac disease. *Best Pract. Res. Clin. Gastroenterol.* **2015**, *29*, 459–468. [CrossRef] [PubMed]

150. Green, P.H.R.; Stavropoulos, S.N.; Panagi, S.G.; Goldstein, S.L.; Mcmahon, D.J.; Absan, H.; Neugut, A.I. Characteristics of adult celiac disease in the USA: Results of a national survey. *Am. J. Gastroenterol.* **2001**, *96*, 126–131. [CrossRef] [PubMed]

151. Farnetti, S.; Zocco, M.A.; Garcovich, M.; Gasbarrini, A.; Capristo, E. Functional and metabolic 876 disorders in celiac disease: New implications for nutritional treatment. *J. Med. Food* **2014**, *17*, 1159–1164. [CrossRef] [PubMed]

152. Hallert, C.; Grant, C.; Grehn, S.; Grännö, C.; Hultén, S.; Midhagen, G.; Strön, M.; Svensson, H.; Valdimarsson, T. Evidence of poor vitamin status in celiac patients on a gluten-free diet for 10 years. *Aliment. Pharmacol. Ther.* **2002**, *16*, 1333–1339. [CrossRef] [PubMed]

153. Dickey, W.; Kearney, N. Overweight in celiac disease: Prevalence, clinical characteristics and effect of a gluten-free diet. *Am. J. Gastroenterol.* **2006**, *101*, 2356–2359. [CrossRef] [PubMed]

154. Valletta, E.; Fornaro, M.; Cipolli, M.; Conte, S.; Bissolo, F.; Danchielli, C. Celiac disease and obesity: Need for nutritional follow-up after diagnosis. *Eur. J. Clin. Nutr.* **2010**, *64*, 1371–1372. [CrossRef] [PubMed]

155. Lanzini, A.; Lanzarotto, F.; Villanacci, V.; Mora, A.; Bertolazzi, S.; Turini, D.; Carella, G.; Malagoli, A.; Ferrante, G.; Cesana, B.M.; *et al.* Complete recovery of intestinal mucosa occurs very rarely in adult coeliac patients despite adherence to gluten-free diet. *Aliment. Pharmacol. Ther.* **2009**, *29*, 1299–1308. [CrossRef] [PubMed]

156. Lebwohl, B.; Granath, F.; Ekbom, A.; Smedby, K.E.; Murray, J.A.; Neugut, A.I.; Green, P.H.R.; Ludvigsson, J.F. Mucosal healing and risk for lymphoproliferative malignancy in celiac disease. *Ann. Intern. Med.* **2013**, *159*, 169–175. [CrossRef] [PubMed]

157. Vreugdenhil, A.C.; Wolters, V.M.; Adriaanse, M.P.; van den Neucker, A.M.; van Bijnen, A.A.; Houwen, R.; Buurman, W.A. Additional value of serum I-FABP levels for evaluating celiac disease activity in children. *Scand. J. Gastroenterol.* **2011**, *46*, 1435–1441. [CrossRef] [PubMed]

158. McNicholl, B.; Egan-Mitchell, B.; Stevens, F.; Keane, R.; Baker, S.; McCarthy, C.F.; Fottrell, P.F. Mucosal recovery in treated childhood celiac disease (gluten-sensitive enteropathy). *J. Pediatr.* **1976**, *89*, 418–424. [CrossRef]

159. Wahab, P.J.; Meijer, J.W.; Mulder, C.J. Histologic follow-up of people with celiac disease on a gluten-free diet: Slow and incomplete recovery. *Am. J. Clin. Pathol.* **2002**, *118*, 459–463. [PubMed]

160. Bardella, M.T.; Velio, P.; Cesana, B.M.; Prampolini, L.; Casella, G.; Di Bella, C.; Lanzini, A.; Gambarotti, M.; Bassotti, G.; Villanacci, V. Coeliac disease: A histological follow-up study. *Histopathology* **2007**, *50*, 465–471. [CrossRef] [PubMed]

161. Tursi, A.; Brandimarte, G.; Giorgetti, G.M.; Elisei, W.; Inchingolo, C.D.; Monardo, E.; Aiello, F. Endoscopic and histological findings in the duodenum of adults with celiac disease before and after changing to a gluten-free diet: A 2-year prospective study. *Endoscopy* **2006**, *38*, 702–707. [CrossRef] [PubMed]

162. Biagi, F.; Vattiato, C.; Agazzi, S.; Balduzzi, D.; Schiepatti, A.; Gobbi, P.; Corazza, G.R. A second duodenal biopsy is necessary in the follow-up of adult coeliac patients. *Ann. Med.* **2014**, *46*, 430–433. [CrossRef] [PubMed]

163. Biagi, F.; Gobbi, P.; Marchese, A.; Borsotti, E.; Zingone, F.; Ciacci, C.; Volta, U.; Caio, G.; Carroccio, A.; Ambrosiano, G.; *et al.* Low incidence but poor prognosis of complicated coeliac disease: A retrospective multicentre study. *Dig. Liver Dis.* **2014**, *46*, 227–230. [CrossRef] [PubMed]

164. Lebwohl, B.; Granath, F.; Ekbom, A.; Montgomery, S.M.; Murray, J.A.; Rubio-Tapia, A.; Green, P.H.R.; Ludvigsson, J.F. Mucosal healing and mortality in coeliac disease. *Alim. Pharmacol. Ther.* **2013**, *37*, 332–339. [CrossRef] [PubMed]

165. Bruins, M.J. The clinical response to gluten challenge: A review of the literature. *Nutrients* **2013**, *5*, 4614–4641. [CrossRef] [PubMed]

166. Dewar, D.H.; Donnelly, S.C.; Mc Laughlin, S.D.; Johnson, M.W.; Ellis, H.J.; Ciclitira, P.J. Celiac disease: Management of persistent symptoms in patients on a gluten-free diet. *World J. Gastroenterol.* **2012**, *18*, 1348–1356. [CrossRef] [PubMed]

Nutrients **2015**, *7*, 8733–8751

167. Mooney, P.D.; Evans, K.E.; Singh, S.; Sanders, D.S. Treatment Failure in Coeliac Disease: A practical guide to investigation and treatment of non-responsive and refractory coeliac disease. *J. Gastrointestin. Liver Dis.* **2012**, *21*, 197–203. [PubMed]

168. Mubarak, A.; Oudshoorn, J.H.; Kneepkens, C.M.F.; Butler, J.C.; Schreurs, M.W.J.; Mulder, C.J.; Houwen, R.H.J. A child with refractory coeliac disease. *J. Pediatr. Gastroenterol. Nutr.* **2011**, *53*, 216–218. [CrossRef] [PubMed]

169. Sigman, T.; Nguyen, V.H.; Costea, F.; Sant'Anna, A.; Seidman, E.G. Ulcerative jejunitis in a child with celiac disease. *BMC Gastroenterol.* **2014**, *14*, 29. [CrossRef] [PubMed]

170. Van Wanrooij, R.L.J.; Müller, D.M.J.; Neefjes-Borst, E.A.; Meijer, J.; Koudstaal, L.G.; Heideman, D.A.M.; Bontkes, H.J.; von Blomberg, B.M.E.; Bouma, G.; Mulder, C.J.J. Optimal strategies to identify aberrant intra-epithelial lymphocytes in refractory coeliac disease. *J. Clin. Immunol.* **2014**, *34*, 828–835. [CrossRef] [PubMed]

171. Malamut, G.; Cellier, C. Refractory coeliac disease. *Curr. Opin. Oncol.* **2013**, *25*, 445–451. [CrossRef] [PubMed]

172. Biagi, F.; Lorenzini, P.; Corazza, G.R. Literature review on the clinical relationship between ulcerative jejunoileitis, coeliac disease, and enteropathy-associated T-cell. *Scand. J. Gastroenterol.* **2000**, *35*, 785–790. [PubMed]

173. Woodward, J. The management of refractory coeliac disease. *Ther. Adv. Chronic Dis.* **2013**, *4*, 77–90. [CrossRef] [PubMed]

174. Corrao, G.; Corazza, G.R.; Bagnardi, V.; Brusco, G.; Ciacci, C.; Cottone, M.; Sategna Guidetti, C.; Usai, P.; Cesari, P.; Pelli, M.A.; *et al.* Mortality in patients with coeliac disease and their relatives: A cohort study. *Lancet* **2001**, *358*, 356–361. [CrossRef]

175. Abdul Sultan, A.; Crooks, C.J.; Card, T.; Tata, L.J.; Fleming, K.M.; West, J. Causes of death in people with coeliac disease in England compared with the general population: A competing risk analysis. *Gut* **2015**, *64*, 1220–1226. [CrossRef] [PubMed]

176. Biagi, F.; Corazza, G.R. Do different patients with coeliac disease have different mortality rates? *Gut* **2015**, *64*, 1187–1188. [CrossRef] [PubMed]

177. Mäki, M.; Mustalahti, K.; Kokkonen, J.; Kulmala, P.; Haapalahti, M.; Karttunen, T.; Ilonen, J.; Laurila, K.; Dahlbom, I.; Hansson, T.; *et al.* Prevalence of celiac disease among children in Finland. *N. Engl. J. Med.* **2003**, *348*, 2517–2524. [CrossRef] [PubMed]

178. Ivarsson, A.; Myléus, A.; Norström, F.; van der Pals, M.; Rosén, A.; Högberg, L.; Danielsson, L.; Halvarsson, B.; Hammarroth, S.; Hernell, O.; *et al.* Prevalence of childhood celiac disease and changes in infant feeding. *Pediatrics* **2013**, *131*, e687–e694. [CrossRef] [PubMed]

179. David, T.J. Transition from the paediatric clinic to the adult service. *JRSM* **2001**, *94*, 373–374.

180. Amaria, K.; Stinson, J.; Cullen-Dean, G.; Sappleton, K.; Kaufman, M. Tools for addressing systems issues in transition. *Healthc. Q.* **2011**, *14*, 72–76. [PubMed]

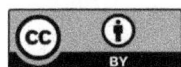

nutrients

MDPI

Review

Seronegative Celiac Disease and Immunoglobulin Deficiency: Where to Look in the Submerged Iceberg?

Floriana Giorgio [1], Mariabeatrice Principi [1], Giuseppe Losurdo [1], Domenico Piscitelli [2], Andrea Iannone [1], Michele Barone [1], Annacinzia Amoruso [1], Enzo Ierardi [1] and Alfredo Di Leo [1,*]

[1] Section of Gastroenterology, University Hospital Policlinico, Department of Emergency and Organ Transplantation, University of Bari, 70124 Bari, Italy; flomic@libero.it (F.G.); b.principi@gmail.com (M.P.); giuseppelos@alice.it (G.L.); ianan@hotmail.it (A.I.); michele.barone@uniba.it (M.B.); annacinzia.amoruso@uniba.it (A.A.); ierardi.enzo@gmail.com (E.I.)

[2] Section of Pathology, University Hospital Policlinico, Department of Emergency and Organ Transplantation, University of Bari, 70124 Bari, Italy; domenico.piscitelli@uniba.it

* Author to whom correspondence should be addressed; alfredo.dileo@uniba.it; Tel.: +39-080-5592-577; Fax: +39-080-5593-088.

Received: 28 May 2015; Accepted: 2 September 2015; Published: 8 September 2015

Abstract: In the present narrative review, we analyzed the relationship between seronegative celiac disease (SNCD) and immunoglobulin deficiencies. For this purpose, we conducted a literature search on the main medical databases. SNCD poses a diagnostic dilemma. Villous blunting, intraepithelial lymphocytes (IELs) count and gluten "challenge" are the most reliable markers. Immunohistochemistry/immunofluorescence tissue transglutaminase (tTG)-targeted mucosal immunoglobulin A (IgA) immune complexes in the intestinal mucosa of SNCD patients may be useful. In our experience, tTG-mRNA was similarly increased in seropositive celiac disease (CD) and suspected SNCD, and strongly correlated with the IELs count. This increase is found even in the IELs' range of 15–25/100 enterocytes, suggesting that there may be a "grey zone" of gluten-related disorders. An immune deregulation (severely lacking B-cell differentiation) underlies the association of SNCD with immunoglobulin deficiencies. Therefore, CD may be linked to autoimmune disorders and immune deficits (common variable immunodeficiency (CVID)/IgA selective deficiency). CVID is a heterogeneous group of antibodies dysfunction, whose association with CD is demonstrated only by the response to a gluten-free diet (GFD). We hypothesized a familial inheritance between CD and CVID. Selective IgA deficiency, commonly associated with CD, accounts for IgA-tTG seronegativity. Selective IgM deficiency (sIgMD) is rare (<300 cases) and associated to CD in 5% of cases. We diagnosed SNCD in a patient affected by sIgMD using the tTG-mRNA assay. One-year GFD induced IgM restoration. This evidence, supporting a link between SNCD and immunoglobulin deficiencies, suggests that we should take a closer look at this association.

Keywords: seronegative celiac disease; tissue-transglutaminase mRNA; common variable immunodeficiency; selective IgA deficiency; selective IgM deficiency; gluten-free diet

1. The Submerged Iceberg of Celiac Disease and the Dilemma of Seronegativity

Celiac disease (CD) is the most common autoimmune enteropathy. In one of the largest screening trials, a prevalence of 1:133 was calculated, meaning that about 1% of the global population is affected [1]. It is characterized by a genetic background in which human leukocyte antigens (HLA) haplotypes DQ2/DQ8 play a major role as predisposing factors [1]. An involvement of some special alleles, such as DQ A1*05 (part of the DQ2 genotype), has been invoked. Nevertheless, these haplotypes are very common in the general population, with a mean prevalence of 20%, and only a minority develops CD [1]. Therefore, the analysis of HLA haplotypes is recommended in CD diagnosis as well as in special situations, such as patients undergoing a serological/histological examination only after having started an empirical gluten-free diet. Despite these evidences, patients with diagnosed CD are much fewer than the estimated prevalence. In Italy, for instance, 600,000 people are estimated to suffer from CD, but only in 150,000 has a firm diagnosis been made [2]. This figure underlines that most affected people could belong to the "submerged iceberg" of undiagnosed CD, such as the seronegative type of disorder (SNCD), characterized by the absence of well-known serological markers (anti-endomysium antibodies (EMA) or anti-tissue transglutaminase (anti-tTG)) [3].

Moreover, the clinical spectrum of CD is extremely wide. Indeed, CD may show extra-intestinal manifestations such as iron deficiency anemia, bone loss, short stature, skin and liver disease [4]. These symptoms, in the absence of classic intestinal involvement, may delay the final diagnosis. Commonly, forms of CD characterized by predominantly extra-intestinal features are regarded as atypical CD, and they may perhaps account for the majority of cases [3,5]. Another reason that may account for the suboptimal detection rate of CD is represented by subclinical features, showing incomplete concordance among the histological, clinical and serological findings. Latent CD is a vague and largely used term indicating various conditions. Sometimes, it may denote a normal villous architecture with abnormalities such as an increased number of intraepithelial lymphocytes (IELs) and/or increased mucosal permeability even in the absence of serological markers. This condition, according to Oslo definition [3], is observed in patients on a gluten containing diet [6,7]. Potential CD is characterized by a positive CD serology and normal small intestinal mucosa [3,8], although often referred to as an increased number of IELs in the villi [9–11]. However, the term (potential) is used also in the case of suspected SNCD. Therefore, atypical, latent and potential CD are part of the submerged iceberg of the disorder and often are linked to SNCD. Currently, a clear indication to assume a gluten free diet does not exist for latent or potential CD.

Seronegativity is a dilemma in CD [12]. SNCD was firstly described by Abrams *et al.* [13], who evaluated the sensitivity and specificity of serology in CD patients with (Marsh 3) or without villous atrophy (Marsh 1 and 2). They found positive EMA in 77% of atrophic and only 33% of non-atrophic lesions. The study also analyzed immunoglobulin A (IgA) anti-tTG. Although only 14 subjects underwent this test, IgA anti-tTG were positive in all the patients with atrophy and absent in those with partial atrophy. Other authors later repeated this experience [14–21], as shown in Table 1, underlining that seronegativity is inversely related to the degree of villous atrophy. Epidemiological data about SNCD are scanty due to its complicated diagnostic frame, but the prevalence ranges from 1.03% among all CD patients [21] to 28% in latent CD [22].

Table 1. Prevalence of anti-tissue transglutaminase (anti-tTG) and endomysium antibodies (EMA) in cases of non-atrophic celiac disease (CD).

Reference	Anti-tTG Positivity	EMA Positivity
Abrams, J.A. *et al.*, 2004 [13]	0%	33%
Tursi, A. *et al.*, 2003 [14]	7.69%	Not tested
Tursi, A. *et al.*, 2003 [15]	17.1%	8.6%
Dickey, W. *et al.*, 2000 [16]	Not tested	79%
Tursi, A. *et al.*, 2001 [17]	Not tested	33%
Rostami, K. *et al.*, 1999 [18]	Not tested	31%
Kurppa, K. *et al.*, 2010 [19]	88%	Not tested
Salmi, T.T. *et al.*, 2006 [20]	28.6%	87.6% (cumulative value including atrophic CD)
Makovicky, P. *et al.*, 2013 [21]	9.1%	0%

Mucosal deposits of anti-tTG and tissue transglutaminase (tTG) may be considered the main feature of SNCD [23]. Although these deposits have been described even in individuals with overt CD, it has been shown that in SNCD, IgA anti-tTG have a great affinity for their antigen, binding strongly to tTG2, and so preventing immunocomplex deposits from being able to pass into the circulation. The strong antigen-antibody connection could explain the negative serological tests [20]. Indeed, the production of auto-antibodies in subjects with CD occurs in the intestinal mucosa, as evidenced by the presence of immune-complexes revealed by immunofluorescence. Usually, auto-antibodies cross the mucosa and enter blood vessels [24]. In SNCD, however, the antibodies may be confined in the lamina propria rather than passing into the bloodstream. Six studies [19,25–29] have investigated such deposits by immunofluorescence, finding amounts ranging from 64.7%–100% in 221 of 307 (72%) potential SNCD patients. Moreover, in a study by Kaukinen *et al.* [30], 41 subjects with IELs at duodenal histology were assigned to a gluten-free or gluten-containing diet, that led to a diagnosis of a gluten-related disorder in 11 of them. Deposits of immunocomplexes, detected by immunohistochemistry, were discovered in 10 of these 11 patients. Interestingly, a study [25] reported that the presence of anti-tTG deposits was a predictor of the subsequent onset of villous atrophy or histological worsening and serological positivization. In a study analyzing the affinity of anti-tTG/tTG [20], Salmi *et al.* demonstrated that after starting a gluten-free diet, the levels of deposits reduced until they were not significantly different from those in controls.

Immunoglobulin deficiencies (ID) are congenital or inherited disorders of humoral immunity characterized by low immunoglobulin titers. They could account for a part of submerged celiac iceberg, since they contribute to a lower CD detection rate, in particular for potential, latent or SNCD.

On these bases, the present narrative review was performed in order to create an overview on the link between SNCD and immunoglobulin deficiencies. For this purpose, we performed a literature search in the main medical databases (PubMed, Scopus, EMBASE and ScienceDirect), by using the following key words: celiac disease, atypical, latent, potential, seronegative, tissue transglutaminase, immunoglobulin deficiency, IgA deficiency, IgM deficiency, common variable immunodeficiency.

2. Immunoglobulin Deficiencies and Celiac Disease

A gastrointestinal involvement is very frequent in ID. Indeed, patients with ID show gastrointestinal symptoms in up to 50% of cases [31], and this may complicate the diagnosis of CD in primary ID. The primary function of the immune system is to protect against viruses, bacteria and non-self antigens. The fact that the gastrointestinal mucosa is the largest contact surface where this process takes place accounts for the very common gastroenterological involvement in ID. Furthermore, ID may cause microscopic alterations in the mucosa that mimic gastrointestinal disorders like CD or inflammatory bowel disease, making a correct differential diagnosis even harder.

Herein, we describe the most common relationships between ID and CD. In detail, selective IgA deficiency (sIgAD), common variable immunodeficiency (CVID) and selective IgM deficiency (sIgMD) are analyzed.

2.1. Selective IgA Deficiency

Selective IgA deficiency (sIgAD) is the most common primary ID, with a prevalence of 1:300–700 individuals. It is defined as serum IgA levels less than 0.07 g/L with normal IgM and IgG levels in people >4 years old [32]. The pathogenic hallmark is a defective regulation of the terminal maturation of B lymphocytes into IgA-secreting plasma cells [33]. sIgAD becomes clinically evident in childhood, because of recurrent respiratory and gastrointestinal infections. Moreover, sIgAD may frequently be associated to atopic or autoimmune disorders such as inflammatory bowel disease, nodular lymphoid hyperplasia, pernicious anemia and CD [34].

The association between CD and sIgAD may be explained by a shared genetic susceptibility. sIgAD, like CD, is strongly associated with the major histocompatibility complex (MHC) region and, in particular, with the human leukocyte antigen (HLA)-B8, DR3, DQ2 haplotype. HLA-DQ/DR is the major immunoglobulin A locus [35,36]. Up to 45% of IgAD patients have at least one copy of this haplotype, compared to 16% in the general population [37].

The prevalence of CD in sIgAD is much more than in the general population, ranging from 6.7%–20.6% as summarized in Table 2 [38–43]. On the other hand, sIgAD is more common in celiac patients, with a prevalence of 1:39 [44].

Serological tests with IgA anti-tTG are not reliable for the diagnosis of CD in sIgAD, because of the lack of IgA production. This is why IgG-tTG tests have been proposed as alternative tools for diagnostic screening [45]. Instead, the histological diagnosis may encounter some pitfalls, since the histopathology of CD in sIgAD is indistinguishable from the pathology in patients with conventional CD. A peculiar feature could be the absence of IgA-secreting plasma cells in biopsy specimens [46]. Moreover, sIgAD patients are at high risk of Giardia spp. infection, which can simulate the histopathology of CD [47]. In doubtful cases, a gluten-free diet (GFD) can be proposed, because CD in sIgAD is promptly responsive to gluten withdrawal, resulting in normalization of the atrophic lesions [48]. In this regard, Valletta, *et al.* [49] reported the case of a nine-year old girl with sIgAD and recurrent diarrhea and abdominal pain, who underwent duodenal biopsy showing partial villous atrophy. Despite seronegativity, a course of GFD was administered and yielded histological resolution of the atrophy, so the diagnosis of SNCD was hypothesized. Four years later, while she was on a gluten-containing diet, serology positivization occurred, confirming the diagnosis of CD. This report strengthens the atypical behavior of CD in ID.

Table 2. Main studies investigating the prevalence of celiac disease (CD) in individuals affected by selective IgA deficiency (sIgAD).

Reference	Prevalence	Test Used for Diagnosis
Bienvenu, F. *et al.*, 2014 [38]	17.7% (8/45)	IgG-tTG, IgG-DGP
Wang, N. *et al.*, 2014 [39]	12.6% (45/356)	IgG-tTG, IgG-DGP and histology
Ludvigsson, J.F. *et al.*, 2014 [40]	6.7% (167/2495)	IgG-tTG, IgG-DGP
Pituch-Noworolska, A. *et al.*, 2013 [41]	20.6% (13/63)	IgG-tTG, IgG-DGP, IgG-EMA
Lenhardt, A. *et al.*, 2004 [42]	8.7% (11/126)	IgG-tTG, IgG-DGP and histology
Korponay-Szabó, I.R. *et al.*, 2003 [43]	9.8% (17/174)	IgG-tTG, IgG-EMA
Total	8% (261/3259)	

tTG, tissue transglutaminase, DGP, deamidated gliadin peptide; EMA, endomysium antibodies.

The observation that subjects with sIgAD have a higher incidence of CD [50] has prompted some authors to look for a "pathogenetic picture" of this patient subset. Borrelli *et al.* [51] discovered that patients with both diseases had higher IEL infiltrates than those with sIgAD alone and controls. In short, an expected finding was observed, *i.e.*, a subset of IELs, the so-called $\gamma\delta$ IELs, were over-expressed in duodenal samples of sIgAD-CD. Moreover, sIgAD-CD had more CD25+ cells (T regulatory lymphocytes) in the lamina propria than isolated sIgAD. Finally, 86% of sIgAD-CD patients showed IgM-tTG deposits, a phenomenon linked to a compensatory overproduction of IgM in response to the lack of IgA. This study represents, to the best of our knowledge, the only one which investigated immune-complexes deposits in sIgAD. This observation may suggest that mucosal immune-complexes characterize SNCD both in the presence and absence of ID. Moreover, sIgAD-CD expressed elevated levels of B-lymphocyte stimulator (BLyS), a molecule that is involved in several autoimmune diseases, while a proliferation-inducing ligand (APRIL) was significantly up-regulated only in isolated sIgAD [52]. Since APRIL promotes IgA production, its increased expression could represent a physiological negative feedback mechanism. BLyS over-expression, instead, may be invoked as a putative mechanism for the increased risk of onset of autoimmune diseases in people with sIgAD. Finally, a cytokine profile of sIgAD-CD was characterized by an enhanced production of inflammatory cytokines (namely interleukin-2, interferon gamma and tumor necrosis factor alpha), which were significantly higher than in CD or sIgAD alone, suggesting a persistent state of activation of pro-inflammatory signals in CD patients, particularly with a coexistent IgAD [53].

In conclusion, all these findings suggest that sIgAD and CD are characterized by signs of an impaired immune activation, which may account for an increased prevalence of seronegative disorder. Although several diagnostic difficulties may be encountered in the detection of SNCD in this group of patients, a strict follow-up, as well as a GFD in selected cases, could offer the best choice to gain a clearer diagnostic perspective for doubtful cases.

2.2. Common Variable Immunodeficiency

Common variable immunodeficiency (CVID) is a heterogeneous group of primary immunoglobulin deficiencies featuring low serum levels of immunoglobulins, a depressed response to specific antigens and high risk of recurrent infections [54]. Although the estimated prevalence is 1:25–50,000, it is considered to be the most common symptomatic ID [54]. The diagnosis relies on reduced levels of IgG and IgA, as well as on an absent or reduced antibody production in response to vaccines. Several pathogenic hypotheses have been made. A single genetic mutation has not been found, but a complex genetic background characterized by mutations and polymorphisms in genes deputed to B lymphocytes development (Inducible T-cell COStimulator: *ICOS*; B-cell activating factor receptor: *BAFF-R*; Cluster of differentiation: *CD20, CD19, CD21, CD81*) has been portrayed [55–58]. Further evidences about a possible common role played by HLA complex in both CD and CVID has been described. Indeed, several common polymorphisms in HLA loci have been detected. As reported, haplotype analysis, linkage disequilibrium, and homozygosity mapping indicated that HLA-DQ/DR is the major immunoglobulin A locus, strongly suggesting an overlapping immune pathogenesis for CVID and CD [59]. Moreover, Viallard *et al.* [60] demonstrated that CVID and CD showed altered expression of HLA-DR on antigen presenting cells (APC), thus hypothesizing that an imbalance in the process of antigen presentation by APC through HLA complex may induce an immunological response shared by CVID and CD.

CVID may show a wide range of immunological manifestations, including autoimmune phenomena, such as cytopenias, megaloblastic anemia/atrophic gastritis, immune thrombocytopenic purpura, autoimmune hemolytic anemia, sarcoidosis-like granulomatous infiltrative disorders, inflammatory bowel disease, autoimmune hepatitis and CD [61].

Gastrointestinal symptoms are very common in CVID, especially persistent diarrhea that manifests in more than 50% of cases. The corresponding histopathological pattern has been described as a sprue-like picture, resembling CD: villous atrophy and IELs infiltrate. However, unlike CD, CVID should be suspected when plasma cells are reduced or absent in the lamina propria [62–64].

For these reasons, patients suffering from both CD and CVID pose a clinical conundrum. It is well known that these diseases may share a common dysregulation of the ICOS molecule [65], and coexistence in the same family of patients with CD and CVID has been described [66]. Although celiac-like lesions can be observed in 30% of CVID patients, the true prevalence of CD in CVID is much lower, as reported in Table 3 [41,63,67–70], being 9.2% overall. Biagi *et al.* [70] have observed that the histologic response to a GFD is the only reliable tool to establish the diagnosis of CD in CVID. Other authors have suggested that human leukocyte antigen (HLA) determination may be helpful, since a DQ2 or DQ8 haplotype was associated with concomitant CD, whilst a "not-at-risk" haplotype in a CVID patient with villous atrophy led them to exclude CD [67]. Indeed, only patients with DQ2/8 responded with a histological and clinical improvement to a GFD and this result may be a further evidence of a link between CD and CVID, mediated by HLA haplotypes. On the other hand, CD serology has shown to be ineffective in CVID due to the high rate of false negatives, caused by the fact that CVID patients cannot mount an appropriate antibody response [71].

Table 3. Main studies investigating the prevalence of celiac disease (CD) in individuals affected by common variable immunodeficiency (CVID).

Reference	Prevalence
Malamut, G. *et al.*, 2010 [63]	4% (2/50)
Pituch-Noworolska, A. *et al.*, 2013 [41]	7% (3/43)
Venhoff, N. *et al.*, 2013 [67]	20% (4/20)
Rodríguez-Negrete, E.V. *et al.*, 2015 [68]	18% (3/18)
Diez, R. *et al.*, 2010 [69]	0% (0/20)
Biagi, F. *et al.*, 2012 [70]	27.3% (3/11)
Total	9.2% (15/162)

The clinicopathologic response to a GFD has been employed only in few case reports to confirm CD in CVID [72–74], but because of the rarity of the disease, larger prospective blinded studies are lacking, and this limits the use of GFD in this setting. Therefore, further studies involving larger sample sizes are warranted in this field.

2.3. Selective IgM Deficiency

Selective IgM deficiency (sIgMD) is a very rare disorder, defined by low levels of IgM—<0.40 g/L according to current guidelines [75]—in the absence of alterations of other immunoglobulin classes. In adults, the prevalence is about 1:15,000 [76].

sIgMD causes a severe alteration in maturation and function of B lymphocytes. Defects in B cell differentiation into IgM-immunoglobulin secreting cells, a reduced number of IgM-secreting B cells with a failure of secreted Igμ chain mRNA synthesis and decreased antigen proliferation IgM responses have been observed [76–81]. Confirming these alterations, Cipe *et al.* [82] found that patients with sIgMD have low levels of non-switched memory B cells.

Clinical manifestations of sIgMD include recurrent viral and bacterial infections resulting in periodic infectious dermatitis, diarrhea, meningitis, upper and lower respiratory infections and sepsis [83]. Autoimmune disorders such as hemolytic anemia, thyroiditis, rheumatoid arthritis systemic lupus erithematosus and CD have been described [83].

Gastrointestinal manifestations occur in 15.7% of patients with sIgMD, and some reports have found an association between these two disorders [84,85]. Interestingly, IgM levels returned to normal levels in most pediatric and adult patients observing a GFD. In this respect, we described the case of a sIgMD patient with SNCD [86]. The 18-year-old patient complained about abdominal pain, diarrhea and weight loss and showed villous atrophy with diffuse immature lymphocytes at duodenal biopsy, despite negative anti-tTG. However, tissue transglutaminase mRNA mucosal levels exhibited a six-fold increase. The patient was assigned to GFD and six months later the symptoms had disappeared, the villous architecture was restored and mucosal tissue transglutaminase mRNA was comparable to that of healthy subjects. A similar result (normalization of increased mucosal tissue transglutaminase mRNA) was obtained by our group in a subset of suspected SNCD patients in an ongoing study. Surprisingly, after one year of GFD, a complete restoration of normal IgM levels was seen. Moreover, we observed that the GFD caused a maturation of lymphocytes. Indeed, the mucosa was populated by numerous lymphocytes before the GFD that turned into plasma cells after starting the diet, thus explaining the increase in IgM levels.

Such secondary forms of sIgMD, occurring concomitantly to CD, could be linked to a decreased immunoglobulin synthesis by a dysfunctional lymphoreticular tissue stimulated by gluten antigen exposure [85,87].

3. Conclusive Remarks

The ID universe is a fascinating field in immunology due to the wide variety of clinical and autoimmune features. Gastrointestinal involvement is common and often resembles primary digestive disorders such as CD. Additionally, the lack of immunoglobulin production often accounts for the absence of serological markers of CD. For this reason, ID could mask CD, and the frequent association between CD and ID is a diagnostic challenge for the clinician, the endoscopist and the pathologist. Apart from gluten-related disorders, indeed, a condition of villous atrophy or duodenal lymphocytosis may be linked to other disorders such as alimentary atopy, inflammatory bowel disease, parasitic or viral infections and drugs such as olmesartan [22,88–90], all conditions demanding differential diagnosis, for which a diagnostic algorithm has been proposed [12]. In Table 4, we summarize the main causes of duodenal lymphocytosis and villous atrophy.

Table 4. Main causes of duodenal lymphocytosis and villous atrophy, classified according to etiological criteria.

Gluten-related	Infectious Causes	Immunological	Drugs	Other
Celiac disease	Virus (Rotavirus, Enterovirus, Adenovirus, Coronavirus)	Immunoglobulin deficiencies	Olmesartan	
Gluten sensitivity	Parasites (*Giardia*)	Food allergy	Non steroidal anti-inflammatory drugs	
Seronegative celiac disease	Bacteria (*Salmonella, Shigella*)	Autoimmune enteritis		
Wheat allergy	Small intestinal bacterial overgrowth	Vasculitides		Irritable bowel syndrome
	Helicobacter pylori	Systemic autoimmune disorders		
		Inflammatory bowel disease		
		Microscopic enteritis		

For these reasons, novel endoscopic advances have been proposed to improve the detection of CD, notably the water-immersion technique and virtual chromoendoscopy [91–94]. It is known that immunohistochemical analysis of T-cell receptor $\gamma\delta$ (TCR$\gamma\delta$) [95] may be effective in discriminating CD from other causes of duodenal lymphocytosis [96–99], especially considering that an increase in IELs may be found even in non-CD conditions [100]. In this regard, Fernández-Bañares *et al.* [101] demonstrated that cytometric analysis of $\gamma\delta$ T-cells in the duodenal mucosa displayed a specificity of 100%, much better than the 87% achieved with anti-TG2 IgA subepithelial deposit analysis. The detection of anti-tTG in the supernatant of cultured enterocytes taken from patients with SNCD has recently been proposed, and has proven to be more effective than serology. Tosco *et al.* [102] found that the measurement of antibodies secreted into culture supernatants has a higher sensitivity and specificity (97.5% and 92.3%, respectively) than the detection of mucosal deposits (77.5% and 80.0%, respectively). Moreover, in a group of 559 CD patients, Picarelli *et al.* [103] showed that anti-tTG and EMA detection in enterocyte culture improved the sensitivity and specificity by about 10% compared to traditional serology. Therefore, we highlight that analysis of the gamma-delta IELs subpopulation yields interesting results in the discrimination between gluten- and non-gluten-related enteropathies [95]. Finally, in our experience [104], tTG-mRNA was similarly increased in seropositive CD and suspected SNCD, and strongly correlated with the IEL count. This increase was found even in the IEL range of 15–25/100 enterocytes, suggesting that there may be a "grey zone" of gluten-related disorders, and that this technique could be helpful in diagnosing doubtful SNCD cases.

Finally, the genetic analysis of the HLA genes has been proposed to support the diagnosis of CD in ID. CD is known to be associated with DQ2 and DQ8 haplotypes. These haplotypes are very common in the general population, with a mean prevalence of 20%, although only a minority would develop CD [105,106]. Due to this, the analysis of HLA haplotypes is recommended [107]. The role of HLA haplotypes may also be a potential tool to recognize CD in patients with ID. Some studies confirmed that a DQ2/DQ8 positivity may be very helpful in doubtful cases [67]. Rare alleles, such as DQ A1*05, have been proven to be linked to some cases of CD (even with seronegativity) [100], but they have not been investigated in patients with ID. However, despite many attempts, a reliable tool for CD detection in ID has not yet been found. Currently, a careful histological analysis by a trained pathologist and a correct clinical study (including the response to a GFD, in particular) are the only available tools. Novel strategies, based on molecular analysis, could offer a "turning point" in this setting [12].

Acknowledgments: We would like to acknowledge Mary Pragnell for linguistic review.

Author Contributions: Alfredo Di Leo and Enzo Ierardi conceived the study. Annacinzia Amoruso, Giuseppe Losurdo, Domenico Piscitelli, Floriana Giorgio, Andrea Iannone and Michele Barone collected the data. Enzo Ierardi, Giuseppe Losurdo and Mariabeatrice Principi wrote the manuscript. All authors read and approved the final version of the manuscript.

Conflicts of Interest: The authors declare no conflict of interest.

References

1. Fasano, A.; Berti, I.; Gerarduzzi, T.; Not, T.; Colletti, R.B.; Drago, S.; Elitsur, Y.; Green, P.H.; Guandalini, S.; Hill, I.D.; *et al.* Prevalence of celiac disease in at-risk and not-at-risk groups in the United States: A large multicenter study. *Arch. Intern. Med.* **2003**, *163*, 286–292. [CrossRef] [PubMed]
2. Italian Celiac Disease Association. Available online: http://www.celiachia.it/AIC/AIC.aspx?SS=351 (accessed on 1 July 2015).
3. Ludvigsson, J.F.; Leffler, D.A.; Bai, J.C.; Biagi, F.; Fasano, A.; Green, P.H.; Hadjivassiliou, M.; Kaukinen, K.; Kelly, C.P.; Leonard, J.N.; *et al.* The Oslo definitions for coeliac disease and related terms. *Gut* **2013**, *62*, 43–52. [CrossRef] [PubMed]
4. Rostami Nejad, M.; Rostami, K.; Pourhoseingholi, M.A.; Nazemalhosseini Mojarad, E.; Habibi, M.; Dabiri, H.; Zali, M.R. Atypical presentation is dominant and typical for coeliac disease. *J. Gastrointestin. Liver Dis.* **2009**, *18*, 285–291. [PubMed]
5. Gasbarrini, G.; Miele, L.; Malandrino, N.; Grieco, A.; Addolorato, G.; Gasbarrini, A.; Gammarota, G.; Bonvicini, F. Celiac disease in the 21st century: Issues of under- and over-diagnosis. *Int. J. Immunopathol. Pharmacol.* **2009**, *22*, 1–7. [PubMed]
6. Moayyedi, P.; O'Mahony, S.; Jackson, P.; Lynch, D.A.; Dixon, M.F.; Axon, A.T. Small intestine in lymphocytic and collagenous colitis: Mucosal morphology, permeability, and secretory immunity to gliadin. *J. Clin. Pathol.* **1997**, *50*, 527–529. [CrossRef] [PubMed]
7. Matysiak-Budnik, T.; Malamut, G.; de Serre, N.P.; Grosdidier, E.; Seguier, S.; Brousse, N.; Caillat-Zucman, S.; Cerf-Bensussan, N.; Schmitz, J.; Cellier, C. Long-term follow-up of 61 coeliac patients diagnosed in childhood: Evolution toward latency is possible on a normal diet. *Gut* **2007**, *56*, 1379–1386. [CrossRef] [PubMed]
8. Ferguson, A.; Arranz, E.; O'Mahony, S. Clinical and pathological spectrum of celiac disease—Active, silent, latent, potential. *Gut* **1993**, *34*, 150–151. [CrossRef] [PubMed]
9. Biagi, F.; Trotta, L.; Alfano, C.; Balduzzi, D.; Staffieri, V.; Bianchi, P.I.; Marchese, A.; Vattiato, C.; Zilli, A.; Luinetti, O.; *et al.* Prevalence and natural history of potential celiac disease in adult patients. *Scand. J. Gastroenterol.* **2013**, *48*, 537–542. [CrossRef] [PubMed]
10. Lionetti, E.; Castellaneta, S.; Pulvirenti, A.; Tonutti, E.; Francavilla, R.; Fasano, A.; Catassi, C.; Italian Working Group of Weaning and Celiac Disease Risk. Prevalence and natural history of potential celiac disease in at-family-risk infants prospectively investigated from birth. *J. Pediatr.* **2012**, *161*, 908–914. [CrossRef] [PubMed]
11. Auricchio, R.; Tosco, A.; Piccolo, E.; Galatola, M.; Izzo, V.; Maglio, M.; Paparo, F.; Troncone, R.; Greco, L. Potential celiac children: 9-Year follow-up on a gluten-containing diet. *Am. J. Gastroenterol.* **2014**, *109*, 913–921. [CrossRef] [PubMed]
12. Ierardi, E.; Losurdo, G.; Piscitelli, D.; Giorgio, F.; Sorrentino, C.; Principi, M.; Montenegro, L.; Amoruso, A.; Di Leo, A. Seronegative celiac disease: Where is the specific setting? *Gastroenterol. Hepatol. Bed Bench* **2015**, *8*, 110–116. [PubMed]
13. Abrams, J.A.; Diamond, B.; Rotterdam, H.; Green, P.H. Seronegative celiac disease: Increased prevalence with lesser degrees of villous atrophy. *Dig. Dis. Sci.* **2004**, *49*, 546–550. [CrossRef] [PubMed]
14. Tursi, A.; Brandimarte, G.; Giorgetti, G.M. Prevalence of antitissue transglutaminase antibodies in different degrees of intestinal damage in celiac disease. *J. Clin. Gastroenterol.* **2003**, *36*, 219–221. [CrossRef] [PubMed]
15. Tursi, A.; Brandimarte, G. The symptomatic and histologic response to a gluten-free diet in patients with borderline enteropathy. *J. Clin. Gastroenterol.* **2003**, *36*, 13–17. [CrossRef] [PubMed]
16. Dickey, W.; Hughes, D.F.; McMillan, S.A. Reliance on serum endomysial antibody testing underestimates the true prevalence of coeliac disease by one fifth. *Scand. J. Gastroenterol.* **2000**, *35*, 181–183. [PubMed]

17. Tursi, A.; Brandimarte, G.; Giorgetti, G.; Gigliobianco, A.; Lombardi, D.; Gasbarrini, G. Low prevalence of antigliadin and anti-endomysium antibodies in subclinical/silent celiac disease. *Am. J. Gastroenterol.* **2001**, *96*, 1507–1510. [CrossRef] [PubMed]

18. Rostami, K.; Kerckhaert, J.; Tiemessen, R.; von Blomberg, B.M.; Meijer, J.W.; Mulder, C.J. Sensitivity of antiendomysium and antigliadin antibodies in untreated celiac disease: Disappointing in clinical practice. *Am. J. Gastroenterol.* **1999**, *94*, 888–894. [CrossRef] [PubMed]

19. Kurppa, K.; Ashorn, M.; Iltanen, S.; Koskinen, L.L.; Saavalainen, P.; Koskinen, O.; Mäki, M.; Kaukinen, K. Celiac disease without villous atrophy in children: A prospective study. *J. Pediatr.* **2010**, *157*, 373–380. [CrossRef] [PubMed]

20. Salmi, T.T.; Collin, P.; Korponay-Szabó, I.R.; Laurila, K.; Partanen, J.; Huhtala, H.; Király, R.; Lorand, L.; Reunala, T.; Mäki, M.; *et al.* Endomysial antibody-negative coeliac disease: Clinical characteristics and intestinal autoantibody deposits. *Gut* **2006**, *55*, 1746–1753. [CrossRef] [PubMed]

21. Makovicky, P.; Rimarova, K.; Boor, A.; Makovicky, P.; Vodicka, P.; Samasca, G.; Kruzliak, P. Correlation between antibodies and histology in celiac disease: Incidence of celiac disease is higher than expected in the pediatric population. *Mol. Med. Rep.* **2013**, *8*, 1079–1083. [CrossRef] [PubMed]

22. DeGaetani, M.; Tennyson, C.A.; Lebwohl, B.; Lewis, S.K.; Abu Daya, H.; Arguelles-Grande, C.; Bhagat, G.; Green, P.H. Villous atrophy and negative celiac serology: A diagnostic and therapeutic dilemma. *Am. J. Gastroenterol.* **2013**, *108*, 647–653. [CrossRef] [PubMed]

23. Gatti, S.; Rossi, M.; Alfonsi, S.; Mandolesi, A.; Cobellis, G.; Catassi, C. Beyond the intestinal celiac mucosa: Diagnostic role of anti-TG2 deposits, a systematic review. *Front. Med. (Lausanne)* **2014**, *1*. [CrossRef] [PubMed]

24. Korponay-Szabó, I.R.; Halttunen, T.; Szalai, Z.; Laurila, K.; Király, R.; Kovács, J.B.; Fésüs, L.; Mäki, M. *In vivo* targeting of intestinal and extraintestinal transglutaminase 2 by coeliac autoantibodies. *Gut* **2004**, *53*, 641–648. [CrossRef] [PubMed]

25. Tosco, A.; Salvati, V.M.; Auricchio, R.; Maglio, M.; Borrelli, M.; Coruzzo, A.; Paparo, F.; Boffardi, M.; Esposito, A.; D'Adamo, G.; *et al.* Natural history of potential celiac disease in children. *Clin. Gastroenterol. Hepatol.* **2011**, *9*, 320–325. [CrossRef] [PubMed]

26. Salmi, T.T.; Collin, P.; Jarvinen, O.; Haimila, K.; Partanen, J.; Laurila, K.; Korponay-Szabo, I.R.; Huhtala, H.; Reunala, T.; Mäki, M.; *et al.* Immunoglobulin A autoantibodies against transglutaminase 2 in the small intestinal mucosa predict forthcoming coeliac disease. *Aliment. Pharmacol. Ther.* **2006**, *24*, 541–552. [CrossRef] [PubMed]

27. Maglio, M.; Tosco, A.; Auricchio, R.; Paparo, F.; Colicchio, B.; Miele, E.; Rapacciuolo, L.; Troncone, R. Intestinal deposits of anti-tissue transglutaminase IgA in childhood celiac disease. *Dig. Liver Dis.* **2011**, *43*, 604–608. [CrossRef] [PubMed]

28. Tosco, A.; Aitoro, R.; Auricchio, R.; Ponticelli, D.; Miele, E.; Paparo, F.; Greco, L.; Troncone, R.; Maglio, M. Intestinal anti-tissue transglutaminase antibodies in potential coeliac disease. *Clin. Exp. Immunol.* **2013**, *171*, 69–75. [CrossRef] [PubMed]

29. Tosco, A.; Maglio, M.; Paparo, F.; Rapacciuolo, L.; Sannino, A.; Miele, E.; Barone, M.V.; Auricchio, R.; Troncone, R. Immunoglobulin A anti-tissue transglutaminase antibody deposits in the small intestinal mucosa of children with no villous atrophy. *J. Pediatr. Gastroenterol. Nutr.* **2008**, *47*, 293–298. [CrossRef] [PubMed]

30. Kaukinen, K.; Peräaho, M.; Collin, P.; Partanen, J.; Woolley, N.; Kaartinen, T.; Nuutinen, T.; Halttunen, T.; Mäki, M.; Korponay-Szabo, I. Small-bowel mucosal transglutaminase 2-specific IgA deposits in coeliac disease without villous atrophy: A prospective and randomized clinical study. *Scand. J. Gastroenterol.* **2005**, *40*, 564–572. [CrossRef] [PubMed]

31. Agarwal, S.; Mayer, L. Diagnosis and treatment of gastrointestinal disorders in patients with primary immunodeficiency. *Clin. Gastroenterol. Hepatol.* **2013**, *11*, 1050–1063. [CrossRef] [PubMed]

32. International Union of Immunological Societies Expert Committee on Primary Immunodeficiencies; Notarangelo, L.D.; Fischer, A.; Geha, R.S.; Casanova, J.L.; Chapel, H.; Conley, M.E.; Cunningham-Rundles, C.; Etzioni, A.; Hammartröm, L.; *et al.* Primary immunodeficiencies: 2009 Update. *J. Allergy Clin. Immunol.* **2009**, *124*, 1161–1178. [CrossRef] [PubMed]

33. Conley, M.E.; Cooper, M.D. Immature IgA B cells in IgA-deficient patients. *N. Engl. J. Med.* **1981**, *305*, 495–497. [CrossRef] [PubMed]

34. Brandtzaeg, P. Update on mucosal immunoglobulin A in gastrointestinal disease. *Curr. Opin. Gastroenterol.* **2010**, *26*, 554–563. [CrossRef] [PubMed]

35. Cunningham-Rundles, C.; Fotino, M.; Rosina, O.; Peter, J.B. Selective IgA deficiency, IgG subclass deficiency, and the major histocompatibility complex. *Clin. Immunol. Immunopathol.* **1991**, *61*, S61–S69. [CrossRef]

36. Olerup, O.; Smith, C.I.; Hammarström, L. Different amino acids at position 57 of the HLA-DQ beta chain associated with susceptibility and resistance to IgA deficiency. *Nature* **1990**, *347*, 289–290. [CrossRef] [PubMed]

37. Mohammadi, J.; Ramanujam, R.; Jarefors, S.; Rezaei, N.; Aghamohammadi, A.; Gregersen, P.K.; Hammarström, L. IgA deficiency and the MHC: Assessment of relative risk and microheterogeneity within the HLA A1 B8, DR3 (8.1) haplotype. *J. Clin. Immunol.* **2010**, *30*, 138–143. [CrossRef] [PubMed]

38. Bienvenu, F.; Anghel, S.I.; Besson Duvanel, C.; Guillemaud, J.; Garnier, L.; Renosi, F.; Lachaux, A.; Bienvenu, J. Early diagnosis of celiac disease in IgA deficient children: Contribution of a point-of-care test. *BMC Gastroenterol.* **2014**, *14*, 186. [CrossRef] [PubMed]

39. Wang, N.; Truedsson, L.; Elvin, K.; Andersson, B.A.; Rönnelid, J.; Mincheva-Nilsson, L.; Lindkvist, A.; Ludvigsson, J.F.; Hammarström, L.; Dahle, C. Serological assessment for celiac disease in IgA deficient adults. *PLoS ONE* **2014**, *9*, e93180. [CrossRef] [PubMed]

40. Ludvigsson, J.F.; Neovius, M.; Hammarström, L. Association between IgA deficiency and other autoimmune conditions: A population-based matched cohort study. *J. Clin. Immunol.* **2014**, *34*, 444–451. [CrossRef] [PubMed]

41. Pituch-Noworolska, A.; Błaut-Szlósarczyk, A.; Zwonarz, K. Occurrence of autoantibodies for gastrointestinal autoimmune diseases in children with common variable immune deficiency and selected IgA deficiency. *Prz. Gastroenterol.* **2013**, *8*, 370–376. [CrossRef] [PubMed]

42. Lenhardt, A.; Plebani, A.; Marchetti, F.; Gerarduzzi, T.; Not, T.; Meini, A.; Villanacci, V.; Martelossi, S.; Ventura, A. Role of human-tissue transglutaminase IgG and anti-gliadin IgG antibodies in the diagnosis of coeliac disease in patients with selective immunoglobulin A deficiency. *Dig. Liver Dis.* **2004**, *36*, 730–734. [CrossRef] [PubMed]

43. Korponay-Szabó, I.R.; Dahlbom, I.; Laurila, K.; Koskinen, S.; Woolley, N.; Partanen, J.; Kovács, J.B.; Mäki, M.; Hansson, T. Elevation of IgG antibodies against tissue transglutaminase as a diagnostic tool for coeliac disease in selective IgA deficiency. *Gut* **2003**, *52*, 1567–1571. [CrossRef] [PubMed]

44. Wang, N.; Shen, N.; Vyse, T.J.; Anand, V.; Gunnarson, I.; Sturfelt, G.; Rantapää-Dahlqvist, S.; Elvin, K.; Truedsson, L.; Andersson, B.A.; *et al.* Selective IgA deficiency in autoimmune diseases. *Mol. Med.* **2011**, *17*, 1383–1396. [CrossRef] [PubMed]

45. Villalta, D.; Tonutti, E.; Prause, C.; Koletzko, S.; Uhlig, H.H.; Vermeersch, P.; Bossuyt, X.; Stern, M.; Laass, M.W.; Ellis, J.H.; *et al.* IgG antibodies against deamidated gliadin peptides for diagnosis of celiac disease in patients with IgA deficiency. *Clin. Chem.* **2010**, *56*, 464–468. [CrossRef] [PubMed]

46. Villalta, D.; Alessio, M.G.; Tampoia, M.; Tonutti, E.; Brusca, I.; Bagnasco, M.; Pesce, G.; Bizzaro, N. Diagnostic accuracy of IgA anti-tissue transglutaminase antibody assays in celiac disease patients with selective IgA deficiency. *Ann. N. Y. Acad. Sci.* **2007**, *1109*, 212–220. [CrossRef] [PubMed]

47. Eren, M.; Saltik-Temizel, I.N.; Yüce, A.; Cağlar, M.; Koçak, N. Duodenal appearance of giardiasis in a child with selective immunoglobulin A deficiency. *Pediatr. Int.* **2007**, *49*, 409–411. [CrossRef] [PubMed]

48. Klemola, T. Immunohistochemical findings in the intestine of IgA-deficient persons: Number of intraepithelial T lymphocytes is increased. *J. Pediatr. Gastroenterol. Nutr.* **1988**, *7*, 537–543. [CrossRef] [PubMed]

49. Valletta, E.; Fornaro, M.; Pecori, S.; Zanoni, G. Selective immunoglobulin A deficiency and celiac disease: Let's give serology a chance. *J. Investig. Allergol. Clin. Immunol.* **2011**, *21*, 242–244. [PubMed]

50. Cataldo, F.; Marino, V.; Ventura, A.; Bottaro, G.; Corazza, G.R. Prevalence and clinical features of selective immunoglobulin A deficiency in coeliac disease: An Italian multicentre study. Italian Society of Paediatric Gastroenterology and Hepatology (SIGEP) and "Club del Tenue" Working Groups on Coeliac Disease. *Gut* **1998**, *42*, 362–365. [CrossRef] [PubMed]

51. Borrelli, M.; Maglio, M.; Agnese, M.; Paparo, F.; Gentile, S.; Colicchio, B.; Tosco, A.; Auricchio, R.; Troncone, R. High density of intraepithelial gammadelta lymphocytes and deposits of immunoglobulin (Ig)M anti-tissue transglutaminase antibodies in the jejunum of coeliac patients with IgA deficiency. *Clin. Exp. Immunol.* **2010**, *160*, 199–206. [CrossRef] [PubMed]

52. Fabris, M.; De Vita, S.; Visentini, D.; Fabro, C.; Picierno, A.; Lerussi, A.; Villalta, D.; Alessio, M.G.; Tampoia, M.; Tonutti, E. B-lymphocyte stimulator and a proliferation-inducing ligand serum levels in IgA-deficient patients with and without celiac disease. *Ann. N. Y. Acad. Sci.* **2009**, *1173*, 268–273. [CrossRef] [PubMed]

53. Cataldo, F.; Lio, D.; Marino, V.; Scola, L.; Crivello, A.; Corazza, G.R. Plasma cytokine profiles in patients with celiac disease and selective IgA deficiency. *Pediatr. Allergy Immunol.* **2003**, *14*, 320–324. [CrossRef] [PubMed]

54. Abolhassani, H.; Sagvand, B.T.; Shokuhfar, T.; Mirminachi, B.; Rezaei, N.; Aghamohammadi, A. A review on guidelines for management and treatment of common variable immunodeficiency. *Expert. Rev. Clin. Immunol.* **2013**, *9*, 561–574. [CrossRef] [PubMed]

55. Grimbacher, B.; Hutloff, A.; Schlesier, M.; Glocker, E.; Warnatz, K.; Dräger, R.; Eibel, H.; Fischer, B.; Schäffer, A.A.; Mages, H.W.; *et al.* Homozygous loss of ICOS is associated with adult-onset common variable immunodeficiency. *Nat. Immunol.* **2003**, *4*, 261–268. [CrossRef] [PubMed]

56. Vences-Catalán, F.; Kuo, C.C.; Sagi, Y.; Chen, H.; Kela-Madar, N.; van Zelm, M.C.; van Dongen, J.J.; Levy, S. A mutation in the human tetraspanin CD81 gene is expressed as a truncated protein but does not enable CD19 maturation and cell surface expression. *J. Clin. Immunol.* **2015**, *35*, 254–263. [CrossRef] [PubMed]

57. Lougaris, V.; Gallizzi, R.; Vitali, M.; Baronio, M.; Salpietro, A.; Bergbreiter, A.; Salzer, U.; Badolato, R.; Plebani, A. A novel compound heterozygous TACI mutation in an autosomal recessive common variable immunodeficiency (CVID) family. *Hum. Immunol.* **2012**, *73*, 836–839. [CrossRef] [PubMed]

58. Van de Ven, A.A.; Compeer, E.B.; Bloem, A.C.; van de Corput, L.; van Gijn, M.; van Montfrans, J.M.; Boes, M. Defective calcium signaling and disrupted CD20-B-cell receptor dissociation in patients with common variable immunodeficiency disorders. *J. Allergy Clin. Immunol.* **2012**, *129*, 755–761. [CrossRef] [PubMed]

59. Kralovicova, J.; Hammarström, L.; Plebani, A.; Webster, A.D.; Vorechovsky, I. Fine-scale mapping at IGAD1 and genome-wide genetic linkage analysis implicate HLA-DQ/DR as a major susceptibility locus in selective IgA deficiency and common variable immunodeficiency. *J. Immunol.* **2003**, *170*, 2765–2775. [CrossRef] [PubMed]

60. Viallard, J.F.; Blanco, P.; André, M.; Etienne, G.; Liferman, F.; Neau, D.; Vidal, E.; Moreau, J.F.; Pellegrin, J.L. CD8+HLA-DR+ T lymphocytes are increased in common variable immunodeficiency patients with impaired memory B-cell differentiation. *Clin. Immunol.* **2006**, *119*, 51–58. [CrossRef] [PubMed]

61. Cunningham-Rundles, C. Autoimmune manifestations in common variable immunodeficiency. *J. Clin. Immunol.* **2008**, *28* (Suppl. S1), S42–S45. [CrossRef] [PubMed]

62. Lougaris, V.; Ravelli, A.; Villanacci, V.; Salemme, M.; Soresina, A.; Fuoti, M.; Lanzarotto, F.; Lanzini, A.; Plebani, A.; Bassotti, G. Gastrointestinal Pathologic Abnormalities in Pediatric- and Adult-Onset Common Variable Immunodeficiency. *Dig. Dis. Sci.* **2015**, *60*, 2384–2389. [CrossRef] [PubMed]

63. Malamut, G.; Verkarre, V.; Suarez, F.; Viallard, J.F.; Lascaux, A.S.; Cosnes, J.; Bouhnik, Y.; Lambotte, O.; Béchade, D.; Ziol, M.; *et al.* The enteropathy associated with common variable immunodeficiency: The delineated frontiers with celiac disease. *Am. J. Gastroenterol.* **2010**, *105*, 2262–2275. [CrossRef] [PubMed]

64. Luzi, G.; Zullo, A.; Iebba, F.; Finaldi, V.; Sanchez Mete, L.; Muscaritoli, M.; Aiuti, F. Duodenal pathology and clinical-immunological implications in common variable immunodeficiency patients. *Am. J. Gastroenterol.* **2003**, *98*, 118–121. [CrossRef] [PubMed]

65. Haimila, K.; Einarsdottir, E.; de Kauwe, A.; Koskinen, L.L.; Pan-Hammarström, Q.; Kaartinen, T.; Kurppa, K.; Ziberna, F.; Not, T.; Vatta, S.; *et al.* The shared CTLA4-ICOS risk locus in celiac disease, IgA deficiency and common variable immunodeficiency. *Genes Immun.* **2009**, *10*, 151–161. [CrossRef] [PubMed]

66. Licinio, R.; Principi, M.; Amoruso, A.; Piscitelli, D.; Ierardi, E.; Di Leo, A. Celiac disease and common variable immunodeficiency: A familial inheritance? *J. Gastrointestin. Liver Dis.* **2013**, *22*, 473. [PubMed]

67. Venhoff, N.; Emmerich, F.; Neagu, M.; Salzer, U.; Koehn, C.; Driever, S.; Kreisel, W.; Rizzi, M.; Effelsberg, N.M.; Kollert, F.; *et al.* The role of HLA DQ2 and DQ8 in dissecting celiac-like disease in common variable immunodeficiency. *J. Clin. Immunol.* **2013**, *33*, 909–916. [CrossRef] [PubMed]

68. Rodríguez-Negrete, E.V.; Mayoral-Zavala, A.; Rodríguez-Mireles, K.A.; Díaz de León-Salazar, O.E.; Hernández-Mondragón, O.; Gómez-Jiménez, L.M.; Moreno-Alcántar, R.; González-Virla, B. Prevalence of gastrointestinal disorders in adults with common variable immunodeficiency at Specialty Hospital Dr. Bernardo Sepulveda. *Rev. Alerg. Mex.* **2015**, *62*, 1–7. (In Spanish) [PubMed]

69. Díez, R.; García, M.J.; Vivas, S.; Arias, L.; Rascarachi, G.; Pozo, E.D.; Vaquero, L.M.; Miguel, A.; Sierra, M.; Calleja, S.; *et al.* Gastrointestinal manifestations in patients with primary immunodeficiencies causing antibody deficiency. *Gastroenterol. Hepatol.* **2010**, *33*, 347–351. (In Spanish) [CrossRef] [PubMed]

70. Biagi, F.; Bianchi, P.I.; Zilli, A.; Marchese, A.; Luinetti, O.; Lougaris, V.; Plebani, A.; Villanacci, V.; Corazza, G.R. The significance of duodenal mucosal atrophy in patients with common variable immunodeficiency: A clinical and histopathologic study. *Am. J. Clin. Pathol.* **2012**, *138*, 185–189. [CrossRef] [PubMed]

71. Daniels, J.A.; Lederman, H.M.; Maitra, A.; Montgomery, E.A. Gastrointestinal tract pathology in patients with common variable immunodeficiency (CVID): A clinicopathologic study and review. *Am. J. Surg. Pathol.* **2007**, *31*, 1800–1812. [CrossRef] [PubMed]

72. Cecinato, P.; Fuccio, L.; Sabattini, E.; Laterza, L.; Caponi, A.; Azzaroli, F.; Mazzella, G. An unusual cause of weight loss in a young Caucasian man. Common variable immunodeficiency (CVI) associated with diffuse enteral nodular lymphoid hyperplasia (NLH) and CD. *Gut* **2014**, *63*, 856–859. [CrossRef] [PubMed]

73. Béchade, D.; Desramé, J.; De Fuentès, G.; Camparo, P.; Raynaud, J.J.; Algayres, J.P. Common variable immunodeficiency and celiac disease. *Gastroenterol. Clin. Biol.* **2004**, *28*, 909–912. (In French) [CrossRef]

74. Bili, H.; Nizou, C.; Nizou, J.Y.; Coutant, G.; Schmoor, P.; Algayres, J.P.; Daly, J.P. Common variable immunodeficiency and total villous atrophy regressive after gluten-free diet. *Rev. Med. Interne* **1997**, *18*, 724–726. (In French) [CrossRef]

75. Dati, F.; Schumann, G.; Thomas, L.; Aguzzi, F.; Baudner, S.; Bienvenu, J.; Blaabjerg, O.; Blirup-Jensen, S.; Carlström, A.; Petersen, P.H.; *et al.* Consensus of a group of professional societies and diagnostic companies on guidelines for interim reference ranges for 14 proteins in serum based on the standardization against the IFCC/BCR/CAP Reference Material (CRM 470). International Federation of Clinical Chemistry. Community Bureau of Reference of the Commission of the European Communities. College of American Pathologists. *Eur. J. Clin. Chem. Clin. Biochem.* **1996**, *34*, 517–520. [PubMed]

76. Ohno, T.; Inaba, M.; Kuribayashi, K.; Masuda, T.; Kanoh, T.; Uchino, H. Selective IgM deficiency in adults: Phenotypically and functionally altered profiles of peripheral blood lymphocytes. *Clin. Exp. Immunol.* **1987**, *68*, 630–637. [PubMed]

77. Inoue, T.; Okumura, Y.; Shirama, M.; Ishibashi, H.; Kashiwagi, S.; Okubo, H. Selective partial IgM deficiency: Functional assessment of T and B lymphocytes *in vitro*. *J. Clin. Immunol.* **1986**, *6*, 130–135. [CrossRef] [PubMed]

78. Kimura, S.; Tanigawa, M.; Nakahashi, Y.; Inoue, M.; Yamamura, Y.; Kato, H.; Sugino, S.; Kondo, M. Selective IgM deficiency in a patient with Hashimoto's disease. *Intern. Med.* **1993**, *32*, 302–307. [CrossRef] [PubMed]

79. Karsh, J.; Watts, C.S.; Osterland, C.K. Selective immunoglobulin M deficiency in an adult: Assessment of immunoglobulin production by peripheral blood lymphocytes *in vitro*. *Clin. Immunol. Immunopathol.* **1982**, *25*, 386–394. [CrossRef]

80. Kondo, N.; Ozawa, T.; Kato, Y.; Motoyoshi, F.; Kasahara, K.; Kameyama, T.; Orii, T. Reduced secreted μ mRNA synthesis in selective IgM deficiency of Bloom's syndrome. *Clin. Exp. Immunol.* **1992**, *88*, 35–40. [CrossRef] [PubMed]

81. Yamasaki, T. Selective IgM deficiency: Functional assessment of peripheral blood lymphocytes *in vitro*. *Intern. Med.* **1992**, *31*, 866–870. [CrossRef] [PubMed]

82. Cipe, F.E.; Doğu, F.; Güloğlu, D.; Aytekin, C.; Plat, M.; Biyikli, Z.; Ikincioğullari, A. B-cell subsets in patients with transient hypogammaglobulinemia of infancy, partial IgA deficiency, and selective IgM deficiency. *J. Investig. Allergol. Clin. Immunol.* **2013**, *23*, 94–100. [PubMed]

83. Goldstein, M.F.; Goldstein, A.L.; Dunsky, E.H.; Dvorin, D.J.; Belecanech, G.A.; Shamir, K. Pediatric selective IgM immunodeficiency. *Clin. Dev. Immunol.* **2008**, *2008*, 624850. [CrossRef] [PubMed]

84. Hobbs, J.R.; Hepner, G.W. Deficiency of γM-globulin in coeliac disease. *Lancet* **1968**, *291*, 217–220. [CrossRef]

85. Brown, D.L.; Cooper, A.G.; Hepner, G.W. IgM metabolism in coeliac disease. *Lancet* **1969**, *1*, 858–861. [CrossRef]

86. Montenegro, L.; Piscitelli, D.; Giorgio, F.; Covelli, C.; Fiore, M.G.; Losurdo, G.; Iannone, A.; Ierardi, E.; Di Leo, A.; Principi, M. Reversal of IgM deficiency following a gluten-free diet in seronegative celiac disease. *World J. Gastroenterol.* **2014**, *20*, 17686–17689. [CrossRef] [PubMed]

87. Blecher, T.E.; Brzechwa-Ajdukiewicz, A.; McCarthy, C.F.; Read, A.E. Serum immunoglobulins and lymphocyte transformation studies in coeliac disease. *Gut* **1969**, *10*, 57–62. [CrossRef] [PubMed]

88. Carroccio, A.; D'Alcamo, A.; Mansueto, P. Nonceliac wheat sensitivity in the context of multiple food hypersensitivity: New data from confocal endomicroscopy. *Gastroenterology* **2015**, *148*, 666–667. [CrossRef] [PubMed]

89. Koot, B.G.; Ten Kate, F.J.; Juffrie, M.; Rosalina, I.; Taminiau, J.J.; Benninga, M.A. Does *Giardia lamblia* cause villous atrophy in children: A retrospective cohort study of the histological abnormalities in giardiasis. *J. Pediatr. Gastroenterol. Nutr.* **2009**, *49*, 304–308. [CrossRef] [PubMed]

90. Ianiro, G.; Bibbò, S.; Montalto, M.; Ricci, R.; Gasbarrini, A.; Cammarota, G. Systematic review: Sprue-like enteropathy associated with olmesartan. *Aliment. Pharmacol. Ther.* **2014**, *40*, 16–23. [CrossRef] [PubMed]

91. Ianiro, G.; Gasbarrini, A.; Cammarota, G. Endoscopic tools for the diagnosis and evaluation of celiac disease. *World J. Gastroenterol.* **2013**, *19*, 8562–8570. [CrossRef] [PubMed]

92. Cammarota, G.; Ianiro, G.; Sparano, L.; La Mura, R.; Ricci, R.; Larocca, L.M.; Landolfi, R.; Gasbarrini, A. Image-enhanced endoscopy with I-scan technology for the evaluation of duodenal villous patterns. *Dig. Dis. Sci.* **2013**, *58*, 1287–1292. [CrossRef] [PubMed]

93. Cammarota, G.; Cazzato, A.; Genovese, O.; Pantanella, A.; Ianiro, G.; Giorgio, V.; Montalto, M.; Vecchio, F.M.; Larocca, L.M.; Gasbarrini, G.; *et al.* Water-immersion technique during standard upper endoscopy may be useful to drive the biopsy sampling of duodenal mucosa in children with celiac disease. *J. Pediatr. Gastroenterol. Nutr.* **2009**, *49*, 411–416. [CrossRef] [PubMed]

94. Singh, R.; Nind, G.; Tucker, G.; Nguyen, N.; Holloway, R.; Bate, J.; Shetti, M.; George, B.; Tam, W. Narrow-band imaging in the evaluation of villous morphology: A feasibility study assessing a simplified classification and observer agreement. *Endoscopy* **2010**, *42*, 889–894. [CrossRef] [PubMed]

95. Lonardi, S.; Villanacci, V.; Lorenzi, L.; Lanzini, A.; Lanzarotto, F.; Carabellese, N.; Volta, U.; Facchetti, F. Anti-TCR gamma antibody in celiac disease: The value of count on formalin-fixed paraffin-embedded biopsies. *Virchows Arch.* **2013**, *463*, 409–413. [CrossRef] [PubMed]

96. Rostami, K.; Aldulaimi, D.; Holmes, G.; Johnson, M.W.; Robert, M.; Srivastava, A.; Fléjou, J.F.; Sanders, D.S.; Volta, U.; Derakhshan, M.H.; *et al.* Microscopic enteritis: Bucharest consensus. *World J. Gastroenterol.* **2015**, *21*, 2593–2604. [CrossRef] [PubMed]

97. Shmidt, E.; Smyrk, T.C.; Faubion, W.A.; Oxentenko, A.S. Duodenal intraepithelial lymphocytosis with normal villous architecture in pediatric patients: Mayo Clinic experience, 2000–2009. *J. Pediatr. Gastroenterol. Nutr.* **2013**, *56*, 51–55. [CrossRef] [PubMed]

98. Aziz, I.; Key, T.; Goodwin, J.G.; Sanders, D.S. Predictors for Celiac Disease in Adult Cases of Duodenal Intraepithelial Lymphocytosis. *J. Clin. Gastroenterol.* **2015**, *49*, 477–482. [CrossRef] [PubMed]

99. Rosinach, M.; Esteve, M.; González, C.; Temiño, R.; Mariné, M.; Monzón, H.; Sainz, E.; Loras, C.; Espinós, J.C.; Forné, M.; *et al.* Lymphocytic duodenosis: Aetiology and long-term response to specific treatment. *Dig. Liver Dis.* **2012**, *44*, 643–648. [CrossRef] [PubMed]

100. Losurdo, G.; Piscitelli, D.; Giangaspero, A.; Principi, M.; Buffelli, F.; Giorgio, F.; Montenegro, L.; Sorrentino, C.; Amoruso, A.; Ierardi, E.; *et al.* Evolution of nonspecific duodenal lymphocytosis over 2 years of follow-up. *World J. Gastroenterol.* **2015**, *21*, 7545–7552. [CrossRef] [PubMed]

101. Fernández-Bañares, F.; Carrasco, A.; García-Puig, R.; Rosinach, M.; González, C.; Alsina, M.; Loras, C.; Salas, A.; Viver, J.M.; Esteve, M. Intestinal intraepithelial lymphocyte cytometric pattern is more accurate than subepithelial deposits of anti-tissue transglutaminase IgA for the diagnosis of celiac disease in lymphocytic enteritis. *PLoS ONE* **2014**, *9*, e101249. [CrossRef] [PubMed]

102. Tosco, A.; Auricchio, R.; Aitoro, R.; Ponticelli, D.; Primario, M.; Miele, E.; Rotondi Aufiero, V.; Discepolo, V.; Greco, L.; Troncone, R.; *et al.* Intestinal titres of anti-tissue transglutaminase 2 antibodies correlate positively with mucosal damage degree and inversely with gluten-free diet duration in coeliac disease. *Clin. Exp. Immunol.* **2014**, *177*, 611–617. [CrossRef] [PubMed]

103. Picarelli, A.; Di Tola, M.; Marino, M.; Libanori, V.; Borghini, R.; Salvi, E.; Donato, G.; Vitolo, D.; Tiberti, A.; Marcheggiano, A.; *et al.* Usefulness of the organ culture system when villous height/crypt depth ratio, intraepithelial lymphocyte count, or serum antibody tests are not diagnostic for celiac disease. *Transl. Res.* **2013**, *161*, 172–180. [CrossRef] [PubMed]

104. Ierardi, E.; Amoruso, A.; Giorgio, F.; Principi, M.; Losurdo, G.; Piscitelli, D.; Buffelli, F.; Fiore, M.G.; Mongelli, A.; Castellaneta, N.M.; *et al.* Mucosal molecular pattern of tissue transglutaminase and interferon gamma in suspected seronegative celiac disease at Marsh 1 and 0 stages. *Saudi J. Gastroenterol.* **2015**, in press.

105. Alarida, K.; Harown, J.; di Pierro, M.R.; Drago, S.; Catassi, C. HLA-DQ2 and -DQ8 genotypes in celiac and healthy Libyan children. *Dig. Liver Dis.* **2010**, *42*, 425–427. [CrossRef] [PubMed]

106. Liu, E.; Lee, H.S.; Aronsson, C.A.; Hagopian, W.A.; Koletzko, S.; Rewers, M.J.; Eisenbarth, G.S.; Bingley, P.J.; Bonifacio, E.; Simell, V.; *et al.* Risk of pediatric celiac disease according to HLA haplotype and country. *N. Engl. J. Med.* **2014**, *371*, 42–49. [CrossRef] [PubMed]
107. Rubio-Tapia, A.; Hill, I.D.; Kelly, C.P.; Calderwood, A.H.; Murray, J.A. ACG clinical guidelines: Diagnosis and management of celiac disease. *Am. J. Gastroenterol.* **2013**, *108*, 656–676. [CrossRef] [PubMed]

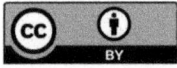

nutrients

Article

Non-Celiac Gluten Sensitivity Has Narrowed the Spectrum of Irritable Bowel Syndrome: A Double-Blind Randomized Placebo-Controlled Trial

Bijan Shahbazkhani [1,2,3], Amirsaeid Sadeghi [1,*], Reza Malekzadeh [2,3], Fatima Khatavi [4], Mehrnoosh Etemadi [4], Ebrahim Kalantri [5], Mohammad Rostami-Nejad [6] and Kamran Rostami [7]

[1] Gastroenterology Unit, Imam Khomeini Hospital, Tehran University of Medical Sciences, Tehran 5715915199, Iran; bijan.shahbaz@gmail.com

[2] Digestive Disease Research Center, Digestive Disease Research Institute, Tehran University of Medical Sciences, Shariati Hospital, Tehran 1599666615, Iran; dr.reza.malekzadeh@gmail.com

[3] Sasan Alborz Biomedical Research Center, Masoud Gastroenterology and Hepatology Clinic, Tehran 14117-13135, Iran

[4] Students' Scientific Research Center, Tehran University of Medical Sciences, Tehran 1449614535, Iran; hototo24@yahoo.com (F.K.); Mehr_etemadi@yahoo.com (M.E.)

[5] Gholhak Medical Laboratory, Tehran 1913913948, Iran; Kalantri@yahoo.com

[6] Gastroenterology and Liver Diseases Research Center, Research Institute for Gastroenterology and Liver Diseases, Shahid Beheshti University of Medical Sciences, Tehran 1985714711, Iran; m.rostamii@gmail.com

[7] Department of Gastroenterology, Alexandra Hospital, Worcestershire B98 7UB, UK; kamran.rostami@nhs.net

* Correspondence: dr.a_sadeghi@yahoo.com; Tel.: +989126156480; Fax: +982166581650

Received: 2 February 2015; Accepted: 26 May 2015; Published: 5 June 2015

Abstract: Several studies have shown that a large number of patients who are fulfilling the criteria for irritable bowel syndrome (IBS) are sensitive to gluten. The aim of this study was to evaluate the effect of a gluten-free diet on gastrointestinal symptoms in patients with IBS. In this double-blind randomized, placebo-controlled trial, 148 IBS patients fulfilling the Rome III criteria were enrolled between 2011 and 2013. However, only 72 out of the 148 commenced on a gluten-free diet for up to six weeks and completed the study; clinical symptoms were recorded biweekly using a standard visual analogue scale (VAS). In the second stage after six weeks, patients whose symptoms improved to an acceptable level were randomly divided into two groups; patients either received packages containing powdered gluten (35 cases) or patients received placebo (gluten free powder) (37 cases). Overall, the symptomatic improvement was statistically different in the gluten-containing group compared with placebo group in 9 (25.7%), and 31 (83.8%) patients respectively ($p < 0.001$). A large number of patients labelled as irritable bowel syndrome are sensitive to gluten. Using the term of IBS can therefore be misleading and may deviate and postpone the application of an effective and well-targeted treatment strategy in gluten sensitive patients.

Keywords: IBS; non-celiac gluten sensitivity; gluten free diet

1. Introduction

Dietary therapies are gaining popularity as evidence of efficacy for specific diets have emerged. The symptoms attributed to irritable bowel syndrome (IBS) seem to have a different etiology, and it has been reported that many patients fulfilling the criteria for IBS have, in fact, a kind of sensitivity to some nutrient components like FODMAP (Fermentable Oligo-Di-Monosaccharides and Polyols), gluten or lactose. Other major groups develop their symptoms related to anxiety, depression and work-related stresses. It is very clear that the spectrum of IBS is narrowing by the recent advances in diagnostic tools [1]. Many conditions that were called IBS 20 years ago, do have a clear and treatable etiology. This is why IBS has a changeable definition in different settings [2]. The major overlooked etiologies that are labelled as irritable bowel syndrome are food sensitivities, anxiety and depression. Due to a lack of proper diagnosis, often depression becomes a part of the natural history in sufferers with symptoms attributed to IBS [3–6]. There are at least three postulated mechanisms by which food components might induce functional gut symptoms in IBS. These three mechanisms are: immune mediated/mast cell pathway (usually referred as "food hypersensitivity"), direct action of bioactive molecules (generally referred as to "food chemicals") and luminal distension [4].

Severe gluten sensitivity without any damage to the intestinal mucosa was reported in some patients fulfilling the criteria for IBS [5]. It is still not very clear how gluten sensitivity causes a range of symptoms in these patients [7]. Some patients who are labelled as post gastroenteritis IBS may in fact have food sensitivity [4].

Recent studies have found that patients with so-called IBS suffer from non-celiac gluten sensitivity and their IBS symptoms improved after six weeks of a gluten-free diet [6–8]. Medical practices only recently started to focus attention on the pathogenicity of some nutrients in causing gastrointestinal symptoms, and it is disappointing that health care professionals receive little formal training in the dietary management of IBS and have traditionally viewed dietary interventions with skepticism. The food sensitivity behind the symptoms caused by changes in motility, visceral sensation, microbiome, permeability, immune activation, and brain-gut interactions are key elements in the pathogenesis of food sensitivity previously attributed to IBS. The role of specific dietary modification in the management of this group of patients has not been rigorously investigated until recently. There is now credible evidence suggesting that targeted dietary carbohydrate exclusion provides clinical benefits in unrecognised food-sensitive patients masked under the diagnosis of IBS. There is emerging evidence to suggest that proteins such as gluten, as well as food chemicals, may play a cardinal role in the symptoms of these patients [9].

We hope, by undertaking the step to evaluate the role of gluten-free diet in patients treated symptomatically under the diagnosis of IBS, to prevent the side effects of medications used for symptomatic relief in those patients who, in fact, are gluten-sensitive.

The aim of this study was thus to evaluate the effects of a gluten-free diet in Iranian patients with a diagnosis of IBS to assess whether dietary intervention has any role in the treatment package of these patients.

2. Materials and Methods

2.1. Study Population

During the years 2011–2013, 148 patients with newly diagnosed IBS based on the Rome III criteria [10] and more than 16 years of age, were recruited in this double-blind randomized placebo-controlled trial study (DBRP). All participants were recruited from a suburban, outpatient, private-practice gastroenterology clinic in Imam Khomeini hospital, Tehran, Iran.

2.2. Inclusion and Exclusion Criteria

From this number 46 patients were excluded from the study because of the following criteria and associations: subjects who had a known diagnosis of celiac disease (CD) and had ever tried a gluten free diet (GFD) and whether this diet was currently in place; patients with self-exclusion of wheat from the diet without a known diagnosis of CD; patients with inflammatory bowel disease and diabetes; those who used any concurrent drugs for depression and/or anxiety; people who used non-steroidal anti-inflammatory drugs; subjects with abnormal levels of: glucose, urea, creatinine, sodium, potassium, hemoglobin, ESR (erythrocyte sedimentation rate) and thyroid function tests; and those who did not sign the consent form to participate in the study.

CD was excluded as a diagnosis in all patients through a combination of serological testing (anti-Tissue transglutaminase antibody (anti-tTG Ab), total IgA levels, and/or anti-endomysial antibody (anti-EMA Ab) positive test) (three cases), and villi atrophy at the duodenal histology (1 case) performed at endoscopy while on a gluten-containing diet. Also those with positive IgE-mediated immuno-allergy tests to wheat were excluded. Only those patients who fulfilled the criteria recently proposed by the experts' meeting on "gluten sensitivity" [11,12] were included in the present study. All were negative for CD serology (anti-endomysial antibody and anti-Tissue transglutaminase antibody of IgA class), wheat allergy tests (specific IgE and skin prick tests) and normal duodenal biopsy with preserved villous architecture performed at the time of endoscopy on a gluten-containing diet.

2.3. Clinical Trial

The gluten free diet was started in 102 IBS patients; 22 patients found it hard and difficult to continue with the gluten-free diet and subsequently were withdrawn from study. Eighty patients responded to the diet and achieved significant improvement. From this group 8/80 did not follow a strict gluten free diet and were unwilling to continue the diet any further, and the remaining 72 patients completed the study. At the end of phase one, 72 patients met the inclusion criteria. From this group, 35 out of 72 were randomized in the gluten group and 37 out of 72 were in the placebo group for six weeks. The mean age in the gluten group was 44.5 ± 10 years and 43.2 ± 17 years in the placebo group. Six patients (17.1%) in the gluten group and 13 in the placebo group (35.1%) were male.

Patients were asked to complete a symptom questionnaire containing the question for the primary outcomes including bloating, abdominal pain, defecation satisfaction, nausea, fatigue and overall symptoms, and scored with visual analogue scale (VAS), with 0 representing no symptoms and 10 indicating severe clinical signs and symptoms.

The patients were randomized according to block randomization method held by an independent observer to either the gluten or the placebo treatment group. Both patients and investigators evaluating patients were blinded to the study treatment. After randomization, serum markers were measured for antibodies to tissue transglutaminase (*i.e.*, tissue transglutaminase IgA) and whole gliadin (IgA and IgG) by ELISA (enzyme-linked immunosorbent assay) using commercially available kits (AESKULISA tTG/AGA, Wendelsheim, Germany). According to the manufacturer's reference ranges, serological results were considered negative when <10 IU/mL; higher values were considered positive.

2.4. Assessment of Dietary Compliance

At each weekly follow-up assessment, dietary adherence was evaluated by a dietitian assessing consumption of any gluten-containing nutrient. Dietary compliance was considered optimal if the consumption of gluten was below 100 mg/day. Those patients (8/80) who did not comply with this policy despite their improvement did not continue with study. After six weeks (phase two) 72/80 patients who complied with the diet optimally and made a significant improvement, agreed to continue with the study and be enrolled in double-blind randomized placebo-controlled trial challenges (Figure 1).

Group A, including 35 patients (the gluten containing group), was given a packet (100 g) containing a gluten meal (free of fermentable oligo di-monosaccharides and polyols and proteins including 2.3% non-gluten, 52% gluten and/or gliadin and 27.7 g glucose). Group B, including 37 patients (placebo group (gluten-free powder)), was given packets (100 g) containing powder of gluten-free foods (rice flour, corn starch and glucose). HLA typing was performed for all patients in both groups.

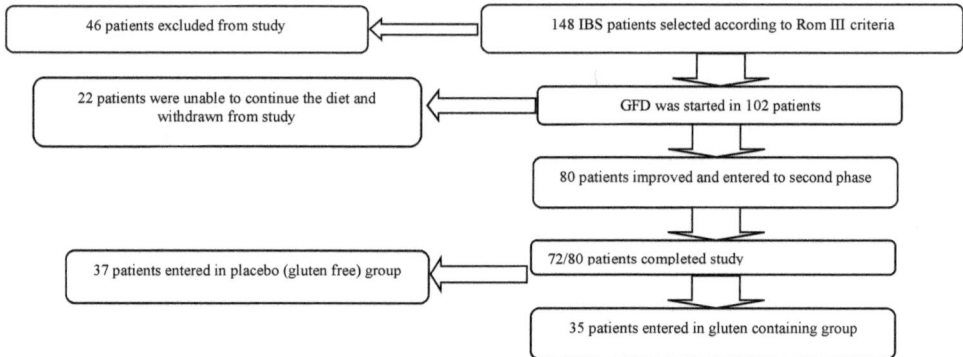

Figure 1. Recruitment pathway and reasons for screen failure and withdrawals.

Patients in both groups consumed powder for six weeks, while both groups were on gluten-free diets. Packages each contained two packs of 50 g powder, each to be poured in a cup containing 150 mL warm water, stirring the emulsion immediately and consuming one with breakfast and one with dinner. Initially, the participants were given complete information about the process of study. The study was approved by the institutional ethics committees of the Gastroenterology Department, Imam Khomeini Hospital, Tehran University of Medical Sciences, Tehran (study number CT711; approval date: 22 November 2012), and all participants signed a written informed consent regarding participation in the research project.

2.5. Statistical Analysis

The results and VAS mean scores were analyzed by χ^2 and Mann-Whitney U test, respectively using SPSS software version 15. Progressions of symptoms in both groups were examined by repeated measurement test. In this study predictive values less than 0.05 was recognized as significant.

3. Results

Seventy-two patients were evaluated into this double-blind randomized placebo-controlled trial. IBS type in the placebo group consisted of constipation type in six patients (16.2%), diarrhea type in 18 (48.6%) and mixed type in 13 (35.1%) patients. On the other hand, type of IBS in the gluten containing group consisted of constipation type in 10 (28.6%), diarrhea type in 19 (54.3%) and mixed type in 6 (17.1%) patients. No statistical differences were detected when the type of IBS in two groups ($p = 0.089$) were compared. The placebo group (62.1%) and gluten-containing group (48.5%) carried either DQ2 or DQ8 haplotypes. Table 1 summarizes the demographic and clinical characteristics of the gluten compared to placebo group. As the result shows there were no statistically significant differences between the groups regarding gender and mean age ($p > 0.05$).

The statistical analysis showed that the differences between gluten-containing and placebo groups in the overall symptoms (placebo (16.2%), gluten (74.3%)) including satisfaction with stool consistency (placebo (8.1%), gluten (77.1%)), tiredness (placebo (8.8%), gluten (60%)), nausea (placebo (5.4%), gluten (8.3%)), bloating (placebo (16.2%), gluten (74.3%)) were statistically significant ($p = 0.001$).

After checking normality and Sphericity assumptions, repeated measurement test was employed to analyse the scores of symptoms, and revealed no statistically significant difference for symptom's score including satisfaction with stool consistency ($p = 0.15$), tiredness ($p = 0.6$), nausea ($p = 0.6$), and bloating ($p = 0.3$) between placebo and gluten groups (See Figure 2).

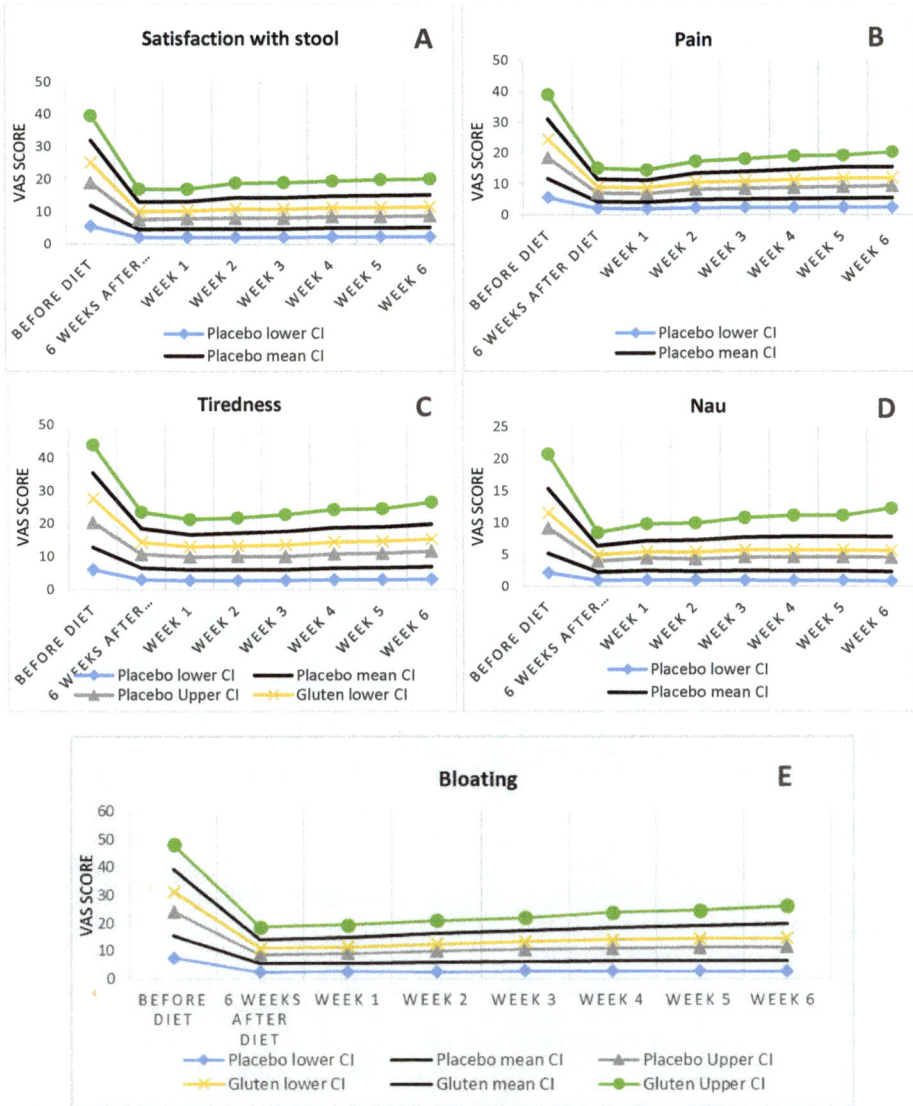

Figure 2. The difference between gluten and placebo groups in the pattern of symptoms. (**A**) Satisfaction with stool consistency; (**B**) Pain; (**C**) Tiredness; (**D**) Nausea; (**E**) Bloating.

After six weeks of the diet, symptoms were controlled only in nine patients (25.7%) in the gluten-containing group, compared to 31 patients (83.8%) in the placebo group, indicating that 26 out of 35 patients in the gluten group became symptomatic on gluten-challenge. Comparison of these ratios indicated that there were significant differences between gluten-containing and placebo group symptoms control ($p < 0.001$). In the gluten-containing group, all symptoms significantly increased especially for bloating and abdominal pain (from 3.1 ± 2.3 to 5.1 ± 2.2) one week after starting the gluten. Mean bloating VAS before starting the gluten-free diet in the gluten group was 8.4 ± 1.5, and after the six-week diet was decreased to 3.1 ± 2.3. Overall time trend analysis revealed statistically significant satisfaction with stool consistency ($p = 0.01$) and bloating ($p = 0.05$) (but no statistically significant difference between the two groups). After a one-week gluten challenge, the mean score was increased to 4 ± 2.1, which was not statistically significant compared with the placebo group. But this symptom continued to increase to 5.1 ± 2.2 in the fifth week.

At the beginning of the study three patients in the placebo and none in the gluten group were positive for anti-gliadin antibodies (AGA) IgG. At the end of six weeks, the patients were tested for anti-gliadin antibodies (IgG and IgA) and tissue transglutaminase antibodies (IgG and IgA) (Table 1). Except for one patient, who had increased anti-gliadin antibodies IgG titer, the titers of the rest of the patients were unchanged, and therefore, no significant differences were seen before and after the regimen in either of the two groups ($p > 0.05$).

Table 1. Demographic and clinical characteristics of the gluten compared to placebo group.

Antibody	Placebo	95% CI [*]	Gluten	95% CI	*p* Value
Number of patients	37		35		–
Age average	43.2 ± 17	37.6–8.8	44.5 ± 10	41.11–47.89	**0.241**
Frequency (%) of male gender	13 (35.1%)	19%–51%	6 (17.1%)	4%–30%	**0.083**
Kind of IBS					
Constipation	6 (16.2%) [4%–28%]		10 (28.6%) [13%–43%]		**0.089**
Diarrhea	18 (48.6%) [32.6%–64.6%]		19 (54.3%) [37%–71%]		
Mixed	13 (35.1%) [20%–50%]		6 (17.1%) [5%–29%]		
Tiredness	(8.8%)		(60%)		
Pain	(16.2%)		(76.3%)		
[1] Anti-tTG IgA	2.3 ± 0.4	2.17–2.43	2.5 ± 0.4	2.37–2.63	**0.259**
Anti-tTG IgG	2 ± 0.3	1.02–2.98	2.2 ± 0.3	2.1–2.3	**0.174**
[2] AGA IgA	2.9 ± 1.8	2.31–3.49	2.6 ± 0.5	2.43–2.77	**0.110**
AGA IgG	2.6 ± 1.4	2.14–3.06	2.4 ± 0.4	2.27–2.53	**0.119**
Positive DQ2/8 [3] HLA	23 (62.1%)	46%–78%	17 (48.5%)	31%–65%	**0.792**

[1] Anti-tTG: anti- tissue transglutaminase antibodies; [2] AGA: anti gliadin antibodies; [3] HLA: human leukocyte antigen; CI: In statistics, a confidence interval (CI) is a type of interval estimate of a population parameter.

4. Discussion

The relationship between nutrition and the gut environment is complex and has been a long-standing subject of intense debate. Although the effects of food allergies such as wheat consumption on gut motility have been well studied, the role of non-allergic, immune hypersensitivity reactions to specific food components is less understood [13–15]. In this study we have clarified that many cases treated symptomatically under the IBS label do have gluten sensitivity. Distinguishing between a non-specific terminology like IBS, and gluten sensitivity is extremely important since the later could be treated specifically and effectively with gluten restriction without implementing a long-term symptomatic drug therapy and having the consequences of drug side effects.

Gluten intolerance in people without celiac disease is a common condition, and most recently was described as "non-celiac gluten sensitivity" [12]. Gastrointestinal signs and symptoms in many patients labelled as IBS seem to be improved after exclusion of gluten from their diet. Basic evidence for such a claim is based on few randomized controlled trials [7,16–18].

This double-blind randomized placebo-controlled trial was performed on the patients with a diagnosis of IBS presenting with intestinal and extra-intestinal symptoms and confirmed that the differences between gluten-containing and placebo groups in the overall symptoms control was statistically significant.

It has become increasingly clear that intestinal inflammation may provide an initial stimulus for a persistent state of visceral hypersensitivity [19]. In fact, it might be that the microenteropathy [20] related to primary or acquired [4] e.g., post gastroenteritis food sensitivity, may cause intestinal irritability.

The role of inflammation in chronic abdominal pain comes from studies evaluating patients with gastroenteritis. Colonic biopsies of patients with persistent symptoms after a gastroenteritis reveal no signs of overt inflammation but show persistent minor increases in epithelial T lymphocytes and mast cells, [21] suggesting that long-term inflammatory changes may be responsible for colonic hypersensitivity.

Identifying and treating this state of hypersensitivity with dietary intervention has opened a new prospect in recognising food sensitivities and bringing IBS to an end as a non-specific and unuseful diagnosis. Unfortunately dietary intervention might not be convenient for every patient in particular in countries where the availability of gluten free products is limited. A significant number of our study group left the study as they were not able to cope with the dietary restrictions.

Abdominal pain was a common presentation in the remaining 72 patients and dietary intervention scored high in resolution of this symptom. Other GI symptoms including bloating and abdominal pain were raised in six patients out of 37 patients in the placebo group and in 26 out of 35 patients in the gluten group. Some studies suggest that pain might be related to wheat's insoluble fibre that may causes increased gas, bloating and cramping after inducing an inflammatory reaction, activating the mast cells in proximity of colonic nerves, and releasing the mediators such as serotonin, histamine and proteases, which are able to activate visceral afferent nerve fibres [22,23]. A correlation might also exist between mast cell degranulation and IgE level in some cases. But the biological activity of some allergen types may also be affected by other parameters [24]. Similar to our finding, Biesiekierski *et al.* [7], reported the reappearance of extra-intestinal symptoms in the group that was re-challenged with gluten than those receiving placebo. It is well known that, besides the intestinal phenotype characterized by IBS-like symptoms, gluten-sensitive patients have plenty of extra-intestinal manifestations, the most frequent being those related to the peripheral and central nervous system, skin and joint/muscle. In contrast to the well-described acknowledgement of extra-intestinal symptoms in cases with gluten-related disorders, extra intestinal symptoms are usually ignored in IBS patients.

Increased "tiredness" by gluten suggests that in addition to the effect of gluten on the intestinal mucosa permeability, it may have a systemic effect in gluten-sensitive patients. Significant difference between gluten-containing and placebo groups regarding this symptom in this study ($p < 0.002$) and also demonstrated in the Biesiekierski study ($p < 0.001$) [7] confirm this hypothesis. The same research group also confirmed in their recent study that the investigated patients remarkably improved on the GFD and their symptoms were well controlled [25].

Despite the difficulties and challenges related to following a gluten-free diet, close communication with participant and support provide by study team facilitated the plan to full compliance with the gluten-free diet. The patients were guided by facilitating access to reliable reference for gluten-free products.

In this study, we did rely only on clinical criteria to evaluate response to regimen, because food sensitivity diagnosis is based on clinical diagnostic criteria and investigation findings are important mainly for ruling out the other intestinal disorders.

There is a need for highly sensitive and specific biomarkers to identify [26] mild inflammation or injury and damages of the intestinal mucosa and systemic inflammation; such biomarkers may help to determine the role and mechanism of gluten in inducing intestinal and extra-intestinal symptoms. A recent study by Valerii *et al.* demonstrates that wheat protein can induce an over-activation of the pro-inflammatory chemokine CXCL10 in peripheral blood mononuclear cell (PBMC) from non-celiac gluten sensitivity patients [27].

Rapid increase of intestinal and extra-intestinal symptoms can occur within hours, days or weeks after the exposure to gluten. Therefore developing symptoms using gluten challenge provides a cardinal criterion of strong reliability for the diagnosis of non-celiac gluten sensitivity.

In our study the antibody titers did not reach statistical differences before and at the end of the dietary intervention similar to others [7].

Identifying the NCGS correctly by using Salerno criteria, would help to differentiate NCGS from IBS [28]. The differentiation between these conditions is important as fermentable carbohydrates delivered to the colon have potential anti carcinogenic and anti-inflammatory actions [29]. Restriction of FODMAPs delivered to the colon might consequently have adverse effects on colonic health. A randomized parallel group study evaluated the effects on fecal microbiota of a dietitian-taught low FODMAP diet compared with those of a habitual diet indicated a reduction of the proportion and concentration of *Bifidobacteria* spp., providing the first evidence for potentially unfavourable effects of the low FODMAP diet [30]. Even though the carbohydrate restriction is much less in GFD compared to the low FODMAP, it has been demonstrated that levels of *Bifidobacteria* and *Lactobacilli* are reduced in CD patients on GFD [31–33]. While effect of GFD on microbiota needs further clarification in NCGS, low FODMAP in the long term seems to be associated with reducing total bacterial abundance in the feces [34], and quite rightly, Halmos *et al.* suggest that the low FODMAP diet should be recommended cautiously and avoided in asymptomatic cases. Therefore, distinguishing between gluten sensitivity and other carbohydrate sensitivities may need to be the starting point in managing patients fulfilling the Rome III criteria as reduced FODMAP delivery to colonic microbiota might have deleterious effects on the growth of bacteria, and thus potentially unfavorable health effects. Implementing low FODMAP perhaps should be restricted to those patients with additional carbohydrate sensitivity induced by FODMAP only.

5. Conclusions

In conclusion, many patients diagnosed as having IBS are clearly gluten-sensitive, and their symptoms could be adequately controlled with a gluten-free diet only. Identifying gluten sensitivity in this group of patients may need to be the first approach. Elimination of other carbohydrates might be considered in non-responders if six weeks of a gluten-free diet proves to be ineffective in controlling the patient's symptoms, as according to Figure 3. Studies with a larger sample size would be needed to determine whether some biomarkers as predictors of response to treatment, may be useful in this subgroup of patients before a gluten-free diet.

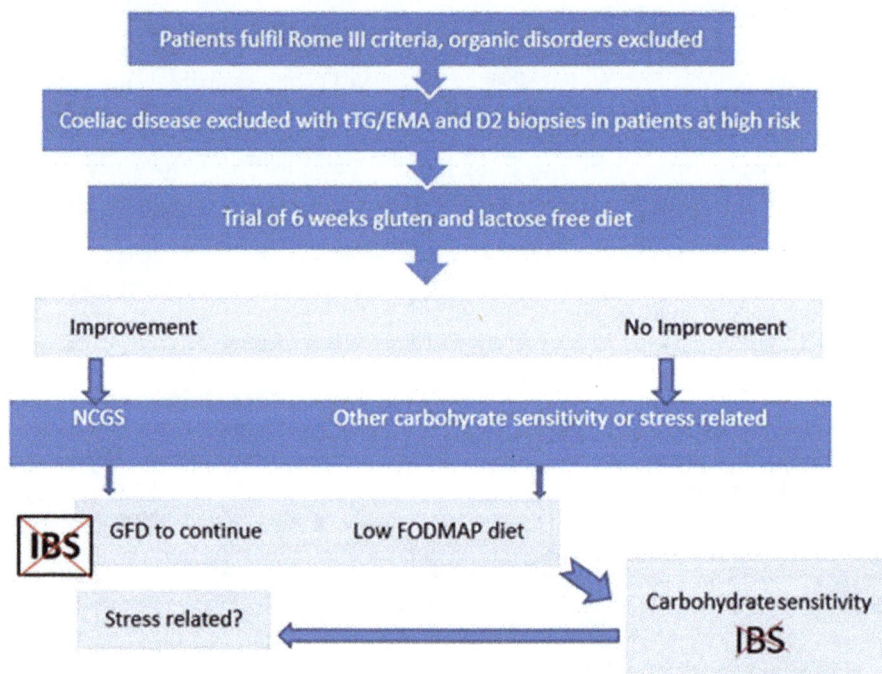

Figure 3. Suggesting algorithm.

Author Contributions: Bijan Shahbazkhani: supervisor of this project and editing the manuscript; Amirsaeid Sadeghi: sample collection, article writing; Reza Malekzadeh: concept and design of the work, final approval; Fatima khatavi: Endoscopy study; Mehrnoosh Etemadi and Ebrahim Kalantri: Sample collection and serological study; Mohammad Rostami-Nejad: analysis and interpretation of data, final approval; and Kamran Rostami: concept and design of the work, article writing, and final approval.

Conflicts of Interest: The authors declare no conflict of interest.

References

1. Thompson, W.G.; Heaton, K.W.; Smyth, G.T.; Smyth, C. Irritable bowel syndrome in general practice: Prevalence, characteristics, and referral. *Gut* **2000**, *46*, 78–82. [CrossRef] [PubMed]

2. Harvey, R.F.; Salih, S.Y.; Read, A.E. Organic and functional disorders in 2000 gastroenterology outpatients. *Lancet* **1983**, *1*, 632–634. [CrossRef]

3. Rostami, K.; Rostami-Nejad, M.; Al Dulaimi, D. Post Gastroenteritis gluten intolerance. *Gastroenterol. Hepatol. Bed Bench* **2015**, *8*, 66–70. [PubMed]

4. Gibson, P.R. Food intolerance in functional bowel disorders. *J. Gastroenterol. Hepatol.* **2011**, *26*, 128–131. [CrossRef] [PubMed]

5. Saito, Y.A.; Locke, G.R.; Talley, N.J.; Zinsmeister, A.R.; Fett, S.L.; Melton, L.J., 3rd. A comparison of the Rome and Manning criteria for case identification in epidemiological investigations of irritable bowel syndrome. *Am. J. Gastroenterol.* **2000**, *95*, 2816–2824. [CrossRef] [PubMed]

6. Ruepert, L.; Quartero, A.O.; de Wit, N.J.; van der Heijden, G.J.; Rubin, G.; Muris, J.W. Bulking agents, antispasmodics and antidepressants for the treatment of irritable bowel syndrome. *Cochrane Database Syst. Rev.* **2011**, *8*. [CrossRef]

7. Biesiekierski, J.R.; Newnham, E.D.; Irving, P.M.; Barrett, J.S.; Haines, M.; Doecke, J.D.; Shepherd, S.J.; Muir, J.G.; Gibson, P.R. Gluten causes gastrointestinal symptoms in subjects without celiac disease: A double-blind randomized placebo-controlled trial. *Am. J. Gastroenterol.* **2011**, *106*, 508–514. [CrossRef] [PubMed]

8. Volta, U.; Tovoli, F.; Cicola, R.; Parisi, C.; Fabbri, A.; Piscaglia, M.; Fiorini, E.; Caio, G. Serological tests in gluten sensitivity (nonceliac gluten intolerance). *J. Clin. Gastroenterol.* **2012**, *46*, 680–685. [CrossRef] [PubMed]

9. Spencer, M.; Chey, W.D.; Eswaran, S. Dietary renaissance in IBS: Has food replaced medications as a primary treatment strategy? *Curr. Treat. Options Gastroenterol.* **2014**, *12*, 424–440. [CrossRef] [PubMed]

10. Longstreth, G.F.; Thompson, W.G.; Chey, W.D.; Houghton, L.A.; Mearin, F.; Spiller, R.C. Functional bowel disorders. *Gastroenterology* **2006**, *130*, 1480–1491. [CrossRef] [PubMed]

11. Troncone, R.; Jabri, B. Celiac disease and gluten-sensitivity. *J. Intern. Med.* **2011**, *269*, 582–590. [CrossRef] [PubMed]

12. Sapone, A.; Bai, J.C.; Ciacci, C.; Dolinsek, J.; Green, P.H.; Hadjivassiliou, M.; Kaukinen, K.; Rostami, K.; Sanders, D.S.; Schumann, M.; *et al.* Spectrum of gluten-related disorders: Consensus on new nomenclature and classification. *BMC Med.* **2012**, *10*. [CrossRef] [PubMed]

13. Verdu, E.F.; Armstrong, D.; Murray, J.A. Between celiac disease and irritable bowel syndrome: The "no man's land" of gluten sensitivity. *Am. J. Gastroenterol.* **2009**, *104*, 1587–1594. [CrossRef] [PubMed]

14. Verdu, E.F.; Huang, X.; Natividad, J.; Lu, J.; Blennerhassett, P.A.; David, C.S.; McKay, D.M.; Murray, J.A. Gliadin-dependent neuromuscular and epithelial secretory responses in gluten-sensitive HLA-DQ8 transgenic mice. *Am. J. Physiol. Gastrointest. Liver. Physiol.* **2008**, *294*, G217–G225. [CrossRef] [PubMed]

15. Natividad, J.M.; Huang, X.; Slack, E.; Jury, J.; Sanz, Y.; David, C.; Denou, E.; Yang, P.; Murray, J.; McCoy, K.D.; *et al.* Host responses to intestinal microbial antigens in gluten-sensitive mice. *PLoS ONE* **2009**, *4*, e6472. [CrossRef] [PubMed]

16. Aziz, I.; Sanders, D.S. The irritable bowel syndrome-celiac disease connection. *Gastrointest. Endosc. Clin. N. Am.* **2012**, *22*, 623–637. [CrossRef] [PubMed]

17. Carroccio, A.; Mansueto, P.; Iacono, G.; Soresi, M.; D'Alcamo, A.; Cavataio, F.; Brusca, I.; Florena, A.M.; Ambrosiano, G.; Seidita, A.; *et al.* Non-celiac wheat sensitivity diagnosed by double-blind placebo-controlled challenge: Exploring a new clinical entity. *Am. J. Gastroenterol.* **2012**, *107*, 1898–1906. [CrossRef] [PubMed]

18. Rodrigo, L.; Blanco, I.; Bobes, J.; de Serres, F.J. Effect of one year of a gluten-free diet on the clinical evolution of irritable bowel syndrome plus fibromyalgia in patients with associated lymphocytic enteritis: A case control study. *Arthritis. Res. Ther.* **2014**, *16*. [CrossRef]

19. Wouters, M.M. Histamine antagonism and postinflammatory visceral hypersensitivity. *Gut* **2014**, *63*, 1836–1837. [CrossRef] [PubMed]

20. Rostami, K. From microenteropathy to villous atrophy: What is treatable? *Dig. Liver. Dis.* **2003**, *35*, 758–759. [CrossRef]

21. Ohman, L.; Simren, M. Pathogenesis of IBS: Role of inflammation, immunity and neuroimmune interactions. *Nat. Rev. Gastroenterol. Hepatol.* **2010**, *7*, 163–173. [CrossRef] [PubMed]

22. Barbara, G.; Stanghellini, V.; de Giorgio, R.; Cremon, C.; Cottrell, G.S.; Santini, D.; Pasquinelli, G.; Morselli-Labate, A.M.; Grady, E.F.; Bunnett, N.W.; *et al.* Activated mast cells in proximity to colonic nerves correlate with abdominal pain in irritable bowel syndrome. *Gastroenterology* **2004**, *126*, 693–702. [CrossRef] [PubMed]

23. Buhner, S.; Li, Q.; Berger, T.; Vignali, S.; Barbara, G.; de Giorgio, R.; Stanghellini, V.; Schemann, M. Submucous rather than myenteric neurons are activated by mucosal biopsy supernatants from irritable bowel syndrome patients. *Neurogastroenterol. Motil.* **2012**, *24*, e1134–e1572. [CrossRef] [PubMed]

24. Bodinier, M.; Brossard, C.; Triballeau, S.; Morisset, M.; Guérin-Marchand, C.; Pineau, F.; de Coppet, P.; Moneret-Vautrin, D.A.; Blank, U.; Denery-Papini, S. Evaluation of an *in vitro* mast cell degranulation test in the context of food allergy to wheat. *Int. Arch. Allergy. Immunol.* **2008**, *146*, 307–320. [CrossRef] [PubMed]

25. Rostami, K.; Aldulaimi, D.; Holmes, G.; Johnson, M.W.; Robert, M.; Srivastava, A.; Fléjou, J.F.; Sanders, D.S.; Volta, U.; Derakhshan, M.H.; *et al.* Microscoppic enteritisis: Bucharest consensus. *World J. Gastroenterol.* **2015**, *21*, 2593–2604. [CrossRef] [PubMed]

26. Biesiekierski, J.R.; Peters, S.L.; Newnham, E.D.; Rosella, O.; Muir, J.G.; Gibson, P.R. No effects of gluten in patients with self-reported non-celiac gluten sensitivity after dietary reduction of fermentable, poorly absorbed, short-chain carbohydrates. *Gastroenterology.* **2013**, *145*, 320–328. [CrossRef] [PubMed]

27. Valerii, M.C.; Ricci, C.; Spisni, E.; di Silvestro, R.; de Fazio, L.; Cavazza, E.; Lanzini, A.; Campieri, M.; Dalpiaz, A.; Pavan, B.; *et al.* Responses of peripheralblood mononucleated cells from non-celiac gluten sensitive patients to variouscereal sources. *Food Chem.* **2015**, *176*, 167–174. [CrossRef] [PubMed]

28. Catassi, C.; Elli, L.; Bonaz, B.; Bouma, G.; Carroccio, A.; Castillejo, G.; Cellier, C.; Cristofori, F.; Magistris, L.D.; Dolinsek, J.; *et al.* How the diagnosis of non celiac gluten sensitivity (NCGS) should be confirmed: The Salerno experts' criteria. *Nutrients* **2015**. submitted.

29. Sengupta, S.; Muir, J.G.; Gibson, P.R. Does butyrate protect from colorectal cancer? *J. Gastroenterol. Hepatol.* **2006**, *21*, 209–218. [CrossRef] [PubMed]

30. Staudacher, H.M.; Lomer, M.C.; Anderson, J.L.; Barrett, J.S.; Muir, J.G.; Irving, P.M.; Whelan, K. Fermentable carbohydrate restriction reduces luminal bifidobacteria and gastrointestinal symptoms in patients with irritable bowel syndrome. *J. Nutr.* **2012**, *142*, 1510–1518. [CrossRef] [PubMed]

31. Di Cagno, R.; de Angelis, M.; de Pasquale, I.; Ndagijimana, M.; Vernocchi, P.; Ricciuti, P.; Gagliardi, F.; Laghi, L.; Crecchio, C.; Guerzoni, M.E.; *et al.* Duodenal and faecal microbiota of celiac children: Molecular, phenotype andmetabolome characterization. *BMC Microbiol.* **2011**, *11*. [CrossRef] [PubMed]

32. Kopecný, J.; Mrázek, J.; Fliegerová, K.; Frühauf, P.; Tucková, L. The intestinal microflora of childhood patients with indicated celiac disease. *Folia Microbiol. (Praha)* **2008**, *53*, 214–216. [CrossRef] [PubMed]

33. De Sousa Moraes, L.F.; Grzeskowiak, L.M.; de Sales Teixeira, T.F.; Gouveia Peluzio Mdo, C. Intestinal microbiota and probiotics in celiac disease. *Clin. Microbiol. Rev.* **2014**, *27*, 482–489. [CrossRef] [PubMed]

34. Halmos, E.P.; Christophersen, C.T.; Bird, A.R.; Shepherd, S.J.; Gibson, P.R.; Muir, J.G. Diets that differ in their FODMAP content alter the colonic luminal microenvironment. *Gut* **2015**, *64*, 93–100. [CrossRef] [PubMed]

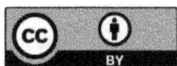

nutrients

MDPI

Article

Cutaneous Manifestations of Non-Celiac Gluten Sensitivity: Clinical Histological and Immunopathological Features

Veronica Bonciolini [1,*], Beatrice Bianchi [1], Elena Del Bianco [1], Alice Verdelli [1] and Marzia Caproni [2]

[1] Department of Surgery and Translational Medicine, Section of Dermatology, University of Florence, Viale Michelangiolo 41, Florence 50125, Italy; beatrice.bianchi@unifi (B.B.); elena.delbianco@unifi (E.D.B.); alice.verdelli@hotmail (A.V.)

[2] Director SOS Skin Immunopathology and Rare Dermatological Diseases Unit, 1st Dermatological Clinic ASF-Piero Palagi, Department of Medical and Surgical Critical Care, Section of Dermatology, University of Florence, Viale Michelangiolo 41, Florence 50125, Italy; marzia.caproni@unifi

* Correspondence: vbonciolini@gmail.com; Tel.: +39-33-8129-2961; Fax: +39-05-5693-9598

Received: 14 June 2015; Accepted: 8 September 2015; Published: 15 September 2015

Abstract: Background: The dermatological manifestations associated with intestinal diseases are becoming more frequent, especially now when new clinical entities, such as Non-Celiac Gluten Sensitivity (NCGS), are identified. The existence of this new entity is still debated. However, many patients with diagnosed NCGS that present intestinal manifestations have skin lesions that need appropriate characterization. Methods: We involved 17 patients affected by NCGS with non-specific cutaneous manifestations who got much better after a gluten free diet. For a histopathological and immunopathological evaluation, two skin samples from each patient and their clinical data were collected. Results: The median age of the 17 enrolled patients affected by NCGS was 36 years and 76% of them were females. On the extensor surfaces of upper and lower limbs in particular, they all presented very itchy dermatological manifestations morphologically similar to eczema, psoriasis or dermatitis herpetiformis. This similarity was also confirmed histologically, but the immunopathological analysis showed the prevalence of deposits of C3 along the dermo-epidermal junction with a microgranular/granular pattern (82%). Conclusions: The exact characterization of new clinical entities such as Cutaneous Gluten Sensitivity and NCGS is an important objective both for diagnostic and therapeutic purposes, since these are patients who actually benefit from a GFD (Gluten Free Diet) and who do not adopt it only for fashion.

Keywords: non-celiac gluten sensitivity; cutaneous gluten sensitivity; skin manifestations; direct immunofluorescence

1. Introduction

The cutaneous manifestations of intestinal bowel diseases have always been an obstacle either for the gastroenterologists or dermatologists. A close collaboration between these practitioners is required because of the wide range of skin diseases that may be associated both with celiac diseases (CD) and the inflammatory bowel diseases (IBD) [1–5]. For a long time, our group has been dedicated to the characterization of specific and non-specific cutaneous manifestations related to bowel diseases, in particular to CD. In a previous article we already described all skin manifestations in patients with celiac disease, adopting the classification of Humbert *et al.* [6], that divided them in two groups: those improved by gluten free diet and those occasionally associated with CD; and in four categories: autoimmune, allergic, inflammatory, and miscellaneous [5].

Recently, the study of Volta *et al.* [7] conducted with the aim to define the clinical picture of this new syndrome and to establish roughly its prevalence compared to CD showed a strong correlation with female gender and adult age. The study reiterated the relationship with the irritable bowel syndrome (IBS). The diagnosis is currently based only on clinical suspicion because of the lack of valid biomarkers and of the gold standard assay dietary elimination of gluten which is followed by a randomized double-blind, placebo-controlled (DBPC) food challenge (even if the last one is difficult to adopt routinely in clinical practice). Confirming our hypothesis of skin involvement, 29% out of 486 patients with suspected Non-Celiac Gluten Sensitivity (NCGS) that took part in the study presented skin rash and 18% of them not well defined dermatitis.

We believe that these cutaneous manifestations should be better defined with a clinical evaluation by expert dermatologists, who may identify specific patterns through finalized immune-histological studies. As it has already happened with CD and dermatitis herpetiformis (DH), also in these patients can be identified a specific skin pattern, which itself may be sufficient to make a diagnosis of bowel disease.

The etiology and the pathophysiology of NCGS is under scrutiny. A lot of people spontaneously adopt a gluten free diet, solving their intestinal and extra-intestinal symptoms such as diarrhea, abdominal discomfort or pain, bloating, flatulence and headache, lethargy, attention-deficit/hyperactivity disorder, ataxia or recurrent oral ulceration. Over the years, the gluten free diet (GFD) has become a fashion, and, due to this, skepticism among some authors in regard to the NCGS has arisen. Nevertheless, scientific papers that describe this new entity are still increasing in number [8], and, in our work experience, skin lesions observed in patients with NCGS are actually sensitive to GFD. In fact, in the Western world, the consumption of wheat that has increased in the last half century, proportionally to the standard of living and life length [9], now has an opposite trend in Europe, Australia, New Zealand and United States of America [10]. However, it is different for the large populations in China and India [11], where currently wheat is more desirable than the rice.

Recently, Hollon J. *et al.* [12] showed that gliadin exposure induced an increase in the intestinal permeability in all individuals, regardless of whether they have CD or not. Their study suggests that the gluten exposure leads to altered barrier function in NCGS patients as well. It results in an exaggerated increase of the intestinal permeability that may confirm the hypothesis of the involvement of an innate immune response to this new syndrome. In respect to this, a US group reported an increased density of CD3 + intra-epithelial T-cells (intra-epithelial lymphocytes IELs) and a higher expression of mucosal Toll-like receptor 2 in NCGS patients compared to controls indicating immune activation in NCGS. The same study showed decreased mucosal level of mRNA for FOXP3 in NCGS patients compared to controls. This can be read as a possible sign of activation of T regulatory cells [13].

At the moment, there are only some hypotheses in regard to the pathogenic mechanisms at the base of this new condition and they still lead to confusion. In part, it is because of their significant impact on the media and socio-economic awareness which has been created. One hypothesis, which is based on what has been demonstrated so far, is that NCGS may be characterized by an activation of innate immunity [13,14], but probably all these symptoms may be the result of an exaggerated response of a normal individual to a meal containing gluten. Indeed, gluten is a component of the more complex protein mixture contained in wheat flour that can cause a significant increase of the intestinal fermentation processes in healthy individuals, through its opioid properties that are naloxone reversible [15]. Moreover, it can induce modifications in the intestinal transit, a possible low degree of intestinal inflammation (in experimental models) [16], and, last but not the least, a *nocebo* effect.

As the previously mentioned association between systemic diseases and cutaneous manifestations is not new, probably this link may be related to the constant communication among the different organ systems of our body.

The purpose of this study is mainly to define the cutaneous manifestations in the course of NCGS and, eventually, to characterize the new pathologic entities known as CGS.

2. Experimental Section

In the collaboration with gastroenterologists and physicians, we enrolled consecutive patients affected by NCGS and with non-specific cutaneous manifestations improved by gluten free diet. In accordance with the new algorithm proposed by Sapone A. *et al.* [17], we excluded other gluten reactions as wheat allergy (WA) and CD performing standard screening. Furthermore, specific skin prick tests and wheat specific serum IgE were done in order to exclude WA. Moreover, serological assay with specific antibodies (anti-tissue transglutaminase antibodies (tTG) IgA and IgG, anti-endomysial antibodies (EMA), anti-gliadin antibodies (AGA), deamidated gliadin peptide (DGP) and total IgA) and esophagogastroduodenoscopy with multiple biopsies served to exclude CD. We enrolled NCGS patients only after dietary elimination of gluten followed by DBPC, also useful to define the time of recurrence of the lesions with the reintroduction of gluten in the diet. We used a special form to collect their clinical data (gender, age, duration, family history of skin and/or intestinal diseases, morphology and localization of cutaneous lesions, gastrointestinal symptoms and other symptoms compatible to NCGS) which allowed us to define the clinical features of CGS and its possible variants (Table S1). We also reported time of resolution of the lesions adopting GFD (Table S1), with the purpose to compare the cutaneous manifestations of other gluten-sensitive diseases such as DH and collected skin samples for histological and direct immunofluorescence studies to define any specific patterns of CGS in the future. A written informed consent was obtained from all patients and procedures were carried out in accordance with the ethical standards of the Committee on Human Experimentation of the Department of the Dermatological Science and the Declaration of Helsinki. For the immunopathological study, skin samples from all the patients and controls were collected and they were immediately frozen at $-80\,°C$ in liquid nitrogen. The frozen specimens were cut into 5 μm thick sections: two of them were layered on each slide and the slides were stored at $-20\,°C$ until being stained. For staining, the sections were warmed to room temperature. Optimally diluted fluorescein isothiocyanate (FITC)—labeled monospecific immunoglobulins (IgG, IgA, IgM, C3 (DakoCytomation, Glostrup, Denmark)) was layered onto the sections and incubated at $37\,°C$ for 45 min–1 h. Then, the sections were washed thrice in PBS (pH 7.2, 0.1 M), mounted in buffered glycerin and finally analyzed under a Nikon C2 confocal microscope (Nikon, Tokyo, Japan) The following features were documented: (a) the nature of the immune deposits: IgG, IgA, IgM, C3; (b) the site of the immune deposits: dermal-epidermal junction (DEJ), intercellular spaces (ICS) or perivascular site; (c) the pattern of the immune deposits: granular, linear or mixed (granular/linear).

3. Results

In this prospective study, we enrolled 17 consecutive patients affected by NCGS after having considered gastroenterology and allergy in order to exclude other forms of gluten sensitivity such as CD and WA. We collected their clinical data in Table S1 (gender, age, duration, family history of skin and/or intestinal diseases, morphology and localization of cutaneous lesions, gastrointestinal or other symptoms compatible with NCGS, time of recurrence of the lesions after gluten re-exposure). The patients involved in the study were between 5 and 69 years old with an average age of 36 and most of them were females (Female: 76%; Male: 24%).

There were only 4 pediatric patients, all female. At the time of our observation the majority of patients reported gastrointestinal symptoms of varying intensity similar to IBS, such as abdominal pain, bloating, flatulence, diarrhea or constipation. Some of them, for example the skin manifestations, generally improved with spontaneously adopted GFD. Ten of the enrolled patients (59%) presented cutaneous manifestations for about one year, while in the others there was much longer disease duration with a typical chronic relapsing course.

Morphologically, the lesions were mainly erythematous, excoriated papular-vesicular and extremely itchy, similar to subacute eczema or DH. Nevertheless, some patients had hyperkeratotic scaly lesions instead overlying mild erythematous infiltrative lesions and they were associated with excoriations similar to chronic psoriasis. In order of frequency, the sites of the lesions were: extensor surfaces of upper limbs (elbows and back of the hands (94% and 6%)), extensor surfaces of lower limbs (knees) (59%), bottom (29%), chest (18%), neck (18%), the palms of the hands (6%), extensor surface of upper limbs (6%) and face (6%) (Figures S1–S5).

The mean time of disappearance of the skin lesions after adoption of GFD was one month or so as it is shown in Table S1.

Given the controversial relationship with NCGS, the serological screening for CD included also AGA, but only three of 17 (18%) patients showed positive results.

Histological features are shown schematically in Table S2. It was possible to outline a specific histological pattern, but it is important to point out the similarity with psoriasis, eczema and DH.

Finally, in Table S3, we reported the immunopathological features obtained by a direct immunofluorescence (DIF) test on a skin biopsy got from a perilesional skin, as it is usual in suspected DH to preserve immunological deposits. We described the type of reactant that forms the immunological deposit (IgG, IgM, IgA, C3 or C1q) and the site (DEJ—Dermoepidermal junction, PV—Perivascular, FB—Fluorescent bodies). The patterns of distribution along the DEJ were microgranular/granular in all patients. For each reactant we calculated (IgG, IgM, IgA, C3 and C1q) in how many patients it appears in different sites (DEJ, PV, FB). This is presented in percentages in Table S3. The C3 fraction of the complement system is the only reactant percentage in more than a half of the patients (82%) localized in particular along the DEJ (Figure S6).

4. Discussion

We are aware of the limitations of this study arising from, the limited number of patients enrolled, but we used very tight exclusion criteria, as we did not include patients with an uncertain diagnosis of NCGS.

The common clinical feature of all the patients involved in this study, as well as the one detached from our clinical experience, was the severe itching. It was difficult to treat with standard topical and systemic therapies, but it showed prompt resolution when GFD was introduced: the reaction was faster than in DH patients. Morphologically, the lesions were polymorphic, in terms of development. In fact, initially they were mainly erythematous and papulo-vesicular like eczema and DH, then later, maybe due to a constant scratching, they appeared psoriatic-like. Furthermore, similar to DH, the lesions were more frequently localized on the extensor surfaces of the limbs, in particular on the elbows (94%), followed by knees (59%), than bottom (29%), chest (18%), neck (18%), the palms and back of the hands (6%), extensor surface of upper limbs (6%) and face (6%).

The mean time of disappearance of the skin lesions after adoption of GFD was about one month in the patients enrolled, much shorter than in DH.

On the contrary to DH, we have not identified a specific histological pattern: the histological characteristics may change during the time just as we said previously about the morphology of the lesions. In particular, in the early stages, lymphocytic infiltrate and spongiosis may be present, while in the later phases hyperkeratosis and mixed infiltrate are prevalent. However, to prove this as certain, we need further research with a larger number of patients.

DH IgA deposits along DEJ with typical reinforcing of the dermal papillae represents either the specific immunological pattern or the gold standard for the diagnosis. This is the reason why we excluded DH in all patients enrolled. In fact, the C3 fraction of the complementary system was the only reactant present in more than a half of the patients (82%) in particular localized along the DEJ in granular or micro-granular pattern, while IgA were present in an insignificant number of patients and still without a specific pattern of distribution. Further studies are needed to define the specificity and sensitivity of the C3 deposits along the DEJ in the diagnosis of CGS. If our partial data should be confirmed, the absence of a biomarker for the diagnosis of NCGS may offset the skin biopsy, at least in those patients with cutaneous manifestations, such as in celiac patients with DH [18]. Furthermore, the involvement of the complementary system may confirm the predominant role of an innate immunity in the pathogenesis of CGS, as suggested for NCGS and the attempt to induce an antigen-specific tolerance resulted in the production of transforming growth factor-beta and interleukin-10 [19].

Even if in our research we have not considered a control after the GFD, all enrolled patients are still in follow-up and they are showing rapid clinical and immunopathological resolution with a disappearance of lesions and deposits only after a month of GFD.

To sum up, in our experience a lot of non-celiac patients with intestinal symptoms compatible with NCGS showed non-specific, often itchy, dermatoses that, in some of the cases, were overlapped by morphology and localization with the DH, the specific cutaneous manifestation of CD. In other patients, instead, it coincided with the eczematoid or psoriasiform appearance. Moreover, if a gluten free diet is adopted to address the intestinal disorders, skin manifestations are resolved or they improve significantly. The histological and immunopathological assays performed on skin samples exclude specific skin diseases of CD and the allergy skin tests exclude sensitization to gluten. Therefore, it is reasonable to assume that there may also appear skin manifestations among the extraintestinal manifestations of NCGS or that "cutaneous gluten sensitivity" (CGS) exists and needs to be characterized and this is the aim of this study. Probably, the late diagnosis in patients we evaluated was due to the lack of knowledge of this new clinical entity and its potential connections with other systems, primarily the skin.

5. Conclusions

At the moment, the results of our study do not allow the exact characterization of a new skin disease related to NCGS. The skin lesions observed were similar both to eczema and psoriasis and did not show a specific histological pattern. Furthermore, no serological marker was useful to identify these patients. The only data common to most of these patients affected by NCGS associated to non-specific skin manifestations are:

1. the itching;
2. the presence of C3 at the dermoepidermal junction;
3. a rapid resolution of lesions when adopting the gluten free diet.

Nevertheless, we want to stress once again the importance of a close collaboration between gastroenterologists and dermatologists, because the gastrointestinal system and the skin may be considered more and more "two sides of the same coin". The exact characterization of new clinical entities such as CGS and NCGS is an important objective both for diagnostic and therapeutic purposes, since these are patients who actually benefit from a GFD and who do not adopt it only for fashion. Therefore, dermatologists must be familiar with the cutaneous manifestations and symptoms of gastrointestinal disorders. An appropriate understanding, work-up, consultation and management will help to identify the important cutaneous—gastrointestinal connection and ensuring that this important gastroenterological disease in patients with skin manifestations is not ignored.

Finally, we suggest an accurate follow-up of all patients who report intense itching and gastrointestinal disorders, even when histology and morphology of the skin lesions do not identify a specific skin disease. We also suggest the adoption of GFD for at least three months assessing any positive effects.

Acknowledgments: The authors thank Emiliano Antiga (Department of Surgery and Translational Medicine, Section of Dermatology, University of Florence, Florence, Italy) and Antonino Calabrò (Gastroenterology Unit, University of Florence, Florence, Italy) for their technical help and expertise.

Author Contributions: Veronica Bonciolini: She contributed to the design of the study, the production, analysis, or interpretation of the results, and preparation of the manuscript. Beatrice Bianchi: She contributed to the analysis of the results. Elena Del Bianco: She contributed to the analysis of the results. Alice Verdelli: She contributed to the production of the results. Marzia Caproni: She contributed to the design of the study, interpretation of the results and preparation of the manuscript.

Conflicts of Interest: The authors declare no conflicts of interest.

References

1. Timani, S.; Mutasin, D.F. Skin manifestations of inflammatory bowel disease. *Clin. Dermatol.* **2008**, *26*, 265–273. [CrossRef] [PubMed]
2. Huang, B.L.; Cahndra, S.; Shih, B.Q. Skin manifestations of inflammatory bowel disease. *Front. Physiol.* **2012**, *3*, 13. [CrossRef] [PubMed]
3. Shah, K.R.; Boland, C.R.; Patel, M.; Thrash, B.; Menter, A. Cutaneous manifestations of gastrointestinal disease: Part I. *J. Am. Acad. Dermatol.* **2013**, *68*, e1–e21. [CrossRef] [PubMed]
4. Marzano, A.V.; Borghi, A.; Stadnicki, A.; Crosti, C.; Cugno, M. Cutaneous manifestations in patients with inflammatory bowel diseases: Pathophysiology, clinical features and therapy. *Inflamm. Bowel Dis.* **2014**, *20*, 213–227. [CrossRef] [PubMed]
5. Caproni, M.; Bonciolini, V.; D'Errico, A.; Antiga, E.; Fabbri, P. Celiac disease and dermatologic manifestations: Many skin clue to unfold gluten-sensitive enteropathy. *Gastroenterol. Res. Pract.* **2012**. [CrossRef] [PubMed]
6. Humbert, P.; Pelletier, F.; Dreno, B.; Puzenat, E.; Aubin, F. Glutenintolerance and skin diseases. *Eur. J. Dermatol.* **2006**, *16*, 4–11. [PubMed]
7. Volta, U.; Bardella, M.T.; Calabrò, A.; Troncone, R.; Corazza, G.R. The Study Group for Non-Celiac Gluten Sensitivity. An Italian prospective multi-center survey on patients suspected of having non-celiac gluten sensitivity. *BMC Med.* **2014**, *12*, 85. [CrossRef] [PubMed]
8. Aziz, I.; Hadjivassiliou, M.; Sanders, D.S. The spectrum of non-celiac gluten sensitivity. *Nat. Rev. Gastroenterol. Hepatol.* **2015**. [CrossRef] [PubMed]
9. Kasarda, D. Can an increase in celiac disease be attributed to an increase in gluten content of wheat as a consequence of wheat breeding? *J. Agric. Food Chem.* **2013**, *61*, 1155–1159. [CrossRef] [PubMed]
10. Makharia, G.; Mulder, C.J.J.; Goh, K.L.; Ahuja, V.; Bai, J.C.; Catassi, C.; Green, P.H.R.; Gupta, S.D.; Lundin, K.E.A.; Ramakrishna, B.S.; *et al.* Issue associated with the emergence of coeliac disease in the Asia-Pacific region: A working party report of the World Gastroenterology Organization and the Asian Pacific Association of Gastroenterology. *J. Gastroenterol. Hepatol.* **2014**, *29*, 666–677. [CrossRef] [PubMed]
11. Lundin, K.E.A. Non-celiac gluten sensitivity-why worry? *BMC Med.* **2014**, *12*, 86. [CrossRef] [PubMed]
12. Hollon, J.; Puppa, E.L.; Greenwald, B.; Goldberg, E.; Guerrerio, A.; Fasano, A. Effect of gliadin on permeability of intestinal biopsy explants from celiac disease patients and patients with non-celiac gluten sensitivity. *Nutrients* **2015**, *7*, 1565–1576. [CrossRef] [PubMed]
13. Sapone, A.; Lammers, K.M.; Casolaro, V.; Cammarota, M.; Giuliano, M.T.; de Rosa, M.; Stefanile, R.; Mazzarella, G.; Tolone, C.; Russo, M.I.; *et al.* Divergence of gut permeability and mucosal immune gene expression in two gluten-associated conditions: Celiac disease and gluten sensitivity. *BMC Med.* **2011**, *9*, 23. [CrossRef] [PubMed]
14. Sapone, A.; Lammers, K.M.; Mazzarella, G.; Mikhailenko, I.; Cartenì, M.; Casolaro, V.; Fasano, A. Differential mucosal IL-17 expression in two gliadin-induced disorders: Gluten sensitivity and the autoimmune enteropathy celiac disease. *Int. Arch. Allergy Immunol.* **2010**, *152*, 75–80. [CrossRef] [PubMed]
15. Corazza, G.R.; Frazzoni, M.; Strocchi, A. Alimentary exorphin actions on motility and hormonal secretion of gastrointestinal tract. In *Opioid Peptides in the Periphery*; Fraioli, F., Isidori, A., Eds.; Elsevier Sciences: Amsterdam, The Netherlands, 1984; pp. 243–247.
16. Verdu, E.F.; Armstrong, D.; Murray, J.A. Between celiac disease and irritable bowel syndrome: The "no man's land" of gluten sensitivity. *Am. J. Gastrenterol.* **2009**, *104*, 1587–1594. [CrossRef] [PubMed]
17. Sapone, A.; Bai, J.C.; Ciacci, C.; Dolinsek, J.; Green, P.H.R.; Hadjivassiliou, M.; Kaukinen, K.; Rostami, K.; Sanders, D.S.; Schumann, M.; *et al.* Spectrum of gluten-related disorders: Consensus of new nomenclature and classification. *BMC Med.* **2012**, *10*, 13. [CrossRef] [PubMed]
18. Caproni, M.; Antiga, E.; Melani, L.; Fabbri, P.; The Italian Group for Cutaneous Immunopathology. Guidelines for the diagnosis and treatment of dermatitis herpetiformis. *J. Eur. Acad. Dermatol. Venereol.* **2009**, *23*, 633–638. [CrossRef] [PubMed]

19. Sohn, J.H.; Bora, P.S.; Suk, H.J.; Molina, H.; Kaplan, H.J.; Bora, N.S. Tolerance is dependent on complement C$_3$ fragment iC$_3$b binding to antigen presenting cells. *Nat. Med.* **2003**, *9*, 206–212. [CrossRef] [PubMed]

nutrients

MDPI

Case Report

Gluten Psychosis: Confirmation of a New Clinical Entity

Elena Lionetti [1,*], Salvatore Leonardi [1], Chiara Franzonello [1], Margherita Mancardi [2], Martino Ruggieri [1] and Carlo Catassi [3,4]

[1] Department of Pediatrics, University of Catania, Via S. Sofia 78, 95124 Catania, Italy; leonardi@unict.it (S.L.); franzo.chiara@gmail.com (C.F.); m.ruggieri@unict.it (M.R.)

[2] Pediatric Neuro-Psychiatric Unit, G. Gaslini Institute, Via Gerolamo Gaslini 5, 16147 Genova, Italy; margheritamancardi@ospedale-gaslini.ge.it

[3] Department of Pediatrics, Marche Polytechnic University, Ancona, Via Corridoni, 11, 60123 Ancona, Italy; c.catassi@univpm.it

[4] The Division of Paediatric Gastroenterology and Nutrition and Center for Celiac Research, MassGeneral Hospital for Children, 55 Fruit Street, Boston, MA 02114, USA

* Author to whom correspondence should be addressed; elenalionetti@inwind.it; Tel.: +39-953-781-782.

Received: 30 May 2015; Accepted: 2 July 2015; Published: 8 July 2015

Abstract: Non-celiac gluten sensitivity (NCGS) is a syndrome diagnosed in patients with symptoms that respond to removal of gluten from the diet, after celiac disease and wheat allergy have been excluded. NCGS has been related to neuro-psychiatric disorders, such as autism, schizophrenia and depression. A singular report of NCGS presenting with hallucinations has been described in an adult patient. We report a pediatric case of a psychotic disorder clearly related to NCGS and investigate the causes by a review of literature. The pathogenesis of neuro-psychiatric manifestations of NCGS is unclear. It has been hypothesized that: (a) a "leaky gut" allows some gluten peptides to cross the intestinal membrane and the blood brain barrier, affecting the endogenous opiate system and neurotransmission; or (b) gluten peptides may set up an innate immune response in the brain similar to that described in the gut mucosa, causing exposure from neuronal cells of a transglutaminase primarily expressed in the brain. The present case-report confirms that psychosis may be a manifestation of NCGS, and may also involve children; the diagnosis is difficult with many cases remaining undiagnosed. Well-designed prospective studies are needed to establish the real role of gluten as a triggering factor in neuro-psychiatric disorders.

Keywords: gluten; hallucinations; non celiac gluten sensitivity; psycosis

1. Introduction

Non-celiac gluten sensitivity (NCGS) is a syndrome diagnosed in patients with symptoms that respond to removal of gluten from the diet, after CD and wheat allergy have been excluded [1,2]. The description of this condition is mostly restricted to adults, including a large number of patients previously labeled with "irritable bowel syndrome" or "psychosomatic disorder" [1].

The "classical" presentation of NCGS is, indeed, a combination of gastro-intestinal symptoms including abdominal pain, bloating, bowel habit abnormalities (either diarrhea or constipation), and systemic manifestations including disorders of the neuropsychiatric area such as "foggy mind", depression, headache, fatigue, and leg or arm numbness [1–3]. In recent studies, NCGS has been related to the appearance of neuro-psychiatric disorders, such as autism, schizophrenia and depression [2,4]. The proposed mechanism is a CD-unrelated, primary alteration of the small intestinal barrier (leaky gut) leading to abnormal absorption of gluten peptides that can eventually reach the central nervous system stimulating the brain opioid receptors and/or causing neuro-inflammation. A singular report of NCGS presenting with hallucinations has also been described in an adult patient showing an indisputable correlation between gluten and psychotic symptoms [5].

Here we report a pediatric case of a psychotic disorder clearly related to NCGS.

2. Case Report

A 14-year-old girl came to our outpatient clinic for psychotic symptoms that were apparently associated with gluten consumption.

The pediatric ethical committee of the Azienda Universitaria Ospedaliera Policlinico Vittorio Emanuele di Catania approved the access to the patient records. Written informed consent was obtained from the parents of the child.

She was first-born by normal delivery of non-consanguineous parents. Her childhood development and growth were normal. The mother was affected by autoimmune thyroiditis. She had been otherwise well until approximately two years before. In May 2012, after a febrile episode, she became increasingly irritable and reported daily headache and concentration difficulties. One month after, her symptoms worsened presenting with severe headache, sleep problems, and behavior alterations, with several unmotivated crying spells and apathy. Her school performance deteriorated, as reported by her teachers. The mother noted severe halitosis, never suffered before. The patient was referred to a local neuropsychiatric outpatient clinic, where a conversion somatic disorder was diagnosed and a benzodiazepine treatment (*i.e.*, bromazepam) was started. In June 2012, during the final school examinations, psychiatric symptoms, occurring sporadically in the previous two months, worsened. Indeed, she began to have complex hallucinations. The types of these hallucinations varied and were reported as indistinguishable from reality. The hallucinations involved vivid scenes either with family members (she heard her sister and her boyfriend having bad discussions) or without (she saw people coming off the television to follow and scare her), and hypnagogic hallucinations when she relaxed on her bed. She also presented weight loss (about 5% of her weight) and gastrointestinal symptoms such as abdominal distension and severe constipation. She was admitted to a psychiatric ward. Detailed physical and neurological examinations, as well as routine blood tests were normal. In order to exclude an organic neuropsychiatric cause of psychosis, the following tests were done: rheumatoid factor, streptococcal antibody tests, autoimmunity profile (including anti-nuclear, anti-double-stranded DNA, anti-neutrophil cytoplasmic, anti-Saccharomyces, anti-phospholipid, anti-mitochondrial, anti-SSA/Ro, anti-SSB/La, anti-transglutaminase IgA (tTG), anti-endomysium (EMA), and anti-gliadin IgA (AGA) antibodies), and screening for infectious and metabolic diseases, but they resulted all within the normal range. The only abnormal parameters were anti-thyroglobulin and thyroperoxidase antibodies (103 IU/mL, and 110 IU/mL; v.n. 0–40 IU/mL). A computed tomography scan of the brain and a blood pressure holter were also performed and resulted normal. Electroencephalogram (EEG) showed mild nonspecific abnormalities and slow-wave activity. Due to the abnormal autoimmune parameters and the recurrence of psychotic symptoms, autoimmune encephalitis was suspected, and steroid treatment was initiated. The steroid led to partial clinical improvement, with persistence of negative symptoms, such as emotional apathy, poverty of speech, social withdrawal and self-neglect. Her mother recalled that she did not return a "normal girl". In September 2012, shortly after eating pasta, she presented crying spells, relevant confusion, ataxia, severe anxiety and paranoid delirium. Then she was again referred to the psychiatric unit. A relapse of autoimmune encephalitis was suspected and treatment with endovenous steroid and immunoglobulins was started. During the following months, several hospitalizations were done, for recurrence of psychotic symptoms. Cerebral and spinal cord magnetic resonance imaging, lumbar puncture, and fundus oculi examination did not show any pathological signs. Several EEG were performed confirming bilateral slow activity. The laboratory tests showed only mild microcytic anemia with reduced levels of ferritin and a slight increase in fecal calprotectin values (350 mg/dL, normal range: 0–50 mg/dL). In September 2013, she presented with severe abdominal pain, associated with asthenia, slowed speech, depression, distorted and paranoid thinking and suicidal ideation up to a state of pre-coma. The clinical suspicion was moving towards a fluctuating psychotic disorder. Treatment with a second-generation anti-psychotic (*i.e.*, olanzapine) was started, but psychotic symptoms persisted. In November 2013, due to gastro-intestinal symptoms and further weight loss (about 15% of her weight in the last year), a nutritionist was consulted, and a gluten-free diet (GFD) was recommended for symptomatic treatment of the intestinal complaints; unexpectedly, within a week of gluten-free diet, the symptoms (both gastro-intestinal and psychiatric) dramatically improved, and the GFD was continued for four months. Despite her efforts, she occasionally experienced inadvertent gluten exposures, which triggered the recurrence of her psychotic symptoms within about four hours. Symptoms took two to three days to subside again. Then, in April 2014 (two years after the onset of symptoms), she was admitted to our pediatric gastroenterology outpatient for suspected NCGS. Previous examinations excluded a diagnosis of CD because serology for CD was negative (*i.e.*, EMA, and tTG). A wheat allergy was excluded due to negativity of specific IgE to wheat, prick test, prick by prick and patch test for wheat resulted negative. Therefore, we decided to perform a double-blind challenge test with wheat flour and rice flour (one pill containing 4 g of wheat flour or rice flour for the first day, following two pills in the second day and 4 pills from the third day to 15 days, with seven days of wash-out between the two challenges). During the administration of rice flour, symptoms were absent. During the second day of wheat flour intake, the girl presented headache, halitosis, abdominal distension, mood disorders, fatigue, and poor concentration, and three episodes of severe hallucinations. After the challenge, she tested negative for: (1) CD serology (EMA and tTG); (2) food specific IgE; (3) skin prick test to wheat (extract and fresh food); (4) atopy patch test to wheat; and (5) duodenal biopsy. Only serum anti-native gliadine antibodies of IgG class and stool calprotectin were elevated.

Due to parental choice, the girl did not continue assuming gluten and she started a gluten-free diet with a complete regression of all symptoms within a week. The adherence to the GFD was evaluated by a validated questionnaire [6]. One month after AGA IgG and calprotectin resulted negative, as well as the EEG, and ferritin levels improved. She returned to the same neuro-psychiatric specialists that now reported a "normal behavior" and progressively stopped the olanzapine therapy without any problem. Her mother finally recalled that she was returned a "normal girl". Nine months after definitely starting the GFD, she is still symptoms-free.

3. Discussion

To our knowledge, this is the first description of a pre-pubertal child presenting with a severe psychotic manifestation that was clearly related to the ingestion of gluten-containing food and showing complete resolution of symptoms after starting treatment with the gluten-free diet.

Until a few years ago, the spectrum of gluten-related disorders included only CD and wheat allergy, therefore our patient would be turned back home as a "psychotic patient" and receive lifelong treatment with anti-psychotic drugs. Recent data, however, suggested the existence of another form of gluten intolerance, known as NCGS [2,4,7]. NCGS is a condition in which symptoms are triggered by gluten ingestion, in the absence of celiac-specific antibodies and of classical celiac villous atrophy, with variable HLA status and variable presence of first generation AGA. Symptoms usually occur soon after gluten ingestion, disappear with gluten withdrawal and relapse following gluten challenge, within hours or few days. No specific blood test is available for diagnosing NCGS [2].

In our case report, the correlation of psychotic symptoms with gluten ingestion and the following diagnosis of NGCS were well demonstrated; the girl was, indeed, not affected by CD, because she showed neither the typical CD-related autoantibodies (anti-tTG and EMA) nor the signs of intestinal damage at the small intestinal biopsy. Features of an allergic reaction to gluten were lacking as well, as shown by the absence of IgE or T-cell-mediated abnormalities of immune response to wheat proteins. The double-blind gluten challenge, currently considered the gold standard for the diagnosis of NCGS, clearly showed that the elimination and reintroduction of gluten was followed by the disappearance and reappearance of symptoms.

Interestingly, a similar case-report of a 23-years-old female with auditory and visual hallucinations that resolved with gluten elimination has been recently reported [5].

The present case-report confirms that: (a) psychotic disorders may be a manifestation of NCGS; (b) neuro-psychiatric symptoms may involve also children with NCGS; and (c) the diagnosis is difficult and many cases may remain undiagnosed.

The possible causes of psychosis in children and young people are not well understood. It is thought to be the result of a complex interaction of genetic, biological, psychological and social factors. However, we still know relatively little about which specific genes or environmental factors are involved and how these factors interact and actually cause psychotic symptoms [8]. Several studies suggested a relationship between gluten and psychosis [9–27] or other neuro-psychiatric disorders [28–31]; however, it remains a highly debated and controversial topic that requires well-designed prospective studies to establish the real role of gluten as a triggering factor in these diseases [2,27].

On the other hand, the pathogenesis of neuro-psychiatric manifestations of NCGS is an intriguing and still poorly understood issue. It has been hypothesized that some neuro-psychiatric symptoms related to gluten may be the consequence of the excessive absorption of peptides with opioid activity that formed from incomplete breakdown of gluten. Increased intestinal permeability, also referred to as "leaky gut syndrome", may allows these peptides to cross the intestinal membrane, enter the bloodstream, and cross the blood brain barrier, affecting the endogenous opiate system and neurotransmission within the nervous system [2,32]. Interestingly, in our case, we observed an elevation of fecal calprotectin that resolved during gluten-free diet, suggesting that a certain degree of gut inflammation may be found in NCGS. The role of stool calprotectin as a biomarker of NCGS requires further evaluation.

Recently, a higher prevalence of antibodies directed toward tTG6 (a transglutaminase primarily expressed in the brain) has been observed in adult patients affected by schizophrenia [26]; this finding suggests that these autoantibodies could have a role in the pathogenesis of the neuro-psychiatric manifestations seen in NCGS. It is possible that gluten peptides (either directly or through activation of macrophages/dendritic cells) may set up an innate immune response in the brain similar to that described in the gut mucosa, causing exposure of tTG6 from neuronal cells. Access of these gluten peptides and/or activated immune cells to the brain may be facilitated by a breach of the blood brain barrier [26]. Evidence from the literature supports the notion that a subgroup of psychotic patients shows increased expression of inflammatory markers including haptoglobin-2 chains α and β [33]. Zonulin is a tight junction modulator that is released by the small intestine mucosa upon gluten stimulation. Interestingly the zonulin receptor, identified as the precursor for haptoglobin-2, has been found in the human brain. Overexpression of zonulin (aka haptoglobin-2) could be involved in the blood brain barrier disruption similarly to the role that zonulin plays in increasing intestinal permeability. This hypothesis is supported by the observation that zonulin analogues can modulate the blood brain barrier by increasing its permability to high molecular weight markers and chemotherapeutic agents. In recent years, there has been a growing emphasis on early detection and intervention of psychotic symptoms in order to delay or possibly prevent the onset of psychosis and schizophrenia [8]. Children and young people with schizophrenia tend to have a shorter life expectancy than the general population, largely because of suicide, injury, or cardiovascular disease, the last partly related to chronic treatment with antipsychotic medication [34]. Moreover, psychotic disorders in children and young people (up to age 17 years) are the leading causes of disability, owing to disruption to social and cognitive development [8]. Shedding light on the possible role of gluten in this context may significantly change the life for a subset of these patients, as shown by the case described in this case-report.

4. Conclusions

The present case report shows that psychosis may be a manifestation of NCGS, and may also involve children; the diagnosis is difficult with many cases remaining undiagnosed. The pathogenesis of neuropsychiatric manifestations of NCGS is an intriguing and still poorly understood issue. Well designed prospective studies are needed to establish the real role of gluten as a triggering factor in these diseases.

Author Contributions: E.L., S.L. and M.R. observed the case and contributed to acquisition of data; E.L. and C.F. performed the review of literature and analyzed the data; E.L. and C.C. wrote the paper; and all authors contributed to revision of the paper.

Conflicts of Interest: Carlo Catassi served as consultant for Menarini diagnostics s.r.l., and for Shaer. Elena Lionetti served as consultant for Heinz Company.

References

1. Sapone, A.; Bai, J.C.; Ciacci, C.; Dolinsek, J.; Green, P.H.; Hadjivassiliou, M.; Kaukinen, K.; Rostami, K.; Sanders, D.S.; Schumann, M.; *et al.* Spectrum of gluten-related disorders: Consensus on new nomenclature and classification. *BMC Med.* **2012**, *10*, 13. [CrossRef] [PubMed]
2. Catassi, C.; Bai, J.C.; Bonaz, B.; Bouma, G.; Calabrò, A.; Carroccio, A.; Castillejo, G.; Ciacci, C.; Cristofori, F.; Dolinsek, J.; *et al.* Non-Celiac Gluten sensitivity: The new frontier of gluten related disorders. *Nutrients* **2013**, *5*, 3839–3853. [CrossRef] [PubMed]
3. Volta, U.; Bardella, M.T.; Calabrò, A.; Troncone, R.; Corazza, G.R.; Study Group for Non-Celiac Gluten Sensitivity. An Italian prospective multicenter survey on patients suspected of having non-celiac gluten sensitivity. *BMC Med.* **2014**, *12*, 85. [CrossRef] [PubMed]
4. Fasano, A.; Sapone, A.; Zevallos, V.; Schuppan, D. Nonceliac gluten sensitivity. *Gastroenterology* **2015**, *148*, 1195–1204. [CrossRef] [PubMed]
5. Biagi, F.; Andrealli, A.; Bianchi, P.I.; Marchese, A.; Klersy, C.; Corazza, G.R. A gluten-free diet score to evaluate dietary compliance in patients with coeliac disease. *Br. J. Nutr.* **2009**, *102*, 882–887. [CrossRef] [PubMed]
6. Genuis, S.J.; Lobo, R.A. Gluten sensitivity presenting as a neuropsychiatric disorder. *Gastroenterol. Res. Pract.* **2014**, *2014*. [CrossRef] [PubMed]
7. Francavilla, R.; Cristofori, F.; Castellaneta, S.; Polloni, C.; Albano, V.; Dellatte, S.; Indrio, F.; Cavallo, L.; Catassi, C. Clinical, serologic, and histologic features of gluten sensitivity in children. *J. Pediatr.* **2014**, *164*, 463–467. [CrossRef] [PubMed]
8. NICE. Psychosis and schizophrenia in children and young people: Recognition and management. In *NICE Clinical Guidance 155*; The British Psychological Society: Leicester, UK; The Royal College of Psychiatrists: London, UK, 2013; Available online: http://www.nice.org.uk/CG155 (accessed on 2 April 2015).
9. Dohan, F.C.; Martin, L.; Grasberger, J.C.; Boehme, D.; Cottrell, J.C. Antibodies to wheat gliadin in blood of psychiatric patients: Possible role of emotional factors. *Biol. Psychiatry* **1972**, *5*, 127–137. [PubMed]
10. Hekkens, W.T.J.M. Antibodies to gliadin in serum of normals, coeliac patients & schizophrenics. In *Biological Basis of Schizophrenia*, 1st ed.; Hemmings, G., Hemmings, W.A., Eds.; MTP Press: Lancaster, PA, USA, 1978; pp. 259–261.
11. Mascord, I.; Freed, D.; Durrant, B. Antibodies to foodstuffs in schizophrenia. *Br. Med. J.* **1978**, *1*, 1351. [CrossRef] [PubMed]
12. Hekkens, W.T.J.M.; Schipperijn, A.J.M.; Freed, D.L.J. Antibodies to wheat proteins in schizophrenia: Relationship or coincidence? In *Biochemistry of Schizophrenia & Addiction*, 1st ed.; Hemmings, G., Ed.; MTP Press: Lancaster, PA, USA, 1980; pp. 125–133.
13. McGuffin, P.; Gardiner, P.; Swinburne, L.M. Schizophrenia, celiac disease, and anti- bodies to food. *Biol. Psychiatry* **1981**, *16*, 281–285. [PubMed]
14. Sugerman, A.A.; Southern, D.L.; Curran, J.F. A study of antibody levels in alcoholic, depressive, and schizophrenic patients. *Ann. Allergy* **1982**, *48*, 166–171. [PubMed]
15. Rix, K.J.B.; Ditchfield, J.; Freed, D.L.J.; Goldberg, D.P.; Hillier, V.F. Food antibodies in acute psychoses. *Psychol. Med.* **1985**, *15*, 347–354. [CrossRef] [PubMed]

16. Rybakowski, J.K.; Chorzelski, T.P.; Sulej, J. Lack of IgA-class endomysial antibodies, the specific marker of gluten enteropathy. *Med. Sci. Res.* **1990**, *18*, 311.

17. Reichelt, K.L.; Landmark, J. Specific IgA antibody increases in schizophrenia. *Biol. Psychiatry* **1995**, *37*, 410–413. [CrossRef]

18. Peleg, R.; Ben-Zion, Z.I.; Peleg, A.; Gheber, L.; Kotler, M.; Weizman, Z.; Shiber, A.; Fich, A.; Horowitz, Y.; Shvartzman, P. "Bread madness" revisited: Screening for specific celiac antibodies among schizophrenia patients. *Eur. Psychiatry* **2004**, *19*, 311–314. [CrossRef] [PubMed]

19. Saetre, P.; Emilsson, L.; Axelsson, E.; Kreuger, J.; Lindholm, E.; Jazin, E. Inflammation- related genes up-regulated in schizophrenia brains. *BMC Psychiatry* **2007**, *7*, 46. [CrossRef] [PubMed]

20. Samaroo, D.; Dickerson, F.; Kasarda, D.D.; Green, P.H.; Briani, C.; Yolken, R.H.; Alaedini, A. Novel immune response to gluten in individuals with schizophrenia. *Schizophr. Res.* **2010**, *118*, 248–255. [CrossRef] [PubMed]

21. Dickerson, F.; Stallings, C.; Origoni, A.; Vaughan, C.; Khushalani, S.; Leister, F.; Yang, S.; Krivogorsky, B.; Alaedini, A.; Yolken, R. Markers of gluten sensitivity and celiac disease in recent-onset psychosis and multi-episode schizophrenia. *Biol. Psychiatry* **2010**, *68*, 100–104. [CrossRef] [PubMed]

22. Cascella, N.G.; Kryszak, D.; Bhatti, B.; Gregory, P.; Kelly, D.K.; mc Evoy, J.P.; Fasano, A.; Willimans, W.W. Prevalence of celiac disease and gluten sensitivity in the United States clinical antipsychotic trials of intervention effectiveness study population. *Schizophr. Bull.* **2011**, *37*, 94–100. [CrossRef] [PubMed]

23. Sidhom, O.; Laadhar, L.; Zitouni, M.; Ben Alaya, N.; Rafrafi, R.; Kallel-Sellami, M.; Makni, S. Spectrum of autoantibodies in Tunisian psychiatric inpatients. *Immunol. Investig.* **2012**, *41*, 538–549. [CrossRef] [PubMed]

24. Jin, S.Z.; Wu, N.; Xu, Q.; Zhang, X.; Ju, G.Z.; Law, M.H.; Wei, J. A study of circulating gliadin antibodies in schizophrenia among a Chinese population. *Schizophr. Bull.* **2012**, *38*, 514–518. [CrossRef] [PubMed]

25. Okusaga, O.; Yolken, R.H.; Langenberg, P.; Sleemi, A.; Kelly, D.L.; Vaswani, D.; Postolache, T.T. Elevated gliadin antibody levels in individuals with schizophrenia. *World J. Biol. Psychiatry* **2013**, *14*, 509–515. [CrossRef] [PubMed]

26. Cascella, N.G.; Santora, D.; Gregory, P.; Kelly, D.L.; Fasano, A.; Eaton, W.W. Increased prevalence of transglutaminase 6 antibodies in sera from schizophrenia patients. *Schizophr. Bull.* **2013**, *39*, 867–871. [CrossRef] [PubMed]

27. Lachance, L.R.; McKenzie, K. Biomarkers of gluten sensitivity in patients with non-affective psychosis: A meta-analysis. *Schizophr. Res.* **2014**, *152*, 521–527. [CrossRef] [PubMed]

28. Lionetti, E.; Francavilla, R.; Pavone, P.; Pavone, L.; Francavilla, T.; Pulvirenti, A.; Giugno, R.; Ruggieri, M. The neurology of coeliac disease in childhood: What is the evidence? A systematic review and meta-analysis. *Dev. Med. Child Neurol.* **2010**, *52*, 700–707. [CrossRef] [PubMed]

29. Hadjivassiliou, M.; Sanders, D.S.; Grünewald, R.A.; Woodroofe, N.; Boscolo, S.; Aeschlimann, D. Gluten sensitivity: From gut to brain. *Lancet Neurol.* **2010**, *9*, 318–330. [CrossRef]

30. Hadjivassiliou, M.; Grunewald, R.A.; Chattopadhyay, A.K.; Davies-Jones, G.A.; Gibson, A.; Jarratt, J.A.; Kandler, R.H.; Lobo, A.; Powell, T.; Smith, C.M. Clinical, radiological, neurophysiological, and neuropathological characteristics of gluten ataxia. *Lancet* **1998**, *352*, 1582–1585. [CrossRef]

31. Dickerson, F.; Stallings, C.; Origoni, A.; Vaughan, C.; Khushalani, S.; Alaedini, A.; Yolken, R. Markers of gluten sensitivity and celiac disease in bipolar disorder. *Bipolar Disord.* **2011**, *13*, 52–58. [CrossRef] [PubMed]

32. Reichelt, K.L.; Seim, A.R.; Reichelt, W.H. Could schizophrenia be reasonably explained by Dohan's hypothesis on genetic interaction with a dietary peptide overload? *Prog. Neuropsychopharmacol. Biol. Psychiatry* **1996**, *20*, 1083–1114. [CrossRef]

33. Yang, Y.; Wan, C.; Li, H.; Zhu, H.; La, Y.; Xi, Z.; Chen, Y.; Jiang, L.; Feng, G.; He, L. Altered levels of acute phase proteins in the plasma of patients with schizophrenia. *Anal. Chem.* **2006**, *78*, 3571–3576. [CrossRef] [PubMed]

34. Hollis, C. Adult outcomes of child and adolescent onset schizophrenia: Diagnostic stability and predictive validity. *Am. J. Psychiatry* **2000**, *157*, 1652–1659. [CrossRef] [PubMed]

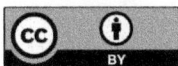

nutrients

MDPI

Article

Recognising and Managing Refractory Coeliac Disease: A Tertiary Centre Experience

Ikram Nasr [1,†], Iman Nasr [2,†], Carl Beyers [3], Fuju Chang [3], Suzanne Donnelly [1] and Paul J. Ciclitira [1,*]

[1] Gastroenterology Department, Guys and St Thomas' Hospital, Westminster Bridge Road, London SE1 7EH, UK; ikramnasr@hotmail.com (I.N.); suzannedonnelly@nhs.uk (S.D.)

[2] Allergy and Immunology Department, Pathology and Pharmacy Building, Royal London Hospital, 80 Newark Street, London E1 2ES, UK; drimannasr@gmail.com

[3] Department of Pathology, Guys and St Thomas' Hospital, Westminster Bridge Road, London SE1 7EH, UK; Carl.Beyers@viapath.co.uk (C.B.); fuju.chang@gstt.nhs.uk (F.C.)

* Correspondence: paul.ciclitira@kcl.ac.uk; Tel.: +44-20-7188-7188 (ext. 82486); Fax: +44-20-7188-2484

† These authors contributed equally to this work.

Received: 22 October 2015; Accepted: 16 November 2015; Published: 1 December 2015

Abstract: Refractory coeliac disease (RCD) is a rare complication of coeliac disease (CD) and involves malabsorption and villous atrophy despite adherence to a strict gluten-free diet (GFD) for at least 12 months in the absence of another cause. RCD is classified based on the T-cells in the intra-epithelial lymphocyte (IEL) morphology into type 1 with normal IEL and type 2 with aberrant IEL (clonal) by PCR (polymerase chain reaction) for T cell receptors (TCR) at the β/γ loci. RCD type 1 is managed with strict nutritional and pharmacological management. RCD type 2 can be complicated by ulcerative jejunitis or enteropathy associated lymphoma (EATL), the latter having a five-year mortality of 50%. Management options for RCD type 2 and response to treatment differs across centres and there have been debates over the best treatment option. Treatment options that have been used include azathioprine and steroids, methotrexate, cyclosporine, campath (an anti CD-52 monoclonal antibody), and cladribine or fluadribine with or without autologous stem cell transplantation. We present a tertiary centre's experience in the treatment of RCD type 2 where treatment with prednisolone and azathioprine was used, and our results show good response with histological recovery in 56.6% of treated individuals.

Keywords: non-responsive coeliac disease (NRCD); refractory coeliac disease (RCD); gluten free diet (GFD); enteropathy associated T-cell lymphoma (EATL); ulcerative jejunitis; villous atrophy; T-cell receptor (TCR); clonality; polymerase chain reaction (PCR); intra-epithelial cell lymphocytes (IEL)

1. Introduction

Enteropathy related to coeliac disease (CD) occurs in genetically predisposed individuals upon exposure to toxic gluten resulting in various gastrointestinal and extra-gastrointestinal manifestations [1]. The symptoms include diarrhoea, bloating, symptoms of malabsorption and anaemia. Diagnosis is based on a positive coeliac serology in addition to duodenal biopsies, which can demonstrate villous atrophy and increased intraepithelial lymphocytes. The latter is considered the gold standard for diagnosis [2]. Most cases respond to a strict elimination of gluten from the diet, which is currently the only accepted treatment for CD. However, a group of patients may continue to exhibit symptoms despite treatment and some describe this as non-responsive coeliac disease (NRCD). The majority of NRCD is related to ongoing gluten ingestion, but in some other cases, the symptoms are not related to coeliac disease and investigation for an alternative diagnosis is recommended. Less frequently, the ongoing symptoms of malabsorption in patients with confirmed CD is secondary to refractory coeliac disease.

RCD is divided into primary (absent response to gluten-free diet (GFD)) or secondary (previously responded to GFD but has now relapsed) [3]. Another classification is type 1 and type 2 based on the clonality of the T-cell receptors. Differentiating between RCD type 1 and RCD type 2 is not easy and requires experience and good diagnostic services. It is necessary to recognize and manage RCD type 2, which has a less predicted response and a poor prognosis due to the associated complications including ulcerative jejunitis and enteropathy associated T-cell lymphoma (EATL). Diagnosing RCD type 1, RCD type 2, ulcerative jejunitis and EATL is frequently complex, requiring small intestinal biopsy histology, intra-epithelial lymphocyte (IEL) phenotype and morphology, and T-cell receptor (TCR) clonality testing using PCR to aid the diagnosis (Table 1) [4]. Treatment options vary due to the low incidence of RCD type 2 resulting in small numbers of randomized clinical trials. Prednisolone combined with a thiopurine has been used in some centres for treatment of RCD type 1 and RCD type 2 with good success [3]. There has been a reported clinical improvement in 75% of patients with RCD type 2 [5]. Malamut *et al.* observed a histologic response in some of the few cases with RCD type 2 following treatment with methotrexate or anti-tumor necrosis factor α [6]. Treatment with cladribine (2-chlorodeoxyadenosine (2-CdA)) was studied in 32 patients and a response noted in 18 cases with a statistically significant increase in survival. Alemtuzumab (an anti CD-52 monoclonal antibody) has been used in single or limited cases with variable success [7,8].

Table 1. Comparison between refractory coeliac disease (RCD) type 1, RCD type 2, ulcerative jejunitis and enteropathy associated T-cell lymphoma (EATL).

Investigations	RCD Type 1	RCD Type 2	Ulcerative Jejunitis	EATL
Histopathology	Identical to any Marsh classification of coeliac disease	Marsh ⩾ II	Mucosal ulceration with villous atrophy and IEL in adjacent mucosa.	Infiltration of medium-sized or large pleomorphic lymphoid cells
Intraepithelial lymphocyte (IEL) phenotype	>70% IEL are surface CD3+ and CD8+	Majority have an aberrant IEL CD3+/CD8− phenotype Rarely have normal CD3+ and CD8+	Mucosal ulceration with villous atrophy and IEL in adjacent mucosa.	Neoplastic cells are CD3+ and large cell variant are CD30+ Background IELs are mostly phenotypically abnormal (CD3+/CD8−)
T-cell receptor gamma gene rearrangement PCR	Polyclonal	Monoclonal	Monoclonal	Monoclonal

We report a single centre retrospective study of all cases of RCD type 2 using the coeliac database in a single centre between 2000 and 2015. We have concluded that Prednisolone combined with azathioprine can be used successfully to treat RCD type 2. Our experience shows it is a safe and successful approach to improve prognosis.

2. Methods

We reviewed the cases of RCD with negative coeliac serology retrospectively over a period of 15 years from 2000 to 2015. The information was collected from patient case notes and the hospital electronic patient records. Thirty-seven patients were diagnosed with RCD type 2 (59% female). The age range was 30–87 (mean age 58). We excluded 7 patients from the study: one was a recent diagnosis and was yet to commence treatment, 2 were diagnosed with RCD type 2 and referred to our centre, but we diagnosed established EATL, one had major comorbidities and opted not to start treatment, and 3 relocated abroad. The human leucocyte antigen (HLA) calls II gene, or HLA-DQ2, which is known to have a strong association with coeliac disease, was found in 86% of the cases. The patients with RCD type 2 (n = 30), were treated with azathioprine and prednisolone (n = 27). The other patients did not tolerate azathioprine and/or prednisolone or had side effects and were given alternative treatment with thioguanine (n = 1), methotrexate (n = 1) or mycophenolate mofetil (n = 1). The initial dose of prednisolone we used was 20 mg daily which is reduced to 15 mg/day, and if necessary to 10 mg/day, if the patients experience side effects. The standard dose of azathioprine used was 2–2.5 mg/Kg per day, but we checked the thiopurine methyltransferase (TPMT) levels to adjust the dose if necessary depending on the patient's methylation activity. Duodenal biopsies were immunostained and PCR of the TCR was performed. The molecular signature of the clones in each repeat biopsy was compared. We looked at the patient clinical outcome after follow up as (1) improvement or (2) remains RCD type 2 on ongoing treatment. We define improvement as conversion from RCD type 2 to RCD type 1 or responsive coeliac disease as indicated by improved symptoms of coeliac disease and malasborption in addition to evidence of downgrading of RCD type 2, including: improved histological Marsh criteria to less than 2, improved CD8 positivity on immunohistochemistery or change of TCR from monoclonal to polyclonal.

3. Results

Eighteen out of 30 patients (60%) completed treatment (Figure 1) and demonstrated improvement as summarized in Table 2. Although the polyclonality was not demonstrated in all the 18 patients, those who completed treatment with improved histological features but remained with a clonal γ-TCR population no longer demonstrated persistent clones (Table 3). The average duration of treatment was 18 to 60 months; 67% were treated for at least 36 months (Figure 2). Four patients were treated for 4 years and two patients required 5 years of treatment. The remaining 12 patients (40%) are on ongoing treatment (Table 4). The duration of treatment ranges between 12 and 78 months.

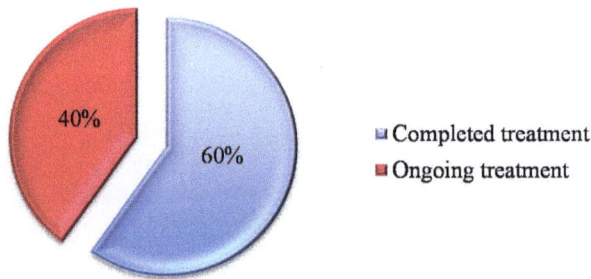

Figure 1. Refractory coeliac disease type 2 on treatment.

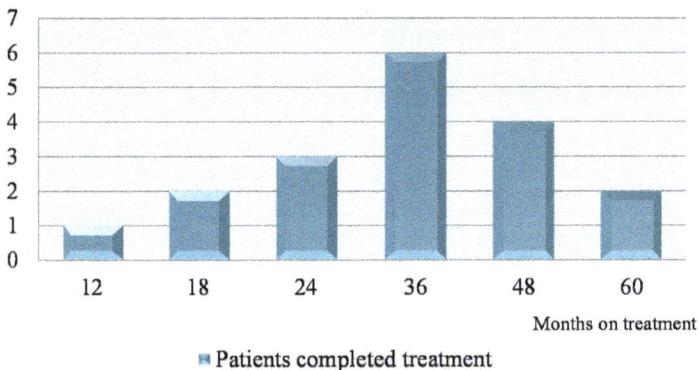

Figure 2. Duration of treatment in patients successfully treated.

Table 2. Baseline and post-treatment follow up data for patients with refractory coeliac disease type 2 who completed treatment.

Gender	Age	PRE-TREATMENT							TREATMENT			POST TREATMETN						Clinical Outcome
		Histology Marsh Grade	IEL Phenotype	T-Cell Receptor Status	Hb (g/dL)	Albumin (g/L)	B12 (ng/L)	Folate (ug/L)	Treatment	Time from Treatment (Months)	Histology Marsh Grade	IEL Phenotype	T-Cell Receptor Status	Hb (g/dL)	Albumin (g/L)	B12 (ng/L)	Folate (ug/L)	
Female	69	3a	CD8 + ve	Clonal	12.9	48	319	20	Azathioprine + Prednisolone	0	1	CD8 + ve	Polyclonal	13.9	52	407	3	Asymptomatic Good quality of life (QOL)
Female	83	3b	CD8 – ve	Clonal	11.7	35	294	17.3	Azathioprine + Prednisolone	6	3a	CD8 – ve	No amplification	11.6	40	495	4	Asymptomatic QOL affected by comorbidities.
Female	80	3b	CD8 – ve	Clonal	11	45	379	3.5	Azathioprine + Prednisolone	12	3a	CD8 – ve	Clonal	11.9	43	>128	4.5	Asymptomatic QOL affected by comorbidities.
Male	49	3b	CD8 + ve	Clonal	14	47	319	14.3	Azathioprine + Prednisolone	14	3a	CD8 – ve	Polyclonal	14.5	46	>128	17.2	Asymptomatic Good QOL
Female	79	3b	CD8 + ve	Clonal	14.8	47	279	4.7	Azathioprine + Prednisolone	18	3a	CD8 + ve	Polyclonal	14.9	49	>1000	7.2	Asymptomatic QOL affected by comorbidities.
Female	74	3c	CD8 – ve	Clonal	11.4	41	1500	6.9	Azathioprine + Prednisolone	20	3b	CD8 + ve	Polyclonal	NA	NA	NA	NA	Asymptomatic Good QOL
Male	50	3a	CD8 + ve	Clonal	14.2	49	177	15.4	Azathioprine + Prednisolone	21	1	CD8 + ve	Polyclonal	13.9	50	70	17.6	Asymptomatic Good QOL
Male	64	3a	CD8 – ve	Clonal	14.7	48	333	3.6	Azathioprine + Prednisolone	26	2	CD8 – ve	Polyclonal	14.9	50	500	3.4	Asymptomatic Good quality of life
Male	45	3a	CD8 – ve	Clonal	13.8	43	177	15.4	Azathioprine + Prednisolone	28	3a	CD8 + ve	Polyclonal	12.1	46	203	13.8	Asymptomatic Good QOL
Female	55	3a	CD8 + ve	Clonal	11.9	41	247	5.1	Azathioprine + Prednisolone	36	3a	CD8 + ve	Equivocal	127	44	198	5.8	Asymptomatic Good QOL
Female	66	3b	CD8 – ve 50%	Clonal	13.7	43	200	9.5	Azathioprine + Prednisolone	36	3a	CD8 + ve 75%	Equivocal	14.1	54	231	12	Asymptomatic Good QOL
Male	63	3a	CD8 – ve	Clonal	16.1	47	140	2	Azathioprine + Prednisolone	36	3a	CD8 – ve	Clonal	15.9	47	195	3.1	Asymptomatic Good QOL
Female	57	3b	CD8 + ve	Clonal	13.5	47	559	4.2	Azathioprine + Prednisolone	36	1	CD8 + ve	Polyclonal	14	46	470	18	Asymptomatic Good QOL
Female	67	3a	CD8 + ve	Clonal	13	46	696	16.8	Mycophenolate mofetil	36	3a	CD8 + ve	Polyclonal	12.9	46	128 (active B12)	5.2	Asymptomatic Good QOL
Male	71	3a	CD8 + ve 50%	Clonal	14.9	36	155	9.5	Azathioprine + Prednisolone	36	1	CD8 + ve 100%	Clonal	12.6	47	339	7.8	Asymptomatic QOL affected by comorbidities.
Male	70	3a	CD8 – ve	Clonal	13.7	48	64 (active B12)	5.2	Azathioprine + Prednisolone	53	1	CD8 – ve 50%	Polyclonal	15	45	68 (active B12)	20	Asymptomatic Good QOL
Female	84	3b	CD8 – ve	Clonal	12.4	38	81	12.3	Azathioprine + Budesonide	54	3b	CD8 + ve	Polyclonal	14.1	40	210	>20	Asymptomatic QOL affected by comorbidities.
Female	74	3b	CD8 – ve	Clonal	13.7	43	287	1.9	Azathioprine + Prednisolone	60	3b	CD8 – ve 50%	Polyclonal	11.7	42	86	2.7	Asymptomatic Good QOL

Table 3. Persistent identical clones observed at the start of treatment and at follow up.

Treatment Outcome	Number of Patients with Identical Clones at the Start of Treatment	Number of Cases with Identical Clones at the End of Treatment or at Latest Follow up
RCD type 2 patient responded to treatment (n = 18)	7 patients with identical clones	0 persistent clones
RCD type 2 who remain on treatment (n = 12)	9 patient identical clones	9 persistent identical clones

Table 4. Baseline and post-treatment follow up data for patients with refractory coeliac disease type 2 who are on ongoing treatment.

Gender	Age	PRE-TREATMENT							TREATMENT		POST TREATMENT						
		Histology Marsh Grade	IEL Phenotype	T-Cell Receptor Status	Hb (g/dL)	Albumin (g/L)	B12 (ng/L)	Folate (ug/L)	Treatment	Time from Treatment (Months)	Histology Marsh Grade	IEL Phenotype	T-Cell Receptor Status	Hb (g/dL)	Albumin (g/L)	B12 (ng/L)	Folate (ug/L)
Male	61	5.2	CD8 – ve	Clonal	12.9	28	42 (active B12)	5.2	Azathioprine + Prednisolone	12	NA	NA	Equivocal	NA	NA	NA	NA
Male	71	7.5	CD8 + ve 50%	Clonal	13.2	28	18	7.5	Azathioprine + Prednisolone	13	3a	CD8 – ve	Polyclonal	15.1	41	40	>20
Female	68	3c	CD8 + ve	Clonal	14.7	47	120	13.4	Thioguanine	21	3b	CD8 + ve	Polyclonal	14.9	49	78	7.7
Female	79	3a	CD8 + ve	Clonal	14.8	47	279	4.7	Azathioprine + Prednisolone	42	1	CD8 + ve	Clonal	NA	NA	NA	NA
Male	48	3b	CD8 – ve	Clonal	11.7	33	207	3.5	Methotrexate	57	3a	CD8 – ve	Clonal	14.8	38	54	12.6
Male	68	3c	CD8 – ve	Clonal	9.7	47	1500	3.6	Azathioprine + Prednisolone	60	0	CD8 + ve	Clonal	11.3	47	1500	8.5
Female	80	3a	CD8 + ve	Clonal	12.4	38	81	12.3	Azathioprine + Prednisolone	72	0	CD8 + ve	Clonal	14.1	40	210	>20
Female	64	3a	CD8 + ve	Clonal	12.4	46	210	2.6	Azathioprine + Prednisolone	72	1	CD8 – ve 50%	Clonal	13	49	127	13.6
Male	54	3a	CD8 + ve	Clonal	14.1	46	171	4.1	Azathioprine + Prednisolone	72	3a	CD8 + ve	Polyclonal	14.8	46	70 (active B12)	7.3
Male	77	3a	CD8 + ve	Clonal	14.6	41	286	3.1	Azathioprine + Prednisolone	74	3a	CD8 + ve	Clonal	14.3	45	123	8.6
Female	67	3a	CD8 + ve	Clonal	13.7	46	157	>20	Azathioprine + Prednisolone	78	3a	CD8 – ve	Clonal	142	45	na	4.5
Female	85	3b	CD8 – ve	Clonal	13.2	46	208	8.9	Azathioprine + Prednisolone	78	2	CD8 – ve	Clonal	134	41	37	18.1

Our data show that treatment of RCD type 2 with steroids and azathioprine show good response with a histological recovery in 16 out of 30 patients (53%). The TCR clonality improved converting to polyclonal in 17/30 (56.6%). None of the patients in our cohort developed ulcerative jejunitis or EATL, providing them with a better 5-year survival.

All patients continued to be on regular follow up after completing their treatment. We observed that all patients who completed treatment were asymptomatic and the percentage of CD8 positivity improved. We also observed persistent clones in the repeat duodenal biopsies of most of the refractory cases not responsive to treatment. Of the 12 patients who have not recovered, nine had persistent identical clones on repeat biopsies. Compared to the group who have completed treatment and improved to either RCD type 1 or responsive coeliac disease (18 patients), seven had identical clones at some point during surveillance (*p*-value 0.017).

4. Discussion

4.1. Non-Responsive Coeliac Disease (NRCD)

NRCD is defined as failure of expected symptomatic response to a GFD and is diagnosed clinically and histologically. Patients frequently complain of continued symptoms including lethargy, abdominal pain and diarrhoea. Laboratory tests often exhibit low iron, B12 and folate levels [2]. On small bowel biopsy, there is evidence of incomplete small intestinal mucosal recovery, although 40% of individuals with CD on GFD will have villous atrophy for over one year [3]. In RCD, there is loss of CD8 and expression of intra-cytoplasmic CD3 by intra-epithelial lymphocytes (IEL). The prevalence of RCD ranges from 1% to 2% of patients with CD and 0.002% in the general population [9], which explains the reason for the small number of affected individuals involved in clinical trials in tertiary referral centres.

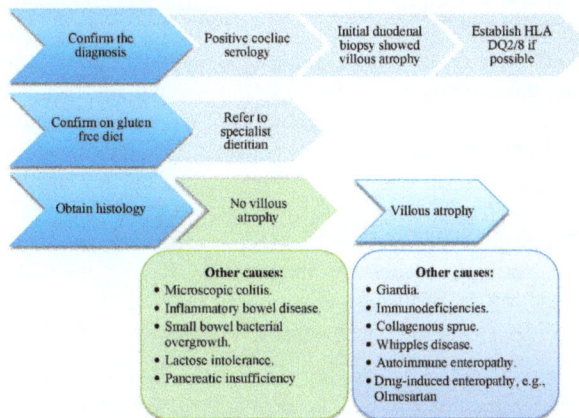

Figure 3. Approach to investigating non-responsive coeliac disease.

Establishing the cause for continued symptoms is the cornerstone for the management of NRCD (Figure 3). When approaching patients who remain symptomatic, it is necessary to classify them based on the history, presentation and investigations into (1) patients not adhering to a gluten-free diet; (2) a second diagnosis other than CD; (3) CD patients with complications; and (4) patients with RCD. RCD type 1 is considered if patients fail to improve after CD has been treated with GFD for one year. The most common cause of a NRCD is non-compliance with the diet or inadvertent gluten ingestion. This is estimated to occur in 90% of cases [10]. It is important when managing NRCD to bear in mind the conditions mimicking coeliac disease such as pancreatic insufficiency, lactose intolerance, small bowel bacterial overgrowth, inflammatory bowel disease, hypo-gammaglobulinemia, tropical sprue, collagenous colitis and adult onset autoimmune enteropathy. Excluding these conditions is, therefore, essential as part of the workup. This involves ensuring the individual is on a strict GFD, endoscopy with small intestinal biopsy for light microscopy, coeliac serology including IgA antibodies to tissue transglutaminase (tTG) and endomysium and polymerase chain reaction for T cell receptor monoclonality. Many centres check the immunoglobulin levels including IgA and IgG titres and subsequently test for IgG antibodies to tTG if there is IgA deficiency. Further testing includes HLA DQ2 and DQ8 status, colonoscopy, lactose and fructose intolerance, small bowel bacterial overgrowth and testing for pancreatic insufficiency. If the diagnosis of coeliac disease is confirmed, other causes for symptoms are ruled out and the patient is on a strict gluten exclusion diet, then the diagnosis of refractory coeliac disease may be entertained. Raised CD serology antibody titres imply continued gluten ingestion, either deliberate or inadvertent.

4.2. Refractory Coeliac Disease (RCD)

RCD is a subset of non-responsive patients with persistent or recurrent malabsorptive symptoms and signs with villous atrophy despite a strict GFD for more than 12 months [11]. Investigations will usually identify no other cause [5]. RCD is classified as primary or secondary based on the time of onset. Primary RCD is described when the individual with coeliac disease is never responsive to a GFD. On the other hand, secondary RCD occurs in patients who developed refractory coeliac having been responsive to a GFD before, months or even decades later.

The other classification is type 1 or type 2 RCD based on the phenotype of intra-epithelial lymphocytes. Type 1 RCD (RCD type 1) has a normal intra-epithelial lymphocyte phenotype whereas type 2 RCD (RCD type 2) has an abnormal clonal population. This classification is important not only to guide treatment but is of prognostic value. RCD type 2 carries a poor prognosis with a five-year mortality in RCD type 2 of about 55% [5]. RCD type 1 carries a much better prognosis with a mortality rate of 7% with aggressive treatment involving strict adherence to a GFD, nutritional support and pharmacologic intervention.

Complications of RCD include ulcerative jejunitis and enteropathy associated T-cell lymphoma (EATL), the latter being the major cause of mortality in these patients. RCD type 2 has a female preponderance with a female to male ration of 3:1, similar to responsive CD, but the ratio is reversed in EATL [6,12,13]. HLA DQ2 homozygosity is a risk factor for RCD type 2 and EATL [14].

4.3. Diagnosis

Diagnosis of RCD may be challenging and is in many cases a diagnosis of exclusion. Clinical assessment, pathological, histological, laboratory and radiological findings all aid in the diagnosis and enable to differentiate between the two subtypes.

In our centre, we follow a strategy when making a diagnosis of RCD type 2:

1. When making the diagnosis, the patient needs to be on a strict GFD with a negative anti-enterocyte antibody result. Dietary assessment of compliance to GFD is key and instruction and education by a specialized dietitian is advised.
2. Upper gastrointestinal endoscopy to obtain small bowel biopsies for tissue analysis. The samples are used for Marsh scoring.
3. Assessment of IEL phenotyping and polymerase chain reaction (PCR) for TCR (T-cell receptor) monoclonality at the β and/or γ loci.

The presence of abnormal (clonal) IEL in the small bowel supports a diagnosis of RCD type 2. Transient TCR clonality can be detected in patients at diagnosis and with poor compliance [15,16]. The TCR (T cell receptor) is a molecule found on the surface of T lymphocytes and is the site for antigen recognition that binds to the major histocompatibility complex (MHC)/CD-toxic gluten complex. The TCR is composed of two different protein chains which in 95% of all T cells comprises an alpha (α) and a beta (β) chain. α/β TCR are present on MHC restricted CD4+ (helper) and CD8+ (cytotoxic) T cells. In the remaining 5% these protein chains comprise the gamma and delta (γ/δ) chains, γ/δ TCR.

The majority of these do not express CD4 or CD8 and are not MHC restricted. They are abundant in epithelial tissues (IEL) where they represent 10% of human intestinal intra-epithelial cells. The role of γ/δ T cells is largely unknown, although they have a number of biologic activities similar to $\alpha/\beta/TCR$ such as cytokine secretion and lysis of target cells. It is hypothesized $\gamma/\delta TCR$ recognise antigens that are frequently encountered at epithelial boundaries between the host and external environment which may initiate immune responses before the recruitment of T cells. Not only do the histological and molecular features help differentiate between RCD type 1 and RCD type 2, but could additionally aid the diagnosis of ulcerative jejunitis and EATL (Table 1).

4. All cases of RCD type 2 should have a capsule endoscopy to exclude EATL (enteropathy associated T cell lymphoma). It is our practice if there is any suggestion of possible EATL to undertake a small bowel magnetic resonance imaging (MRI) in the first instance to exclude an obstructing lesion, which would be a contra-indication to capsule endoscopy. The capsule endoscopy should be repeated after a year to exclude the development of EATL in view of the high risk. It has been proposed that RCD type 2 should be renamed pre-EATL [17]. Double balloon enteroscopy may be required depending on the findings on capsule endoscopy in order to make a better assessment of an abnormality and obtain samples if required.

5. Cross sectional imaging including small bowel MRI, computed tomography (CT) scan and positron emission tomography (PET) scan are recommended when suspecting EATL. This can identify abnormal areas within the bowel, abnormal lymph nodes and other organ involvement.

Patients with RCD presenting with abdominal pain, weight loss or evidence of malnutrition should undergo urgent investigation. Cross-sectional imaging by CT $+/-$ PET or MRI for the presence of lymphadenopathy or intestinal tumours should be carried out and capsule or balloon enteroscopy should be performed to diagnose any cases of EATL [18].

4.4. Management of RCD Type 2

Several approaches to management of RCD type 2 have been trialed in different centres (Table 5). Treatment with budesonide alone has been reported to provide a good clinical response in refractory coeliac disease, but the effects on prognosis is not clear [19–22]. Treatment with a thiopurine, including azathioprine, mercaptopurine or thioguanine, combined with prednisolone has been used in our practice with good results. Some centres report an unfavourable response to this regimen, such as the Mulder group who reported a 52% progression to EATL [5]. It is our view that factors that may affect our positive results with treatment include early detection of RCD type 2 cases, close monitoring of the patients, adherence to treatment and a multidisciplinary approach in patient care. The latter involves an expert dietitian, histopathologist with knowledge of RCD and the availability of a molecular pathology TCR PCR service, that allows close monitoring. The percentage of aberrant IEL and the percentage of clonal TCR population may additionally play a role.

There have been other reports of different treatment options, some with limited cases and variable results. Methotrexate has been used as a single agent [5] or in combination with cyclosporine [23] in a few cases with good results. Campath (anti CD-52 monoclonal antibody) has been used on single or limited cases with variable success [8]. Cladribine or fluadribine with or without autologous stem cell transplantation has been another area of interest [24]. Mulder *et al.* reported 32 patients treated with cladribine, of whom 18 had a good response [25]. Cyclosporine has also been used in RCD type 2 [26–28]. Wahab *et al.* reported 61% histological improvement with this treatment in a group of 13 patients with RCD type 2 [29]. There have been single cases of successful treatment with infliximab, although some of these reported cases were used to treat RCD type 1 [30–32]. A multicenter study on the effect of anti-TNF treatment on RCD is required to establish the value of this treatment in RCD type 2.

Table 5. Treatment options in RCD type 2.

Treatment Option	Recommended Dose	Outcome	References
Budesonide	9 mg (range 6–12 mg)	Good Clinical response. Also used in maintenance of clinical remission in collagenous colitis	Brar *et al.* [19]. Daum *et al.* [20]. Miehlke *et al.* [21]. Bonderup *et al.* [22].
Combination thiopurine, including azathioprine, mercaptopurine or thioguanine, combined with prednisolone		52% progression to EATL within 4–6 years	Al-Toma *et al.* [12].
Alemtuzumab (anti CD-52 monoclonal antibody)	30 mg twice a week per 12 weeks	Not effective	Verbeek *et al.* [8].
		Effective	Vivas *et al.* [7].
Cladribine	0.1 mg/kg/day for 5 days	Thirty-two patients treated with cladribine, of whom 18 had a good response	Tack *et al.* [25].
		Six of 17 patients had clinical and histologic improvement Clinical improvement (36%), histological improvement (59%), and significant decrease in the number of clonal intraepithelial lymphocytes (35%). However, up to 41% developed EATL and died despite cladribine therapy.	Al-Toma *et al.* [33]
Cyclosporin A	5 mg/kg/day	Case report of histological and clinical improvement in a 45 year old lady with RCD type 2	Longstreth *et al.* [26].
		Single cases reported to show improvement of clinical parameters and mucosal abnormalities during treatment with cyclosporine	Bernstein *et al.* [27]. Eijsbouts *et al.* [28].
		61% histological improvement with this treatment in a group of 13 patients with RCD type 2	Wahab *et al.* [29].
Combination of pentostatin (4 mg/m² every two weeks per 24 weeks) and budesonide	Pentostatin (4 mg/m² every two weeks per 24 weeks)	Clinical and histological response as well as a decrease but not disappearance of clonal intraepithelial lymphocytes in 1 case	Dray *et al.* [34].
High-dose chemotherapy followed by ASCT has been explored for RCD type 2 in a pilot study from a single center		All 7 patients: Significant reduction in the aberrant T cells in duodenal biopsies associated with improvement 1 out of the 7 died of progressive neurosypillis	Al-Toma *et al.* [35].
		Out of the 4 patients with EATL, 1 patient sustained remission 32 months after ASCT. Three patients died from relapse within few months after ASCT.	Al-Toma *et al.* [36].

5. Conclusions

Prednisolone combined with azathioprine can be used successfully to treat RCD type 2. Our experience shows it is a safe and successful approach to improve prognosis. We successfully treated 18 out of 30 patients with RCD type 2 with this regimen, converting either to RCD type 1 or responsive coeliac disease. Where azathioprine and/or steroids are not tolerated or patients experience side effects, alternatives may be used. In our cohort, we used methotrexate ($n = 1$), thioguanine ($n = 1$) or mycophenolate mofetil ($n = 1$); the latter responded to treatment and converted to RCD type 1. Our data show improved outcomes with this management, which could be that we may be seeing affected subjects earlier through the UK tertiary referral system such that they may be less ill. In some centres, RCD type 2 patients are seen to have a serum albumin that we do not see. This suggests the patients that are referred to us are earlier in the disease process, and this may explain the improved outlook with less risk of developing EATL. In the azathioprine/steroid group, we block the aberrant immune response to gluten proteins that occurs in coeliac disease resulting in a better outcome than using other drugs with a different mechanism of action. The percentage of CD8 negative cells and/or the presence of persistent identical clones may have a role in persistent features of RCD type 2. Further studies are required to confirm this. The immunophenotyping is less sensitive than PCR TCR clonality testing. However, immunostains for CD3/CD8 are easier to be carried out in a routine pathology laboratory and almost always available in non-tertiary centres. This method can be used as a screening tool. Although the majority of IELs in RCD type 2 show an abnormal CD3+/CD8− immunophenotype, a normal CD3+/CD8+ phenotype has been seen in up to 52% of RCD type 2 cases [37]. However, some authors have questioned the reliability of this method. For instance, Goerres *et al.* found that only one out of eight RCD type 2 patients showed a loss of CD8 expression and concluded that other more sensitive ancillary tests such as flow cytometry may be necessary in the diagnosis of some RCD2 patients [19]. In flow cytometry, it is suggested that the percentage of aberrant IEL can differentiate between RCD type 1 and type 2, with type 1 exhibiting < 20% aberrant IEL and type 2 > 20%. Therefore, in our practice we used TCR clonality testing as an additional tool to confirm the diagnosis of RCD type 2. No reports appear to suggest a better prognosis of RCD2 patients with a CD3+/CD8+ immunophenotype. This could be an interesting area to explore in the future.

Acknowledgments: This manuscript was prepared using data obtained from the laboratory database with the help of Carl Beyers who also contributed to writing the article, particularly in relation to TCR data. Fuju Chang reviewed the histopathology specimens in addition to external specimens that were sent to him for second opinion. He has also contributed in writing, especially covering areas relating to histopathology and immunohistochemistry.

Author Contributions: Carl Beyers collected the patient data and provided the results for the TCR PCR. Fuju Chang reviewed the histopathology specimens and performed the immunohistochemistry. Paul Ciclitira supervised the process and provided the references. Ikram Nasr, Iman Nasr and Suzanne Donnelly analyzed the data, collected the patient results, summarized the outcomes and wrote up the manuscript.

Conflicts of Interest: The authors declare no conflict of interest.

References

1. Nasr, I.; Nasr, I.H.; Ciclitira, P.J. Patient management: Coeliac disease. *Found. Years J.* **2015**, *9*, 26–29.
2. Nasr, I.; Leffler, D.A.; Ciclitira, P.J. Management of celiac disease. *Gastrointest. Endosc. Clin. N. Am.* **2012**, *22*, 695–704. [CrossRef] [PubMed]
3. Woodward, J. The management of refractory coeliac disease. *Ther. Adv. Chronic Dis.* **2013**, *4*, 77–90. [CrossRef] [PubMed]
4. Cellier, C.; Delabesse, E.; Helmer, C.; Patey, N.; Matuchansky, C.; Jabri, B.; Macintyre, E.; Cerf-Bensussan, N.; Brousse, N.; the French Coeliac Disease Study Group. Refractory sprue, coeliac disease, and enteropathy-associated T-cell lymphoma. *Lancet* **2000**, *356*, 203–208. [CrossRef]
5. Rubio-Tapia, A.; Murray, J.A. Classification and management of refractory celiac disease. *Gut* **2010**, *59*, 547–557. [CrossRef] [PubMed]

6.   Malamut, G.; Afchain, P.; Verkarre, V.; Lecomte, T.; Amiot, A.; Damotte, D. Presentation and long term follow up of refractory coeliac disease: Comparison of type I with type II. *Gastroenterology* **2009**, *136*, 81–90. [CrossRef] [PubMed]

7.   Vivas, S.; de Morales, J.; Ramos, R.; Suárez-Vilela, D. Alemtuzumab for refractory celiac disease in a patient at risk for enteropathy-associated T-cell lymphoma. *N. Engl. J. Med.* **2006**, *354*, 2514–2515. [CrossRef] [PubMed]

8.   Verbeek, W.H.M.; Mulder, C.J.J.; Zweegman, S. Alemtuzumab for refractory celiac disease. *N. Engl. J. Med.* **2006**, *355*, 1396–1397. [PubMed]

9.   Di Sabatino, A.; Biagi, F.; Gobbi, P.G.; Corazza, G.R. How I treat enteropathy-associated T-cell lymphoma. *Blood* **2012**, *119*, 2458–2468. [CrossRef] [PubMed]

10. Dewar, D.H.; Donnelly, S.C.; McLaughlin, S.D.; Johnson, M.W.; Ellis, H.J.; Ciclitira, P.J. Coeliac disease: Management of persistent symptoms in patients on a gluten-free diet. *World J. Gastroenterol.* **2012**, *18*, 1348–1356. [CrossRef] [PubMed]

11. Ludvigsson, J.F.; Leffler, D.A.; Bai, J.; Biagi, F.; Fasano, A.; Green, P.H.; Hadjivassiliou, M.; Kaukinen, K.; Kelly, C.P.; Leonard, J.N.; *et al.* The Oslo definitions for coeliac disease and related terms. *Gut* **2013**, *62*, 43–52. [CrossRef] [PubMed]

12. Al-Toma, A.; Verbeek, M.; Hadithi, M.; von Blomberg, B.; Mulder, C. Survival in refractory coeliac disease and enteropathy-associated T-cell lymphoma: Retrospective evaluation of single centre experience. *Gut* **2007**, *56*, 1373–1378. [CrossRef] [PubMed]

13. Rubio-Tapia, A.; Kelly, D.; Lahr, B.; Dogan, A.; Wu, T.; Murray, J. Clinical staging and survival in refractory coeliac disease: A single center experience. *Gastroenterology* **2009**, *136*, 99–107. [CrossRef] [PubMed]

14. Al-Toma, A.; Goerres, M.S.; Meijer, J.W.; Peña, A.S.; Crusius, J.B.; Mulder, C.J. Human leukocyte antigen-DQ2 homozygosity and the development of refractory celiac disease and enteropathy-associated T-cell lymphoma. *Clin. Gastroenterol. Hepatol.* **2006**, *4*, 315–319. [CrossRef] [PubMed]

15. Prisco, A.; Troncone, R.; Mazzarella, G.; Gianfrani, C.; Auricchio, S.; Even, J. Identical T-cell receptor beta chain rearrangements are present in T cells infiltrating the jejunal mucosa of untreated coeliac patients. *Hum. Immunol.* **1997**, *55*, 22–33. [CrossRef]

16. Ubiali, A.; Villanacci, V.; Facchetti, F.; Lanzini, A.; Lanzarotto, F.; Rindi, G. Is TCRgamma clonality assay useful to detect early coeliac disease? *J. Clin. Gastroenterol.* **2007**, *41*, 275–279. [CrossRef] [PubMed]

17. Nijeboer, P.; Malamut, G.; Bouma, G.; Cerf-Bensussan, N.; Koning, F.; van Bergen, J.; Cellier, C.; Mulder, C.J.J. Therapy in RCDII: Rationale for combination strategies? *Dig. Dis.* **2015**, *33*, 227–230. [CrossRef] [PubMed]

18. Van Weyenberg, S.; Meijerink, M.; Jacobs, M.; van Kuijk, C.; Mulder, C.; van Waesberghe, J. MR enteroclysis in refractory coeliac disease: Proposal and validation of a severity scoring system. *Radiology* **2011**, *259*, 151–161. [CrossRef] [PubMed]

19. Brar, P.; Lee, S.; Lewis, S.; Egbuna, I.; Bhagat, G.; Green, P. Budesonide in the treatment of refractory celiac disease. *Am. J. Gastroenterol.* **2007**, *97*, 2016–2021. [CrossRef] [PubMed]

20. Daum, S.; Ipczynski, R.; Heine, B.; Schulzke, J.D.; Zeitz, M.; Ullrich, R. Therapy with budesonide in patients with refractory sprue. *Digestion* **2006**, *73*, 60–68. [CrossRef] [PubMed]

21. Miehlke, S.; Maddish, A.; Karimi, D.; Wonschik, S.; Kuhlisch, E.; Beckmann, R.; Morgner, A.; Mueller, R.; Greenwald, R.; Seitz, G.; *et al.* Budesonide is effective in treating lymphocytic colitis: A randomized double-blind placebo-controlled study. *Gastroenterology* **2009**, *136*, 2092–2100. [CrossRef] [PubMed]

22. Bonderup, O.K.; Hansen, J.B.; Birket-Smith, L.; Vestergaard, V.; Teglbjærg, P.S.; Fallingborg, J. Long-term budesonide treatment of collagenous colitis: A randomised, double-blind, placebo-controlled trial. *Gut* **2003**, *52*, 248–251. [CrossRef] [PubMed]

23. Malamut, G.; Meresse, B.; Verkarre, V.; Kaltenbach, S.; Montcuquet, N.; van Huyen, J.P.D.; Callens, C.; Lenglet, J.; Rahmi, G.; Samaha, E.; *et al.* Large granular lymphocytic leukemia: A treatable form of refractory coeliac disease. *Gastroenterology* **2012**, *143*, 1470–1472. [CrossRef] [PubMed]

24. Tack, G.J.; Wondergem, M.J.; al-Toma, A.; Verbeek, W.H.M.; Schmittel, A.; Machado, M.V.; Perri, F.; Ossenkoppele, G.J.; Huijgens, P.C.; Schreurs, M.W.J.; *et al.* Auto-SCT in refractory celiac disease type II patients unresponsive to cladribine therapy. *Bone Marrow Transpl.* **2011**, *46*, 840–846. [CrossRef] [PubMed]

25. Tack, G.J.; Verbeek, W.H.; al-Toma, A.; Kuik, D.J.; Schreurs, M.W.; Visser, O.; Mulder, C. Evaluation of Cladribine treatment in refractory celiac disease type II. *World J. Gastroenterol.* **2011**, *17*, 506–513. [CrossRef] [PubMed]

26. Bernstein, E.F.; Whitington, P.F. Successful treatment of atypical sprue in an infant with cyclosporin. *Gastroenterology* **1988**, *95*, 199–204. [PubMed]

27. Eijsbouts, A.M.M.; Witteman, B.J.M.; de Sevaux, R.G.L. Undefined malabsorption syndrome with villous atrophy successfully reversed by treatment with cyclosporin. *Eur. J. Gastroenterol. Hepatol.* **1995**, *7*, 803–806. [PubMed]

28. Wahab, P.J.; Crusius, J.B.; Meijer, J.W.; Uil, J.J.; Mulder, C. Cyclosporin in the treatment of adults with refractory coeliac disease—An open pilot study. *Aliment. Pharmacol. Ther.* **2000**, *14*, 767–774. [CrossRef] [PubMed]

29. Dray, X.; Joly, F.; Lavergne-Slove, A.; Treton, X.; Bouhnik, Y.; Messing, B. A severe but reversible refractory sprue. *Gut* **2006**, *55*, 1210–1211. [CrossRef] [PubMed]

30. Turner, S.M.; Moorghen, M.; Probert, C.S. Refractory coeliac disease: Remission with infliximab and immunomodulators. *Eur. J. Gastroenterol. Hepatol.* **2005**, *17*, 667–669. [CrossRef] [PubMed]

31. Rawal, N.; Twaddell, W.; Fasano, A.; Blanchard, S.; Safta, A. Remission of refractory coeliac disease with infliximab in a pediatric patient. *ACG Case Rep. J.* **2015**, *2*, 121–123. [PubMed]

32. Al-Toma, A.; Goerres, M.S.; Meijer, J.W.; von Blomberg, B.M.; Wahab, P.J.; Kerckhaert, J.A.; Mulder, C.J. Cladribine therapy in refractory celiac disease with aberrant T cells. *Clin. Gastroenterol. Hepatol.* **2006**, *4*, 1322–1327. [CrossRef] [PubMed]

33. Longstreth, G.F. Successful treatment of refractory sprue with cyclosporine. *Ann. Intern. Med.* **1993**, *119*, 1014–1016. [CrossRef] [PubMed]

34. Al-Toma, A.; Visser, O.J.; van Roessel, H.M.; von Blomberg, B.M.; Verbeek, W.H.; Scholten, P.E.; Ossenkoppele, G.J.; Huijgens, P.C.; Mulder, C.J. Autologous hematopoietic stem cell transplantation in refractory coeliac disease with aberrant T cells. *Blood* **2007**, *109*, 2243–2249. [CrossRef] [PubMed]

35. Al-Toma, A.; Verbeek, W.H.; Visser, O.J.; Kuijpers, K.C.; Oudejans, J.J.; Kluin-Nelemans, H.C.; Mulder, C.J.; Huijgens, P.C. Disappointing outcome of autologous stem cell transplantation for enteropathy-associated T-cell lymphoma. *Dig Liver Dis.* **2007**, *39*, 634–641. [CrossRef] [PubMed]

36. Gillett, H.R.; Arnott, I.D.; McIntyre, M.; Campbell, S.; Dahele, A.; Priest, M.; Jackson, R.; Ghosh, S. Successful infliximab treatment for steroid-refractory coeliac disease: A case report. *Gastroenterology* **2002**, *22*, 800–805. [CrossRef]

37. Patey-Mariaud de Serre, N.; Cellier, C.; Jabri, B. Distinction between coeliac disease and refractory sprue: A simple immunohistochemical method. *Histopathology* **2000**, *37*, 70–77. [CrossRef] [PubMed]

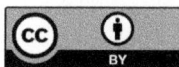

Section 3:
Treatment and Follow-Up

nutrients MDPI

Article

The Effects of Reduced Gluten Barley Diet on Humoral and Cell-Mediated Systemic Immune Responses of Gluten-Sensitive Rhesus Macaques

Karol Sestak [1,*], Hazel Thwin [1], Jason Dufour [2], Pyone P. Aye [2,3], David X. Liu [3] and Charles P. Moehs [4,*]

[1] Division of Microbiology, Tulane National Primate Research Center, Covington, LA 70433, USA; hthwin@tulane.edu

[2] Division of Veterinary Resources, Tulane National Primate Research Center, Covington, LA 70433, USA; jdufour@tulane.edu (J.D.); paye@tulane.edu (P.P.A.)

[3] Division of Comparative Pathology, Tulane National Primate Research Center, Covington, LA 70433, USA; dliu1@tulane.edu

[4] Arcadia Biosciences Inc., Seattle, WA 98119, USA; max.moehs@arcadiabio.com

* Correspondence: ksestak@tulane.edu (K.S.); max.moehs@arcadiabio.com (C.P.M.);
Tel.: +1-985-871-6409 (K.S.); +1-206-903-0262 (C.P.M.); Fax: +1-985-871-6248

Received: 20 January 2015; Accepted: 27 February 2015; Published: 6 March 2015

Abstract: Celiac disease (CD) affects approximately 1% of the general population while an estimated additional 6% suffers from a recently characterized, rapidly emerging, similar disease, referred to as non-celiac gluten sensitivity (NCGS). The only effective treatment of CD and NCGS requires removal of gluten sources from the diet. Since required adherence to a gluten-free diet (GFD) is difficult to accomplish, efforts to develop alternative treatments have been intensifying in recent years. In this study, the non-human primate model of CD/NCGS, e.g., gluten-sensitive rhesus macaque, was utilized with the objective to evaluate the treatment potential of reduced gluten cereals using a reduced gluten (RG; 1% of normal gluten) barley mutant as a model. Conventional and RG barleys were used for the formulation of experimental chows and fed to gluten-sensitive (GS) and control macaques to determine if RG barley causes a remission of dietary gluten-induced clinical and immune responses in GS macaques. The impacts of the RG barley diet were compared with the impacts of the conventional barley-containing chow and the GFD. Although remission of the anti-gliadin antibody (AGA) serum responses and an improvement of clinical diarrhea were noted after switching the conventional to the RG barley diet, production of inflammatory cytokines, e.g., interferon-gamma (IFN-γ), tumor necrosis factor (TNF) and interleukin-8 (IL-8) by peripheral CD4+ T helper lymphocytes, persisted during the RG chow treatment and were partially abolished only upon re-administration of the GFD. It was concluded that the RG barley diet might be used for the partial improvement of gluten-induced disease but its therapeutic value still requires upgrading—by co-administration of additional treatments.

Keywords: celiac; gluten; barley; gluten-free; NCGS; AGA; T cell; enteritis

1. Introduction

CD is an autoimmune disease that affects approximately 3 million people in the United States (US) [1], although only a small fraction has been diagnosed. Furthermore, a non-autoimmune NCGS affects an estimated additional 6% of the population e.g., 20 million in the US [2,3]. Both CD and NCGS are characterized by sensitivity to dietary gluten. High prevalence of CD and NCGS in cereal grain-consuming societies highlights the need for novel treatments for gluten sensitivity and illustrates how many people may benefit from the successful outcome of related research.

Nutrients **2015**, *7*, 1657–1671

A number of novel pharmacological strategies are currently being explored for the treatment of CD. These strategies include experimental drugs that reduce intestinal permeability, inhibitors of intestinal tissue transglutaminase (TG2), as well as major histocompatibility class II blockers [4]. Most of these therapies are still far from the clinic. An alternative therapy for CD and NCGS may include cereals whose storage proteins are modified to reduce the accumulation of the immunotoxic gluten epitopes [5]. The endosperm in cereals such as barley and wheat consists of 8%–14% protein; these storage proteins are prolamins and glutenins known colloquially as "gluten". The major CD-eliciting epitopes have been found in the S-rich and S-poor prolamins [6–8]. Several groups have explored the natural variation present in wheat, barley and oats germplasm to determine if conventional plant-breeding approaches could be used to develop reduced gluten (RG) cereals [9–13]. Additionally, a transgenic approach to developing RG wheat was taken by Gil-Humanes and colleagues who down-regulated α, γ, and ω classes of wheat gliadins using the RNAi hairpin constructs of conserved gliadin sequences. The resulting transformed wheat had 10–20-fold lower content of immunotoxic epitopes [14–16].

Our group is focusing on a similar approach. Using a known RG barley mutant [17,18], the potential therapeutic benefits are evaluated in gluten-sensitive rhesus macaques. The barley mutant *lys3a* (RISØ 1508) was first identified in the early 1970s at an agricultural station in Denmark during the course of mutagenesis studies aimed at increasing the lysine content of barley, to enhance its nutritional value as animal feed [18]. This was successful; the lysine content was increased by 44% and follow-up experiments with rats and pigs confirmed superior nutritional properties of this mutant [19,20]. The increase in lysine in the *lys3a* mutant is due to a decrease in the accumulation of lysine-poor hordeins with a concomitant increase in the accumulation of more lysine-rich albumins and globulins [21]. These effects of the mutation resulted in a gluten content in the *lys3a* barley that is approximately 1% of that in the parental cultivar (Bomi). Here, we report the effects of conventional and RG barley-based primate diets (containing 10% by weight of Bomi or *lys3a* whole grain barley flour) in our gluten-sensitive rhesus macaque model.

2. Experimental Section

2.1. Ethics Approval

This study was performed with non-human primates. Ethics approval for veterinary procedures was obtained from the Tulane University Animal Care and Use Committee, Animal Welfare Assurance A-4499-01. All procedures were in accordance with the recommendations of the Guide to the Care and Use of Laboratory Animals (NIH) 78–23 (Revised, 1996).

2.2. Pre-Screening and Selection of Rhesus Macaques for the Study

The 200 young (1–3 years-old) rhesus macaques (*Macaca mulatta*) of Indian origin, belonging to Tulane National Primate Research Center breeding colony, were tested for the presence of serum anti-gliadin antibodies (AGA) as well as anti-TG2 antibodies as previously described [22] to identify suitable study subjects: Three AGA and TG2 antibody-negative macaques, without a clinical history of diarrheal illness (controls) and three AGA and TG2-positive macaques, with past histories of chronic diarrhea (gluten-sensitive e.g., GS) were assigned to the study. All six animals were Specific Pathogen-Free (SPF) e.g., negative for simian retrovirus type D, seronegative for simian T lymphotropic virus type 1, simian immunodeficiency virus and herpes B viruses, and free of selected enteric pathogens [23]. Tuberculin skin tests, performed semi-annually, were negative for each animal involved.

2.3. Diets Used

Upon assignment to the study animals were placed on a strict GFD, as described before [24], in order to accomplish immunological and clinical remission in GS macaques, characterized by baseline levels of AGA and TG2 serum antibodies and absence of diarrhea. The two barley-based diets were formulated in collaboration with Purina Inc., consistent with primate diet requirements. Conventional (variety Bomi) and RG barley (*lys3a*-derived from Bomi by mutagenesis) were obtained from the ARS National Small Grains Collection, Aberdeen, ID (http://www.ars.usda.gov/main/docs.htm?docid= 2884). Both varieties were grown in southern California in the winter of 2013/2014 and harvested in the spring of 2014. The barley seeds were de-husked and milled to flour; gluten levels in the barley flours and the monkey chows were determined by Bia Diagnostics (http://www.biadiagnostics.com/) by the commercial immunoassay (R5 ELISA). Conventional and RG barley chows were manufactured by Purina Test-Diet. Barley flour was incorporated at 10% w/w of the chow. As measured by R5 ELISA, the conventional barley flour exhibited gluten levels between 175,000 and 240,000 parts per million (ppm) (mg/kg) while the RG barley flour ranged between 2000 and 3000 ppm. The gluten levels in conventional barley chow were approximately 16,000 ppm while in RG barley chow they were 200 ppm. Thus, both the RG barley flour and the corresponding chow contained approximately 1% of the gluten of conventional barley. Subsequently, gluten sources of traditional non-human primate chow (5K63) were replaced in Purina's mixing facility with conventional barley flour (5BQF) and RG barley flour (5BQG). Respective chow pellets were color-coded brown and green. Based on amount of chow eaten daily (160–320 g of chow/day) and the level of gluten in the conventional and RG barley chow, we estimate that conventional barley chow delivered a dose of 2.5–5 g of gluten/day, while the RG barley chow led to an intake of approximately 32–64 mg of gluten/day.

2.4. Dietary Time Periods and Samples Collected

The six study macaques were kept on identical diets, during four periods, each period lasting approximately 2 months, in the following order: (1) GFD; (2) conventional barley-derived diet; (3) RG barley-derived diet and (4) GFD. Macaques were stationed in a Biosafety Level 2 (BSL2) facility, separated from the rest of the colony, to prevent contamination of their diet with gluten sources. When fed conventional barley chow, all six macaques had also access to a wheat bread. Five milliliters of EDTA blood and 1 g of stool were collected every two weeks from each animal to extract the serum and peripheral blood mononuclear cells (PBMC) as described [25] and to confirm the enteric pathogen-free status of studied animals [23]. Individual records of animal well-being and stool consistency (diarrhea) were recorded daily. Based on assessment of healthy control animals, diarrhea clinical scores were scaled in a range of 0–1, with values of >0.4 indicating diarrhea. To simplify and to summarize the scores, the animal group averages were calculated for every week.

2.5. Histopathological Evaluation, AGA, TG2 and Anti-Hordein Antibody (AHA) Serum Responses

A small intestinal biopsy sample (distal duodenum or proximal jejunum) was collected once every dietary period from each animal, as described [22,25]. The AGA and TG2 antibody-specific immunoassays were also performed [24,26]. In addition, an AHA immunoassay was used to determine if AGA responses overlapped with barley-induced AHA responses. Briefly, 10 mg/mL of pepsin-trypsin digested (PT)-gliadin was replaced with PT-hordein (Arcadia Bio.) as the coating antigen in AHA immunoassay to measure the AHA serum levels [26]. Histopathological evaluation of collected small intestinal biopsy samples was also done as previously described [24,26].

2.6. Fluorescent-Activated Cell Sorting (FACS) of Cytokine-Producing PBMCs

The FACS was performed according to standard protocols [27]. Briefly, PBMCs were stained with a mix of fluorescent antibodies from BD Pharmingen (San Diego, CA) unless otherwise noted: CD3 (SP34-2), CD4 (OKT4, Bio Legend, San Diego, CA), CD8 (SK1), CD20 (2H7, Bio Legend), CD152 e.g., CTLA-4 (BN13), TNF (MAb11), IFN-γ (4S.B3), IL-8 (G265-8, BD Horizon, San Jose, CA, USA) and IL-10 (JES3-9D7, Bio Legend). In order to detect the TNF, IFN-γ, IL-8 and IL-10 intracellular cytokines, lymphocytes were stimulated *in vitro* with 0.1 µM PMA and 0.5 µg/mL ionomycin (Sigma, St. Louis, MO, USA) and processed as described [27]. Samples were resuspended in BD Stabilizing Fixative (BD

Biosciences, San Jose, CA, USA) and data acquired on FACSAria flow cytometer (BD Biosciences). Data were analyzed by the use of Flowjo software (Tree star, Ashland, OR, USA).

2.7. Statistical Analysis

The individual cytokine responses (proportions of parent peripheral lymphocytes secreting each of the pro- or anti-inflammatory cytokines) were compared between the control and GS groups of macaques by the use of Student T test. The probability *p < 0.05* was considered as significantly different.

3. Results

3.1. Serum Antibody Responses, Intestinal Histopathology and Diarrhea

In order to accomplish the immunological and clinical remission in GS macaques and to maintain the consistency between the diets of control and GS animals, all six macaques were first placed on a GFD. Two out of three GS animals (KF97 and JR67) responded well to the GFD and within one month decreased their AGA (as well as TG2, not shown) serum antibody levels to a base-range (Figure 1).

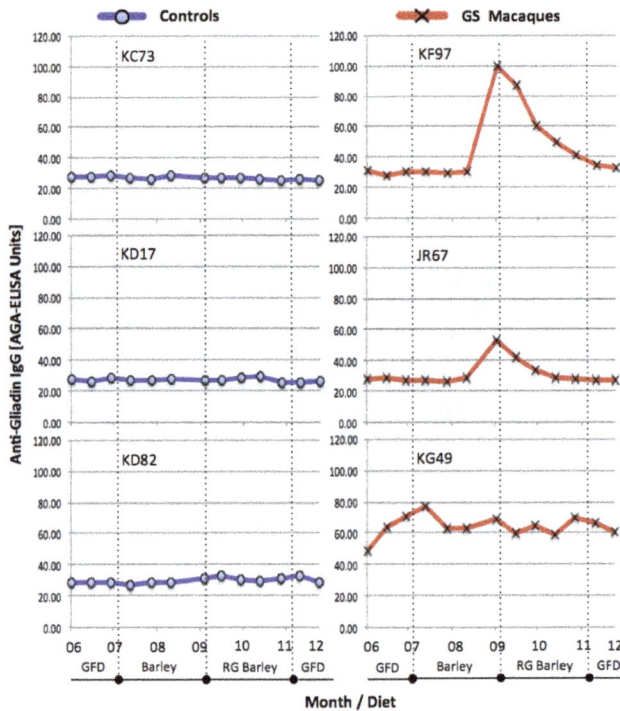

Figure 1. The kinetics of serum AGA antibody levels in three control (KC73, KD17 and KD82) and three GS (KF97, JR67 and KG49) macaques during the periods of (1) immunological remission e.g., GFD; (2) conventional barley diet; (3) RG barley diet and (4) GFD. Vertical, dotted lines indicate borders between different diets. Only the GS animals but not the healthy controls seroconverted to dietary gluten. The two GS macaques (KF97 and JR67) responded to its presence (AGA increase) as well as withdrawal (AGA decrease). KG49 macaque remained with elevated AGAs throughout the entire period of experiment regardless of dietary changes. AGA-ELISA cut-off = 40 Units.

The third GS macaque (KG49) remained, despite the GFD treatment, with elevated AGAs suggesting that a longer GFD period might be required to remit AGAs of this animal. As anticipated, none of the healthy control macaques showed any AGAs before and during the study, regardless of dietary gluten intake (Figure 1). Upon introduction of conventional barley diet to GS macaques, KF97 and JR67, both animals responded with elevated AGAs while RG barley diet had the reverse effects (Figure 1). The AGA serum responses were followed by anti-hordein antibody (AHA) responses (not shown), confirming that measured serum antibody responses were, at least in part, induced by barley-derived prolamins.

The AGA responses in GS macaques were paralleled with histopathological manifestations of gluten-sensitive enteropathy (Figure 2) as well as with clinical manifestations of diarrhea (Supplementary Figure S1). Although the effects of conventional barley diet were not as severe in GS macaques as previously described effects of wheat diet [24,25], both histopathological and clinical manifestations of villous atrophy and diarrhea were clearly present. Replacement of conventional barley with RG barley diet had beneficial effects not only on intestinal architecture (Figure 2C) but also for the improvement of clinical diarrhea scores (Supplement Figure S1). Despite these beneficial effects of RG barley diet, after two months on this diet mild enteritis and soft stools were still persisting in GS macaques. Such an incomplete remission of gluten-induced disease is in agreement with our past results when a wheat-free but not completely gluten-free diet was fed to GS macaques [24]. In this study, an incomplete remission of gluten-induced disease became more obvious when dissecting the expression of pro- and anti-inflammatory factors by peripheral CD4+ T helper cells (Figures 3 and 4).

3.2. Production of Pro- and Anti-Inflammatory Cytokines by Peripheral T and B Lymphocytes

The populations of peripheral blood CD3+CD4+ T helper, CD3+CD8+ T and CD3-CD20+ B lymphocytes of control and GS macaques were identified (Supplementary Figure S2) and evaluated for the production of pro- and anti-inflammatory cytokines (Figure 3).

Selected time points representing the GFD, conventional barley, RG barley and GFD periods were included with the objective to illustrate the effects of RG barley diet on peripheral T and B cell cytokine responses. As anticipated, the baseline, associated with consumption of GFD, was characterized with very few cytokine-secreting cells of interest, namely the CD4+ T helper cells (Figure 3A). High proportions of CD8+IFN-γ+ T and CD20+IL-10+ B cells persisted throughout the experiment in both groups of macaques (Figure 3A–D), indicating that the presence of these cells was not due to dietary gluten changes. The two inflammatory cytokines that were affected by dietary gluten exposure were TNF and IFN-γ (Figure 3B–D). While there were no consistent differences between the control and GS groups with respect to TNF production, the IFN-γ-positive cells were consistently higher in the GS group. This difference became statistically significant by day 64 of the conventional barley diet (Figure 3B). Such a result indirectly corroborates the prominent role IFN-γ plays in pathogenesis of gluten-sensitive enteropathy e.g., GSE [28–30]. With the transition from the conventional barley to the RG barley diet, a transient decrease of TNF production by all three types of studied lymphocytes was observed regardless of group affiliation (Figure 3C). No further decrease of inflammatory cytokine-producing cells after feeding the RG barley diet continuously for two months (not shown) indicated that even the minute quantities of gluten contained in RG barley (200 ppm) were able to prevent remission of inflammatory cytokine production to baseline. Only when the animals were placed again on the GFD did cytokine production very slowly start returning to lower levels (Figure 3D).

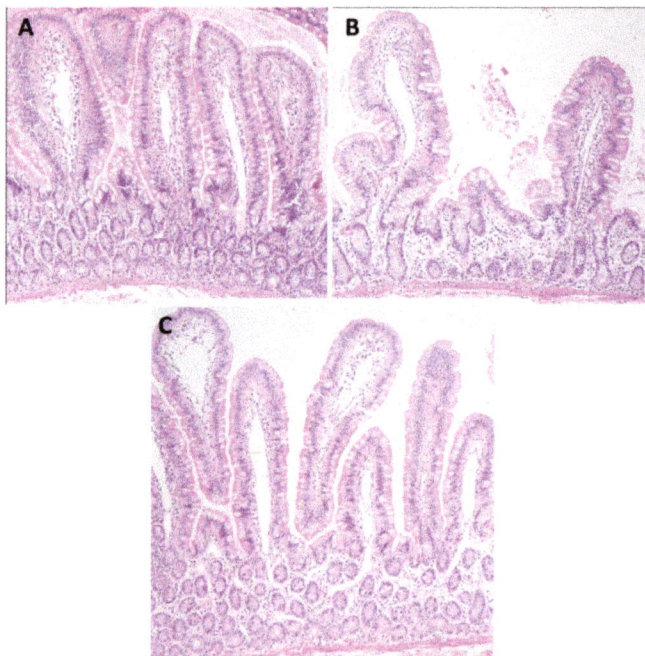

Figure 2. The effects of conventional and RG barley diets on small intestinal tissue architecture of control and GS macaques (H & E staining, jejunum, 100×). After being on conventional barley diet for 64 days, jejunum of control macaque (KD17) looks normal, unaffected, with only minimal lacteal dilatation (**A**) while GS macaque (KF97) jejunum is showing shortened villi e.g., villous atrophy (**B**). Multifocally, KF97's lamina propria is moderately expanded by lymphoid aggregates. The lacteals are mildly dilated (lymphangiectasia). The submucosa is expanded by edema containing infiltrates of small number of neutrophils, eosinophils, lymphocytes and plasma cells (**B**). Follow-up treatment of KF97 with RG barley diet for 56 days resulted in an improvement: Jejunum became close to normal, with only moderate lymphangiectasia (**C**).

3.3. Expression of CD152 by Peripheral CD4+ Cells e.g., Enumeration of CD4+CTLA-4+ T Helper Cells

CTLA-4 is normally expressed on the surface of CD4+ T helper cells from where it transmits immunoregulatory signals that in general suppress T cell mediated immune responses. Clinical significance of CTLA-4 agonists was implicated in the context of several autoimmune diseases including CD. In this study, the proportions of peripheral CD3+CD4+CD152+ T helper cells were assessed in GS and control macaques. It was hypothesized that increased numbers of these cells would indicate that GS hosts need to counter-balance the gluten-induced T cell responses. Thus, peripheral CD4+ T cell populations from control and GS macaques were evaluated for CD152 expression (Figure 4). While CD152 was only poorly expressed during the remission period (<1%), a robust increase of CD3+CD4+CD152+ cells was measured at days 14 and 64 of the conventional barley diet (Figure 4). Despite that a significant increase in CD152 expression was measured in both groups of macaques, no differences between the control and GS macaques were detected. With increasing time on the gluten-containing diet, the fraction of CD4+CD152+ to CD4+IFN-γ+ cells (anti- and pro-inflammatory T helper cells) started shifting in favor of IFN-γ cells in the GS macaque(s), while in the controls, this fraction was in favor of the CD4+CD152+ cells (Supplementary Figure S3). Reintroduction of the GFD had the expected effect—expression of both CD152 and IFN-γ dropped to levels closer to baseline (Figures 3 and 4).

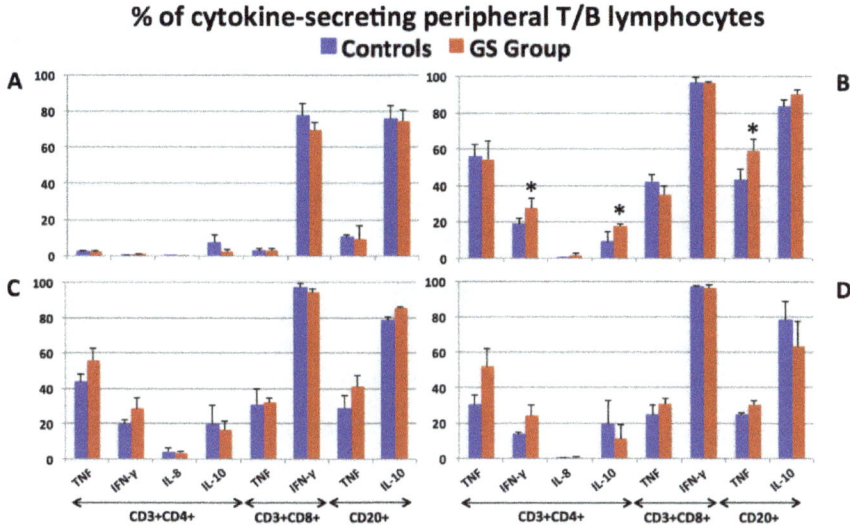

Figure 3. The production of inflammatory (IFN-γ, IL-8 and TNF) and anti-inflammatory (IL-10) cytokines by peripheral T helper (CD3+CD4+), cytotoxic T (CD3+CD8+) and B (CD3-CD20+) lymphocytes from control and GS macaques is shown at four selected time points. While only the minimal cytokine production by CD4+ T helper cells was measured at the stage of immunological remission induced by GFD (**A**), the use of conventional barley diet was characterized with significantly increased cytokine production: Day 64 is shown (**B**) with differentially increased cytokine production (*). An introduction of RG barley diet and its continuous administration for two months led only to transient decrease of TNF production by CD3+CD8+ T and CD20+ B cells in all animals (**C**). Upon reintroduction of GFD for one month, a further but still transient decrease of inflammatory cytokine-producing cells was noted (**D**) indicating the necessity of more sustained treatment.

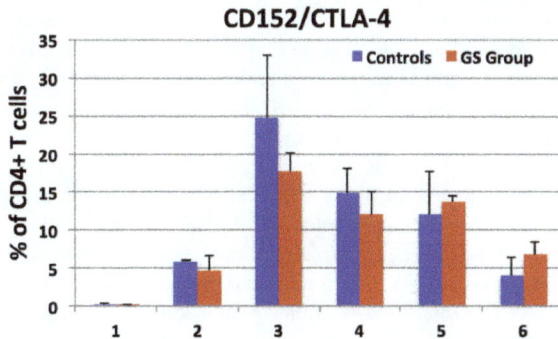

Figure 4. The proportions of CD152 (marker of T cell inhibition) expression by peripheral CD3+CD4+ T cells from control (C = blue columns) and gluten-sensitive (GS = red columns) macaques were evaluated. Six selected time points are shown including the GFD day 28 (X axis value 1); conventional barley diet days 14 (2) and 43 (3); RG barley diet days 28 (4) and 42 (5); followed again by GFD day 13 (6). While only the minimal expression of CD152 was measured during the first GFD period, an introduction of conventional barley diet led to an increased expression of CD152 by day 14, and further increase by day 43 in both groups. Replacement of conventional barley with RG barley diet did result in transiently lower % of CD3+CD4+CD152+ T cells. No significant differences in CD152 expression were observed between the two groups.

4. Discussion

This study was conducted with the objective to evaluate the treatment potential of RG barley-based diet. A GS rhesus macaque model was used to study the effects of RG diet, including humoral and T cell mediated immune responses. Consistent with past studies, experimental macaques were selected based on positive serum AGA and TG2 antibodies as well as clinical histories of chronic diarrhea of non-infectious etiology [22,25]. After being placed on a GFD for one month, both AGA and TG2 antibodies in two of the GS macaques dropped to baseline levels while the third GS animal was not responsive to GFD. This is in agreement with reports involving CD patients, according to which not all celiac patients respond promptly to GFD [31,32]. Consistent with our unpublished data, once the immunological remission is accomplished in GS rhesus macaques and dietary gluten is re-introduced, relapse of serum antibodies is faster in the case of AGA than TG2 auto-antibodies. This might be due to fundamentally different mechanisms of how AGA *vs.* TG2 antibodies are generated [31,33,34]. GS macaques chosen for this study were identified as both AGA and TG2 antibody-positive, however, since AGAs were more responsive to dietary gluten changes than the TG2 antibodies, AGA rather than TG2 antibody responses are presented in this manuscript to reflect the kinetics of the experimental diets.

Following the replacement of the GFD with the conventional barley diet, the two GS macaques that responded to dietary gluten withdrawal (KF97 and JR67), also responded to its re-introduction—with increased AGAs (Figure 1). These AGA responses were followed by serum anti-hordein antibody (AHA) responses (not shown), confirming that AGA responses were, at least in part, caused by barley-derived prolamins [35,36]. While AHAs were detected in serum from both control and GS animals, AGAs were only detected in GS macaques but not in controls. Seed storage proteins from related grasses including the gliadins from wheat and hordeins from barley share a number of proline and glutamine-rich epitopes; these are likely being recognized by both AGAs and AHAs [8]. Small intestinal histopathology and clinical diarrhea scores (Figure 2 and Supplementary Figure S1) corroborated the AGA results and provided additional clues: While all of the GS macaques showed evidence of GSE upon administration of the conventional barley diet, only partial remission of GSE was accomplished in these animals by the administration of the RG barley diet. This incomplete disease remission became even more apparent when comparing the numbers of pro- and anti-inflammatory peripheral blood lymphocytes at different time points (Figures 3 and 4).

Because of their demonstrated and suspected involvement in CD and/or NCGS pathogenesis, the following factors were studied: IFN-γ, IL-10, IL-8, TNF and CD152/CTLA-4 [28–30,37–45]. The cells that were the subject of above analysis were peripheral lymphocytes including CD4+ T helper cells, CD8+ T cells and CD20+ B cells. It is important to underscore that all of the selected factors are known to play roles also in other inflammatory and autoimmune diseases [29]. Thus, to establish their order of significance in the GS macaques fed RG barley was the secondary objective of this study. In the case of human CD, a prominent role of IFN-γ was established due to its capability to activate the TG2 [30]. Therefore, an inhibition of the phosphatidylinositol-3-kinase pathway was suggested as a potential CD therapy [30]. Of the factors investigated in this study, the expression of pro-inflammatory IFN-γ by CD4+ T cells, followed by its IL-10 antagonist, reflected the dietary gluten changes more closely than the other studied factors. At several time points, the expression of IL-8, TNF and CTLA-4 were influenced by dietary gluten changes, however, without significant differences between the control and GS macaques. These results suggest that dietary gluten also affects to some extent healthy individuals. Interestingly and in contrast to AGA and cytokine responses, there was no significant trend for differences in CTLA-4 expression between the two groups of macaques. One consideration that could simplify observed effects in future studies is the use of genetically pre-selected macaques. In this study, GS subjects were selected by their TG2/AGA/clinical phenotype, without consideration of their *MHC II*, e.g., *Mamu II* characteristics. We recently showed that specific *Mamu II* alleles might predispose rhesus macaques to GS, analogous to the role played by human DQ2/8 alleles [25]. For the upcoming studies with novel CD therapeutic approaches, it would be beneficial to establish a genetically and phenotypically defined colony of CD and NCGS rhesus macaques, to initiate studies without the need to pre-screen large numbers of animals.

The results reported here demonstrate that the RG diet leads to a partial amelioration of gluten-induced symptoms in GS macaques. These results provide direction for the future use of RG barley. Despite its 100-fold lower content of dietary gluten, administration of RG barley still appears to trigger inflammatory responses in GS macaques.

The RG barley used, namely a mutant in the *lys3a* gene induced by a DNA alkylating agent, results in the simultaneous reduction of several classes of hordeins, including B and C hordeins. The molecular nature of the mutation is unknown, although it is hypothesized to be a lesion in a 5-methylcytosine DNA glycosylase enzyme that de-methylates DNA [46]. The altered DNA methylation of several hordein gene promoters in mutant endosperm compared to non-mutant parental endosperm has been found in the mutant [47]. An independent mutant, Riso 56, that contains a large deletion of B hordein genes [48], has been crossed with the *lys3a* mutant to create Ultra Low Gluten barley 2.0 (ULG), indicating that there is a potential to reduce barley gluten even further [49]. While ULG was reported to stimulate the *in vitro* reactivity of T cells 20-fold less than conventional barley [49], it has not yet been tested *in vivo*.

Other therapies that are being developed to treat CD such as glutenase enzymes with strong gluten degrading activity may be envisioned to synergize with a RG cereal to help break down the residual gluten [50–53]. Even if not yet appropriate for GS patients, the development of RG barley and other RG cereals may have additional benefits, such as increased content of the lysine in the grain. Future studies could also include morphometric end-points of macaques' GSE, as described [24]. The future use of improved RG grains may ultimately contribute to a reduction in the incidence of gluten sensitivities.

5. Conclusions

This study was performed with the highly sensitive rhesus macaque model of gluten sensitivity to test the hypothesis that a RG barley mutant is less deleterious than its parental counterpart. Upon switching from the conventional to a RG barley diet, GS macaques exhibited an improvement in symptoms of gluten-induced disease, including GSE and diarrhea. Nevertheless, persisting production of inflammatory cytokines by peripheral lymphocytes indicated that complete remission could not be accomplished by the RG barley diet alone. Future studies should therefore focus on additional approaches to detoxifying the residual gluten.

Acknowledgments: The authors wish to thank Carol Coyne, Monica Mayer, Julie Bruhn, Calvin Lanclos, Cecily Conerly, William J. Austill, Cate McGuire, Paul Gallawa and Meir Gadisman for their excellent technical support. For assistance with milling the barley grain we are grateful to Craig Morris and his staff at the ARS Western Wheat Quality Lab in Pullman, WA. We also thank Huanbin Xu for his help with FACS multicolor panel design. This work was funded by the National Institute of Diabetes and Digestive and Kidney Diseases of the National Institutes of Health under Award Number R42DK097976. The authors alone are responsible for the content of this article and this work does not necessarily represent the views of the National Institutes of Health. This study was completed as part of the collaboration between Arcadia Biosciences and Tulane University.

Author Contributions: Karol Sestak wrote the manuscript, coordinated the overall work, participated in work related to multi-color flow cytometry and analyzed the data. Hazel Thwin assisted with work coordination, processed and distributed samples from rhesus macaques and participated in execution and analysis of laboratory immunoassays. Jason Dufour provided veterinary care, executed surgical procedures and helped with coordination of primate diets. Pyone P. Aye helped with statistical analysis and interpretation of generated results. David X. Liu performed veterinary pathology procedures and was responsible for evaluation of intestinal biopsy samples. Charles P. Moehs was responsible for growth and characterization of the barley varieties and preparation of the experimental diets as well as for the study's overall coordination and manuscript preparation.

Conflicts of Interest: The authors declare no conflict of interest.

References

1. Catassi, C.; Fasano. Celiac disease. *Curr. Opin. Gastroenterol.* **2008**, *24*, 687–691. [CrossRef]

2. Sapone, A.; Bai, J.C.; Ciacci, C.; Dolinsek, J.; Green, P.H.; Hadjivassiliou, M.; Kaukinen, K.; Rostami, K.; Sanders, D.S.; Schumann, M.; *et al.* Spectrum of gluten-related disorders: consensus on new nomenclature and classification. *BMC Med.* **2012**, *10*, 1–12. [CrossRef] [PubMed]

3. Sestak, K.; Fortgang, I. Celiac and non-celiac forms of gluten sensitivity: Shifting paradigms of an old disease. *Br. Microb. Res. J.* **2013**, *3*, 585–589. [CrossRef]

4. Sollid, L.M.; Khosla, C. Novel therapies for coeliac disease. *J. Int. Med.* **2011**, *269*, 604–613. [CrossRef]

5. Sollid, L.M.; Khosla, C. Future therapeutic options for celiac disease. *Nat. Clin. Pract. Gastroenterol. Hepatol.* **2005**, *2*, 140–147. [CrossRef] [PubMed]

6. Shan, L.; Molberg, O.; Parrot, I.; Hausch, F.; Filiz, F.; Gray, G.M.; Sollid, L.M.; Khosla, C. Structural basis for gluten intolerance in celiac sprue. *Science* **2002**, *297*, 2275–2279. [CrossRef] [PubMed]

7. Shan, L.; Qiao, S.W.; Arentz-Nansen, H.; Molberg, O.; Gray, G.M.; Sollid, L.M.; Khosla, C. Identification and analysis of multivalent proteolytically resistant peptides from gluten: Implications for celiac sprue. *J. Proteom. Res.* **2005**, *4*, 1732–1741. [CrossRef]

8. Tye-Din, J.A.; Stewart, J.A.; Dromey, J.A.; Beissbarth, T.; van Heel, D.A.; Tatham, A.; Henderson, K.; Mannering, S.I.; Gianfrani, C.; Jewell, D.P. Comprehensive, quantitative mapping of T cell epitopes in gluten in celiac disease. *Sci. Transl. Med.* **2010**, *2*. [CrossRef]

9. Molberg, O.; Uhlen, A.K.; Jensen, T.; Flaete, N.S.; Fleckenstein, B.; Arentz-Hansen, H.; Raki, M.; Lundin, K.E.A.; Sollid, L.M. Mapping of gluten T-cell epitopes in the bread wheat ancestors: Implications for celiac disease. *Gastroenterology* **2005**, *128*, 393–401. [CrossRef] [PubMed]

10. Spaenij-Dekking, L.; Kooy-Winkelaar, Y.; van Veelen, P.; Wouter-Drijhout, J.; Jonker, H.; van Soest, L.; Smulders, M.J.M.; Bosch, D.; Gilissen, L.J.W.J.; Koning, F. Natural variation in toxicity of wheat: Potential for selection of nontoxic varieties for celiac disease patients. *Gastroenterology* **2005**, *129*, 797–806. [CrossRef] [PubMed]

11. Van den Broeck, H.; van Herpen, T.; Schuit, C.; Salentijn, E.; Dekking, L.; Bosch, D.; Hamer, R.; Smulders, M.; Gilissen, L.; van der Meer, I. Removing celiac disease-related gluten proteins from bread wheat while retaining technological properties: a study with Chinese Spring deletion lines. *BMC Plant Biol.* **2009**, *9*, 41. [CrossRef] [PubMed]

12. Comino, I.; Real, A.; de Lorenzo, L.; Cornell, H.; Lopez-Casado, M.A.; Barro, F.; Lorite, P.; Torres, M.I.; Cebolla, A.; Sousa, C. Diversity in oat potential immunogenicity: Basis for the selection of oat varieties with no toxicity in coeliac disease. *Gut* **2011**, *60*, 915–922. [CrossRef] [PubMed]

13. Comino, I.; Real, A.; Gil-Humanes, J.; Piston, F.; de Lorenzo, L.; Moreno, M.L.; Lopez-Casado, M.A.; Lorite, P.; Cebolla, A.; Torres, M.I.; *et al.* Significant differences in coeliac immunotoxicity of barley varieties. *Mol. Nutr. Food Res.* **2012**, *56*, 1697–1707. [CrossRef] [PubMed]

14. Gil-Humanes, J.; Piston, F.; Tollefsen, S.; Sollid, L.M.; Barro, F. Effective shutdown in the expression of celiac disease-related wheat gliadin T-cell epitopes by RNA interference. *Proc. Natl. Acad. Sci. USA* **2010**, *107*, 17023–17028. [CrossRef] [PubMed]

15. Piston, F.; Gil-Humanes, J.; Rodriguez-Quijano, M.; Barro, F. Down-regulating γ-gliadins in bread wheat leads to non-specific increases in other gluten proteins and has no major effects on dough gluten strength. *PLoS One* **2011**, *6*, e24754. [CrossRef] [PubMed]

16. Gil-Humanes, J.; Piston, F.; Altamirano-Fortoul, R.; Real, A.; Comino, I.; Sousa, C.; Rosell, C.M.; Barro, F. Reduced-gliadin wheat bread: an alternative to the gluten-free diet for consumers suffering gluten-related pathologies. *PLoS One* **2014**, *9*, e90898. [CrossRef] [PubMed]

17. Doll, H. Inheritance of the high-lysine character of a barley mutant. *Hereditas* **1973**, *74*, 293–294. [CrossRef] [PubMed]

18. Doll, H.; Koie, B.; Eggum, B. Induced high lysine mutants in barley. *Radiat. Bot.* **1974**, *14*, 73–80. [CrossRef]

19. Jorgensen, H.; Gabert, V.M.; Fernandez, J.A. Influence of nitrogen fertilization on the nutritional value of high-lysine barley determined in growing pigs. *Anim. Feed Sci. Technol.* **1999**, *79*, 79–91. [CrossRef]

20. Newman, C.; Overland, M.; Newman, R.; Bang-Olsen, K.; Pedersen, B. Protein quality of a new high-lysine barley derived from Riso 1508. *Canad. J. Anim. Sci.* **1990**, *70*, 279–285. [CrossRef]

21. Munck, L.; Pram Nielsen, J.; Moller, B.; Jacobsen, S.; Sondergaard, I.; Engelsen, S.; Norgaard, L.; Bro, R. Exploring the phenotypic expression of a regulatory proteome-altering gene by spectroscopy and chemometrics. *Analyt. Chim. Acta* **2001**, *446*, 169–184. [CrossRef]

22. Mazumdar, K.; Alvarez, X.; Borda, J.T.; Dufour, J.; Martin, E.; Bethune, M.T.; Khosla, C.; Sestak, K. Visualization of transepithelial passage of the immunogenic 33-residue peptide from α-2 gliadin in gluten-sensitive macaques. *PLoS One* **2010**, *5*, e10228. [CrossRef] [PubMed]

23. Sestak, K.; Merritt, C.K.; Borda, J.; Saylor, E.; Schwamberger, S.R.; Cogswell, F.; Didier, E.S.; Didier, P.J.; Plauche, G.; Bohm, R.P.; *et al.* Infectious agent and immune response characteristics of chronic enterocolitis in captive rhesus macaques. *Infect. Immun.* **2003**, *71*, 4079–4086. [CrossRef] [PubMed]

24. Bethune, M.T.; Borda, J.T.; Ribka, E.; Liu, M.X.; Phillipi-Falkenstein, K.; Jandacek, R.J.; Doxiadis, G.G.M.; Gray, G.M.; Khosla, C.; Sestak, K. A non-human primate model for gluten sensitivity. *PLoS One* **2008**, *3*, e1614. [CrossRef] [PubMed]

25. Xu, H.; Feely, S.L.; Wang, X.; Liu, D.X.; Borda, J.T.; Dufour, J.; Li, W.; Aye, P.P.; Doxiadis, G.G.; Khosla, C.; *et al.* Gluten-sensitive enteropathy coincides with decreased capability of intestinal T cells to secrete IL-17 and IL-22 in a macaque model for celiac disease. *Clin. Immunol.* **2013**, *147*, 40–49. [CrossRef] [PubMed]

26. Bethune, M.T.; Ribka, E.; Khosla, C.; Sestak, K. Transepithelial transport and enzymatic detoxification of gluten in gluten-sensitive rhesus macaques. *PLoS One* **2008**, *3*, e1857. [CrossRef] [PubMed]

27. Xu, H.; Wang, X.; Liu, D.X.; Rasmussen, T.; Lackner, A.A.; Veazey, R.S. IL-17-producing innate lymphoid cells are restricted to mucosal tissues and are depleted in SIV-infected macaques. *Mucos. Immunol.* **2012**, *5*, 658–669. [CrossRef]

28. Anderson, R.P.; van Heel, D.A.; Tye-Din, J.A.; Barnardo, M.; Salio, M.; Jewell, D.P.; Hill, A.V.S. T cells in peripheral blood after gluten challenge in coeliac disease. *Gut* **2005**, *54*, 1217–1223. [CrossRef] [PubMed]

29. Abadie, V.; Sollid, L.M.; Barreiro, L.B.; Jabri, B. Integration of genetic and immunological insights into a model of celiac disease pathogenesis. *Annu. Rev. Immunol.* **2011**, *29*, 493–525. [CrossRef] [PubMed]

30. DiRaimondo, T.R.; Klock, C.; Khosla, C. Interferon-γ activates transglutaminase 2 via a phosphatidylinositol-3-kinase-dependent pathway: Implications for celiac sprue therapy. *J. Pharmacol. Exp. Therapeut.* **2012**, *341*, 104–114. [CrossRef]

31. Schuppan, D.; Junker, Y.; Barisani, D. Celiac disease: From pathogenesis to novel therapies. *Gastroenterology* **2009**, *137*, 1912–1933. [CrossRef] [PubMed]

32. Spatola, B.N.; Kaukinen, K.; Collin, P.; Maki, M.; Kagnoff, M.F.; Daugherty, P.S. Persistence of elevated deamidated gliadin peptide antibodies on a gluten-free diet indicates nonresponsive coeliac disease. *Aliment. Pharmacol. Ther.* **2014**, *39*, 407–417. [CrossRef] [PubMed]

33. Troncone, R.; Jabri, B. Coeliac disease and gluten sensitivity. *J. Intern. Med.* **2011**, *269*, 582–590. [CrossRef] [PubMed]

34. Klock, C.; DiRaimondo, T.R.; Khosla, C. Role of transglutaminase 2 in celiac disease pathogenesis. *Semin. Immunopathol.* **2012**, *34*, 513–522. [CrossRef] [PubMed]

35. Tanner, G.J.; Blundell, M.J.; Colgrave, M.L.; Howitt, C.A. Quantification of hordeins by ELISA: The correct standard makes a magnitude of difference. *PLoS One* **2013**, *8*, e56456. [CrossRef] [PubMed]

36. Tanner, G.J.; Colgrave, M.L.; Blundell, M.J.; Goswami, H.P.; Howitt, C.A. Measuring hordein (gluten) in beer-A comparison of ELISA and mass spectrometry. *PLoS One* **2013**, *8*, e56452. [CrossRef] [PubMed]

37. Meresse, B.; Curran, S.A.; Ciszewski, C.; Orbelyan, G.; Setty, M.; Bhagat, G.; Lee, L.; Tretiakova, M.; Semrad, C.; Kistner, E.; *et al.* Reprogramming of CTLs into natural killer-like cells in celiac disease. *J. Exp. Med.* **2006**, *203*, 1343–1355. [CrossRef] [PubMed]

38. Sollid, L.M.; Jabri, B. Triggers and drivers of autoimmunity: Lessons from coeliac disease. *Nat. Rev. Imunol.* **2013**, *13*, 294–302. [CrossRef]

39. Forsberg, G.; Hernell, O.; Melgar, S.; Israelsson, A.; Hammarstrom, S.; Hammarstrom, M.L. Paradoxical coexpression of proinflammatory and down-regulatory cytokines in intestinal T cells in childhood celiac disease. *Gastroenterology* **2002**, *123*, 667–678. [CrossRef] [PubMed]

40. Forsberg, G.; Hernell, O.; Hammarstrom, S.; Hammarstrom, M.L. Concomitant increase of IL-10 and pro-inflammatory cytokines in intraepithelial lymphocyte subsets in celiac disease. *Internat. Immunol.* **2007**, *19*, 993–1001. [CrossRef]

41. Diosdado, B.; Wijmenga, C. Molecular mechanisms of the adaptive, innate and regulatory immune responses in the intestinal mucosa of celiac disease patients. *Expert Rev. Mol. Diagn.* **2005**, *5*, 681–700. [CrossRef] [PubMed]

42. Tack, G.J.; van Wanrooij, R.L.; Von Bloomberg, B.M.; Amini, H.; Coupe, V.M.; Bonnet, P.; Mulder, C.J.; Schreurs, M.W. Serum parameters in the spectrum of coeliac disease: Beyond standard antibody testing—A cohort study. *BMC Gastroenterol.* **2012**, *12*, 159. [CrossRef] [PubMed]

43. Brottveit, M.; Beitnes, A.C.; Tollefsen, S.; Bratlie, J.E.; Jahnsen, F.L.; Johansen, F.E.; Sollid, L.M.; Lundin, K.E. Mucosal cytokine responses after short-term gluten challenge in celiac disease and non-celiac gluten sensitivity. *Am. J. Gastroenterol.* **2013**, *108*, 842–850. [CrossRef] [PubMed]

44. Bjorck, S.; Lindehammer, S.R.; Fex, M.; Agardh, D. Serum cytokine pattern in young children with screening detected celiac disease. *Clin. Exp. Immunol.* **2015**, *179*, 230–235. [CrossRef] [PubMed]

45. Pesce, G.; Auricchio, R.; Bagnasco, M.; Saverino, D. Oversecretion of soluble CTLA-4 in various autoimmune diseases overlapping celiac disease. *Genet. Test. Mol. Biomark.* **2014**, *18*, 8–11. [CrossRef]

46. Wen, S.; Wen, N.; Pang, J.; Langen, G.; Brew-Appiah, R.A.; Mejias, J.H.; Osorio, C.; Yang, M.; Gemini, R.; Moehs, C.P.; *et al.* Structural genes of wheat and barley 5-methylcytosine DNA glycosylases and their potential applications for human health. *Proc. Natl. Acad. Sci. USA* **2012**, *109*, 20543–20548. [CrossRef] [PubMed]

47. Sorensen, M.B. Methylation of B-hordein genes in barley endosperm is inversely correlated with gene activity and affected by the regulatory gene Lys3. *Proc. Natl. Acad. Sci. USA* **1992**, *89*, 4119–4123. [CrossRef] [PubMed]

48. Kreis, M.; Shewry, P.; Forde, B.; Rahman, S.; Miflin, B. Molecular analysis of a mutation conferring the high-lysine phenotype on the grain of barley (*Hordeum. vulgare*). *Cell* **1983**, *34*, 161–167. [CrossRef] [PubMed]

49. Tanner, G.; Howitt, C.; Forrester, R.; Campbell, P.; Tye-Din, J.; Anderson, R. Dissecting the T-cell response to hordeins in coeliac disease can develop barley with reduced immunotoxicity. *Aliment. Pharmacol. Ther.* **2010**, *32*, 1184–1191. [CrossRef] [PubMed]

50. Stepniak, D.; Spaenij-Dekking, L.; Mitea, C.; Moester, M.; de Ru, A.; Baak-Pablo, R.; van Veelen, P.; Edens, L.; Koning, F. Highly efficient gluten degradation with a newly identified prolyl endoprotease: Implications for celiac disease. *Am. J. Physiol. Gastrointest Liver Physiol.* **2006**, *291*, G621–G629. [CrossRef] [PubMed]

51. Tack, G.J.; van de Water, J.M.; Bruins, M.J.; Kooy-Winkelaar, E.M.; van Bergen, J.; Bonnet, P.; Vreugdenhil, A.C.; Korponay-Szabo, I.; Edens, L.; von Blomberg, B.M.E. Consumption of gluten with gluten-degrading enzyme by celiac patients: A pilot study. *World J. Gastroenterol.* **2013**, *19*, 5837–5847. [CrossRef] [PubMed]

52. Toft-Hansen, H.; Rasmussen, K.S.; Staal, A.; Roggen, E.L.; Sollid, L.M.; Lillevang, S.T.; Barington, T.; Husby, S. Treatment of both native and deamidated gluten peptides with an endo-peptidase from *Aspergillus niger* prevents stimulation of gut-derived gluten-reactive T cells from either children or adults with celiac disease. *Clin. Immunol.* **2014**, *153*, 323–331. [CrossRef] [PubMed]

53. Lahdeaho, M.-L.; Kaukinen, K.; Laurila, K.; Vuotikka, P.; Koivurova, O.-P.; Karja-Lahdensuu, T.; Marcantonio, A.; Adekman, D.C.; Maki, M. Glutenase ALV003 attenuates gluten-induced mucosal injury in patients with celiac disease. *Gastroenterology* **2014**, *146*, 1649–1658. [CrossRef] [PubMed]

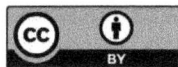

nutrients

MDPI

Article

Sourdough Fermentation of Wheat Flour does not Prevent the Interaction of Transglutaminase 2 with α_2-Gliadin or Gluten

Niklas Engström *, Ann-Sofie Sandberg and Nathalie Scheers

Division of Food and Nutrition Science, Department of Biology and Biological Engineering, Chalmers University of Technology, S-412 96 Gothenburg, Sweden; ann-sofie.sandberg@chalmers.se (A.-S.S.); nathalie.scheers@chalmers.se (N.S.)

* Correspondence: niklas.engstrom@chalmers.se; Tel.: +46-31-772-3845; Fax: +46-31-772-3830

Received: 15 October 2014; Accepted: 19 March 2015; Published: 25 March 2015

Abstract: The enzyme transglutaminase 2 (TG2) plays a crucial role in the initiation of celiac disease by catalyzing the deamidation of gluten peptides. In susceptible individuals, the deamidated peptides initiate an immune response leading to celiac disease. Several studies have addressed lactic fermentation plus addition of enzymes as a means to degrade gluten in order to prevent adverse response in celiacs. Processing for complete gluten degradation is often harsh and is not likely to yield products that are of comparable characteristics as their gluten-containing counterparts. We are concerned that incomplete degradation of gluten may have adverse effects because it leads to more available TG2-binding sites on gluten peptides. Therefore, we have investigated how lactic acid fermentation affects the potential binding of TG2 to gluten protein in wheat flour by means of estimating TG2-mediated transamidation in addition to measuring the available TG2-binding motif QLP, in α_2-gliadin. We show that lactic fermentation of wheat flour, as slurry or as part of sourdough bread, did not decrease the TG2-mediated transamidation, in the presence of a primary amine, to an efficient level (73%–102% of unfermented flour). Nor did the lactic fermentation decrease the available TG2 binding motif QLP in α_2-gliadin to a sufficient extent in sourdough bread (73%–122% of unfermented control) to be useful for celiac safe food.

Keywords: celiac disease; gluten intolerance; lactic fermentation; sourdough; G12 antibody; tissue transglutaminase; TG2; QLP; α_2-gliadin

1. Introduction

1.1. Celiac Disease

Celiac disease (CD) is a disease with an autoimmune component in tissue transglutaminase, which is initiated by the ingestion of gluten proteins in wheat and related proteins in barley (hordeins) and rye (secalins) in genetically predisposed individuals. Exposure will lead to various degrees of inflammation and damage to the small intestine [1]. The majority of patients will experience an improvement in their physical and psychological condition after starting on a gluten-free diet, which to date is the only treatment available [2]. The main genetic risk factors for developing CD are the genotypes encoding for the HLA class II molecules HLA-DQ2 and HLA-DQ8, where the majority of patients carry the DQ2 heterodimer [3,4]. However, roughly one third of the population in Europe carries the DQ2 heterodimer, which means that there are other factors contributing to disease development [5]. Other factors thought to increase the risk for developing CD are various types of infections and the age of gluten introduction [6–9]. CD can be diagnosed at any age but it is most commonly discovered at early childhood, following the introduction of gluten in the diet, and at around the age of 40 and 50 for women and men, respectively [10,11].

1.2. Deamidation of Gluten Initiates Celiac Disease

The enzyme transglutaminase 2, also referred to as tissue transglutaminase (TG2, EC 2.3.2.13), plays a crucial role in the initiation of CD [9,12,13]. As reviewed by Park *et al.* (2010), TG2 is expressed ubiquitously and can be found in, e.g. the cytoplasm, the nucleus, on the extracellular cell surface as well as in the extracellular matrix [14]. It is present in the mucosa of the small intestine and more highly expressed in untreated CD patients [9,15]. TG2 is a member of a family of Ca^{2+}-dependent enzymes that catalyze transamidation or deamidation reactions of, e.g. gluten peptides. In the first step of the enzymatic reaction, the γ-carboxamide of a peptide-bound glutamine acts as an acyl donor that binds to a cysteine at the active site of TG2, resulting in the formation of a γ-glutamylthioester bond and the release of ammonia. In the second part of the reaction, the enzyme is deacylated either by aminolysis or hydrolysis. In the deacylation reaction, a primary amine, such as peptide-bound lysine, acts as acyl acceptor forming an amide bond (transamidation). Transamidated gluten does not result in a celiac response. In the hydrolysis reaction, water acts as acyl acceptor leading to the deamidation of glutamine into glutamic acid [16–18]. The deamidated gluten has a much higher affinity for the HLA-DQ2 and DQ8 heterodimers on antigen-presenting cells [9,12,13]. Once the deamidated gluten peptides are presented to $CD4^+$ T-cells they produce pro-inflammatory cytokines and the subsequent inflammation leads to the degradation of the extracellular matrix and apoptosis of enterocytes leading to the celiac lesion [19]. $CD4^+$ T-cells also activate B-cells, which differentiate into plasma cells that produce antibodies against both gluten and TG2 [19].

1.3. Potential Use of Sourdough in Bread Making to Decrease the Celiac Response

Several studies address the possibility of sourdough fermentation as a means to reduce the level of gluten proteins in bread [20–25]. However, to accomplish this, stringent methods are often used that are sometimes impractical or unrealistic to be able to yield products that are of comparable characteristics, quality and price as their gluten-containing counterparts. Full degradation of gluten requires long fermentations with a combination of several strains of different lactic acid bacteria and/or with the addition of a suitable peptidase. By fully degrading wheat gluten, the viscoelastic properties are lost, which reduces the benefit of the process. Incomplete degradation may lead to the retention of part of the beneficial properties but we are concerned that the protein breakdown may lead to more available TG2-binding sites on gluten peptides and thus increase deamidation reactions by TG2, which would increase the intra-tissue accumulation of antigen and thus potentiate the immune response in celiacs.

Therefore, we have investigated the effect of lactic acid fermentation on potential binding of TG2 to gluten proteins in wheat flour and breads made under similar conditions as industrially baked sourdough breads available on the consumer market. We used two methods: (1) a commercial antibody-based assay that recognizes the TG2-binding motif QLP present in α_2-gliadin, considered to be the most immunogenic peptide derived from gluten proteins during digestion. The assay was used to indicate how many QLP motives remain available for TG2 binding after lactic fermentation and *in vitro* digestion; (2) a transamidation assay that indicates the interaction of TG2 with gluten proteins as an estimate of the interaction of *any* binding site, independent of the identity of gluten proteins. A primary amine is added in the assay to favor transamidation instead of deamidation reactions, which are undetectable in the present conditions. The experiments were made with three lactic acid bacterial strains (*L. plantarum*, *L. pentosus* and *L. brevis*) independently.

2. Materials and Methods

2.1. Sample Preparation

2.1.1. Strains and Culture Conditions

Three *lactobacillus* subspecies (*L. brevis*, *L. plantarum*, and *L. pentosus*) were cultivated in M.R.S. broth (Oxoid Ltd., Hampshire, UK; 37 °C, 150 rpm). Overnight cultures inoculated at $OD_{600} = 0.5$ were prepared for the wheat flour fermentations (American Biosciences Ultrospec 10 cell density meter, Blauvelt, NY, USA). Colony forming units (CFU; Tryptone glucose extract agar, Sharlau SL, Barcelona, Spain; 24–48 h, 30 °C) were done to estimate bacteria concentration and to check for contamination. The cultures were washed by centrifugation (5 min, 1000 g) and re-suspended in NaCl-solution (0.9%) followed by a second centrifugation (5 min, 1000 g) and re-suspension in NaCl-solution (0.9%).

2.1.2. Lactic Fermentation of Wheat Flour

Wheat flour (extraction rate 80%; Saltå Kvarn, Järna, Sweden) was fermented using the three different lactic acid bacteria. Flour (5 g) was mixed with water (MQ; 70 mL) and respective strain in NaCl-solution (0.9%, 5 M) resulting in a final OD_{600} of approximately 0.5. The flour slurries were allowed to ferment during shaking (21 h, 37 °C, 150–200 rpm). The samples were immediately frozen (−20 °C). The control was made in the same way but without the fermentation step.

2.1.3. Sourdough Bread Making

Each *Lactobacillus* strain was transferred, in NaCl-solution (0.9%, 5 mL), to a mixture of equal amounts (w/w) of wheat flour and tap water, which was let to ferment 24 h in ambient temperature (sourdough). The sourdough (175 g) was mixed with fresh flour (350 g), tap water (200 g), commercial baker's yeast (12.5 g; Kronjäst, Rotebro, Sweden), olive oil (10 g; Zeta Originale, Stockholm, Sweden) and NaCl (7.5 g; Santa Maria Bordssalt, Mölndal, Sweden). The sourdough constituted 20% of the total flour used for the bread. All the ingredients were mixed and kneaded in a KitchenAid (10 min, speed 2; Benton Harbor, MI, USA). The dough was leavened for 2 h in the bowl and was then divided into two parts which each were manually kneaded for approximately 1 min before left to rise for another 2 h. The breads were put on a hot baking plate and baked until reaching satisfactory crust coloration (18–25 min, approx. 220 °C). After baking the breads were freeze-dried (Heto DW6-55 Drywinner, Allerød, Denmark) and ground.

2.1.4. *In Vitro* Digestion of Wheat Flour and Sourdough Bread

In order to simulate the impact of the gastric and proximal duodenal digestion, an *in vitro* digestion procedure using pepsin was conducted for all samples. The reasoning for terminating the digestion at early duodenal phase is that the digesta may come in contact with TG2 before the secretion of pancreatic enzymes. The fermented wheat flour samples (5 g) were mixed with water (MQ; 50 mL). The freeze-dried sourdough bread samples (0.34 g) were mixed with water (MQ; 54.76 mL) and NaCl-solution (0.9%, 0.34 mL), to correspond to the water content in the slurry of the fermented wheat flour. The simulated gastric digestion was started by lowering the pH to approximately 2.1 with HCl (5 M) and adding pepsin (porcine pepsin, Sigma Aldrich, St. Louis, MO, USA) dissolved in HCl (0.1 M, 1.5 mL, 406400 U/mL) and incubated (1 h, 37 °C, 150 rpm). The digestion was terminated by raising the pH to approximately 7 with NaOH (0.5 M). The samples were stored at −20 °C until further analysis. All samples were centrifuged (15 min, 5000 g) before assay analysis.

2.2. Detection of the TG2 Binding Motif QLP in α_2-Gliadin

An antibody-based assay was done according to the instructions provided with the kit (GlutenTox ELISA Competitive; Biomedal Diagnostics, Sevilla, Spain), with a few modifications. The sample extraction was done at room temperature during 5 minutes with constant mild agitation, after which the samples were centrifuged (5 min, 2500 g). The sample dilution was 1:250. In brief, the samples were incubated with the G12-HRP conjugated antibody, which specifically recognizes the amino acid sequence QPQLPY that is present in α_2-gliadin [26]. The sample-antibody mixture was added to a 96-well plate coated with gliadin, to capture residual antibodies. After washing, the gliadin-bound G12-HRP was allowed to react with the substrate, before adding H_2SO_4 (1 M) and measuring the absorbance at 450 nm.

2.3. TG2-Mediated Transamidation Assay

The transamidation assay was done according to Skovbjerg *et al.* [27] with a few modifications. Sample proteins were coated on 96 well plates onto which TG2 incorporated 5-(biotinamido) pentylamine; Eu-labeled streptavidin was subsequently added to bind to biotin; after which the chelated europium was measured by time-resolved fluorescence (345 nm excitation; 617 nm emission; Safire2; Tecan Group Ltd.; Männedorf; Switzerland). Tris-HCl (5 mM, pH 7.5; Gibco, Life Technologies, Stockholm, Sweden) and bovine serum albumin (BSA; 1%; Pierce/Thermo Scientific, Life Technologies, Stockholm, Sweden) were used as negative controls.

2.4. Statistics

For the fermented wheat flour, four separate fermentations were made for each strain and the control. For the sourdough bread, three breads were prepared for each strain and the control. When detecting the QLP binding motif, two replicates were made for each trial ($n = 8$–12 measurements). In the transamidation assay five to eight replicates were made for each trial ($n = 27$–32 measurements)). Two-tailed student's *t*-test was used for significance testing (IBM SPSS Statistics 22). Differences were considered to be significant at $p < 0.05$.

3. Results

3.1. The Fermentation Process

The lactic fermented wheat flour samples showed no visible growth of other microorganisms as observed by examination of streaked TGE-agar plates. The starting pH of the controls was 6.3 and 6.0–6.2 for the samples. At the end of the fermentations (24 h), the pH was 3.2–3.8. Approximately 4×10^7–9×10^8 cells/mL dough was added to each sourdough as estimated by the CFU count. After *in vitro* digestion, all samples were between pH 6.9–7.2.

3.2. Fermentation with L. plantarum Significantly Increases Available QLP Motives on α_2-Gliadin

Lactic fermentation of wheat flour with *L. plantarum* significantly increased available QLP sites on α_2-gliadin ($22\% \pm 18\%$, $p = 0.047$, Figure 1) while the other *lactobacilli* subspecies reduced the binding motif either significantly (*L. pentosus*; $27\% \pm 21\%$, $p = 0.027$) or insignificantly (*L. brevis*; $8\% \pm 15\%$, $p = 0.317$) compared to unfermented wheat flour. Since α_2-gliadin is considered to be the most immunogenic peptide in gluten, fermentation of wheat flour with *L. plantarum* may thus potentiate the toxicity of gluten to celiacs. Although, *L. pentosus* decreased the available TG2 binding sites on α_2-gliadin, the extent ($27\% \pm 21\%$) is not sufficient to be of any importance in the aim to use lactic fermentation as a means to detoxify gluten in wheat flour.

3.3. Fermentation with L. plantarum Slightly Decreased TG2-Mediated Transamidation of Gluten

By measuring the TG2-mediated transamidation, we get a measure of TG2 interaction with all gluten peptides in the flour sample, as in opposition to the antibody based assay, in which we focus on the interaction of TG2 with α_2-gliadin (33 amino acid-long peptide, often referred to as the 33-mer). Fermentation of wheat flour with *L. plantarum* significantly decreased the transamidation of gluten ($27\% \pm 18\%$, $p < 0.001$, Figure 2), while fermentation with *L. brevis and L. pentosus* did not affect the transamidation significantly (decrease of $18\% \pm 22\%$, $p = 0.073$ and increase of $2\% \pm 25\%$, $p = 0.564$, respectively). Important to remember is that despite that *L. plantarum* decreased, the total interaction of TG2 with gluten, the available binding sites on the most immunogenic peptide in gluten, was significantly increased.

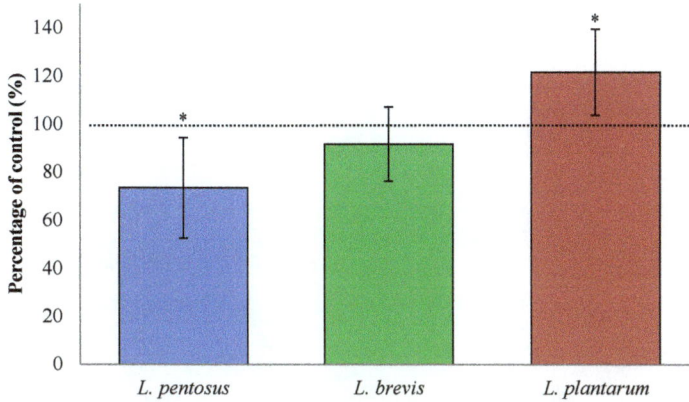

Figure 1. This bar graph shows the change in number of the TG2 binding motif QLP, specific to α_2-gliadin, which remains available for TG2 binding after lactic fermentation and *in vitro* digestion of wheat flour. Wheat flour fermented with *L. brevis*, *L. pentosus*, or *L. plantarum* was compared to unfermented breads (control = 100%). Data are presented as means ± SD (n = 8–12) and shows the change 73%–122% of control. The asterisk indicates a significant change ($p < 0.05$) from control.

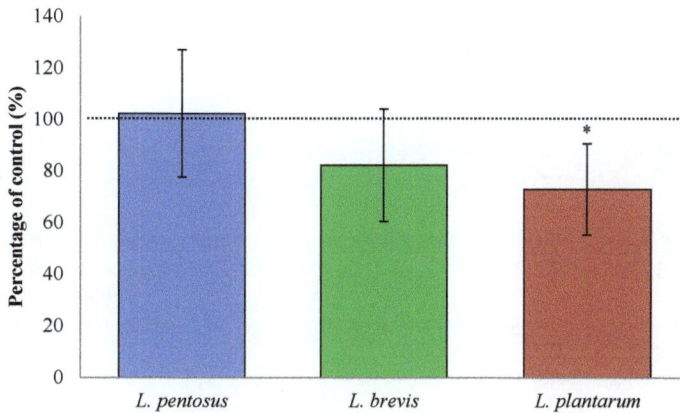

Figure 2. TG2-mediated transamidation of *in vitro* digested, fermented and unfermented, wheat flour in the presence of a primary amine indicates the interaction of TG2 and various binding sites on gluten protein. The change in transamidation caused by lactic fermentation was 73%–102% of the control. Data are presented as means ± SD (n = 27–32). The asterisk indicates a significant change ($p < 0.05$) from control.

3.4. Sourdough Fermentation with L. plantarum Decreased Available QLP Motives in α_2-Gliadin

In digested sourdough bread in which the sourdough part (20%) was fermented with *L. plantarum*, the available TG2 binding sites were decreased (19% ± 15%, $p = 0.042$; Figure 3) compared to control breads, leavened with baker's yeast only. Sourdough fermented with *L. pentosus* and *L. brevis* did not significantly decrease available TG2 binding sites (8% ± 16%, $p = 0.359$ and 6% ± 12%, $p = 0.390$, respectively). The *L. plantarum* fermented wheat flour was fermented for 24 h while the *L. plantarum* fermented sourdough was fermented for 4 h (20% of total bread weight was fermented for 24 h), which suggests that a longer fermentation time produces more celiac toxic α_2-gliadin peptides, than a shorter time.

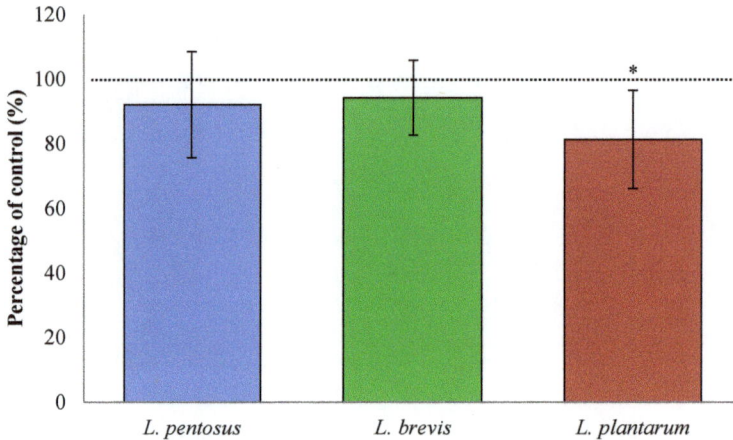

Figure 3. The change in the number of TG2 binding motif QLP in α_2-gliadin from *in vitro* digested sourdough breads. The sourdough was fermented with *L. brevis*, *L. pentosus*, or *L. plantarum*. Changes were compared to those from unfermented control breads (control = 100%). Data are presented as means $\pm$ SD (n = 8–12). The asterisk indicates a significant change ($p < 0.05$) from control. Data show changes in the range 81%–94% of control.

4. Discussion

4.1. Is It Beneficial to Degrade Gluten?

Several studies have shown that fermentation with multiple selected strains of lactic acid bacteria and/or the use of specific enzymes may successfully degrade gluten [20–23,28,29]. These studies do not address if the processing affects the TG2 binding or the formation of deamidation products by TG2. Total degradation of wheat gluten would eliminate the viscoelastic properties, which are responsible for, e.g., the leavening capacity of bread or other baked products. Bread baked of wheat flour with no gluten will be perceived as inferior compared to a gluten-containing wheat bread. Wheat flour rendered gluten free by lactic fermentation and/or enzymatic treatment may, however, be used together with naturally gluten free flours and structuring agents to make products of similar quality as gluten-containing counterparts [21,22,25]. Full degradation of gluten requires long fermentation times (~24 h), often in combination of several strains of different lactic acid bacteria and with the addition of peptidases. Long fermentation times and addition of enzymes also mean higher production costs for the final product. Verification of the degradation is important, since a partial degradation of gluten may lead to an increased number of available TG2-binding sites as we observed in the present study. The increased interaction of TG2 with gluten or gluten-derived peptides may increase the load of deamidation products in the gastrointestinal tissues and thus potentiate or initiate the immune response in celiacs.

4.2. Evaluation of Methods for TG2 and Gluten Interactions

We have evaluated the use of different methods for estimating the interactions of TG2 with gluten, such as measuring the level of (1) deamidation and transamidation, (2) the ammonia release upon binding of TG2 to gluten, and (3) the specific recognition of an antibody to TG2 binding motifs. After evaluation and optimization, we dismissed two of the methods due to poor reproducibility, namely the ammonia release and deamidation measurements. The ammonia release predicts the total binding of TG2 to gluten since ammonia is released upon the formation of γ-glutamylthioester bonds during a SN_2 substitution reaction between TG2 and glutamine side chains in gluten. This gives us the total binding of TG2 to gluten, regardless of the subsequent transamidation or deamidation reaction. Which of these reactions will follow depends on the availability of primary amines. If no such amine is present, TG2 uses water instead to deamidate the substrate [19]. However, due to the low levels and volatile nature of ammonia, it proved difficult to obtain reliable results with this method. We also analyzed the samples for the deamidation product glutamate using a commercial deamidation assay (Glutamate Colorimetric Assay Kit, BioVision, San Francisco, CA, USA). The enzyme mix supplied with the assay uses glutamate as a substrate leading to color development, which can be measured spectrophotometrically. However, this assay proved not to be suitable for our samples.

5. Conclusions

We conclude that lactic fermentation of wheat flour does not sufficiently prevent TG2 interaction with gluten or decrease available TG2 binding sites on α_2-gliadin, compared to unfermented flour. Prolonged fermentation times with *L. plantarum* (24 h) even increased available TG2 binding sites on α_2-gliadin, indicating that lactic fermentation may not be an appropriate method for making celiac safe products.

Acknowledgments: We would like to acknowledge the work of the B. Sc. Students Josefine Alphonce, Karin Bäcksten, Josefin Klangefjäll, Olivia Larsson, and Fanny Taborsak (the Biotechnology program at Chalmers University of Technology) for their initial work on the transamidation assay. This work was funded by research grant no. 2012-4131 from the Swedish Research Council (Vetenskapsrådet).

Author Contributions: N. Engström, N. Scheers and A.-S. Sandberg designed the research, N. Engström collected data and performed statistical analyses, N. Engström wrote the manuscript draft, N. Engström, N. Scheers and A.-S. Sandberg revised the manuscript. All authors read and approved the final manuscript.

Conflicts of Interest: The authors declare no conflict of interest.

References

1. Ludvigsson, J.F.; Leffler, D.A.; Bai, J.C.; Biagi, F.; Fasano, A.; Green, P.H.R.; Hadjivassiliou, M.; Kaukinen, K.; Kelly, C.P.; Leonard, J.N.; *et al.* The oslo definitions for coeliac disease and related terms. *Gut* **2013**, *62*, 43–52. [CrossRef] [PubMed]

2. Fabiani, E.; Catassi, C.; Villari, A.; Gismondi, P.; Pierdomenico, R.; Ratsch, I.; Coppa, G.; Giorgi, P. Dietary complience in screening-detected coeliac disease adolescents. *Acta Paediatr.* **1996**, *85*, 65–67. [CrossRef]

3. Sollid, L.M.; Markussen, G.; Ek, J.; Gjerde, H.; Vartdal, F.; Thorsby, E. Evidence for a primary association of celiac disease to a particular hla-dq alpha/beta heterodimer. *J. Exp. Med.* **1989**, *169*, 345–350. [CrossRef] [PubMed]

4. Spurkland, A.; Sollid, L.M.; Polanco, I.; Vartdal, F.; Thorsby, E. Hla-dr and -dq genotypes of celiac disease patients serologically typed to be non-dr3 or non-dr5/7. *Hum. Immunol.* **1992**, *35*, 188–192. [CrossRef] [PubMed]

5. Di Sabatino, A.; Corazza, G. Coeliac disease. *Lancet* **2009**, *373*, 1480–1493. [CrossRef] [PubMed]

6. Agostoni, C.; Decsi, T.; Fewtrell, M.; Goulet, O.; Kolacek, S.; Koletzko, B.; Michaelsen, K.F.; Moreno, L.; Puntis, J.; Rigo, J.; *et al.* Complementary feeding: A commentary by the espghan committee on nutrition. *J. Pediatr. Gastroenterol. Nutr.* **2008**, *46*, 99–110. [CrossRef]

7. Sandberg-Bennich, S.; Dahlquist, G.; Källén, B. Coeliac disease is associated with intrauterine growth and neonatal infections. *Acta Pædiatr.* **2002**, *91*, 30–33. [CrossRef] [PubMed]

8. Plot, L.; Amital, H. Infectious associations of celiac disease. *Autoimmun. Rev.* **2009**, *8*, 316–319. [CrossRef] [PubMed]

9. Molberg, O.; McAdam, S.N.; Korner, R.; Quarsten, H.; Kristiansen, C.; Madsen, L.; Fugger, L.; Scott, H.; Noren, O.; Roepstorff, P.; *et al.* Tissue transglutaminase selectively modifies gliadin peptides that are recognized by gut-derived t cells in celiac disease. *Nat. Med.* **1998**, *4*, 713–717. [CrossRef] [PubMed]

10. Tack, G.; Verbeek, W.; Schreurs, M.; Mulder, C. The spectrum of coeliac disease: Epidemiology, clinical aspects and treatment. *Nat. Rev. Gastroenterol. Hepatol.* **2010**, *7*, 204–213. [CrossRef] [PubMed]

11. Abadie, V.; Sollid, L.; Barreiro, L.; Jabri, B. Integration of genetic and immunlogical insights into a model of celiac disease pathogenesis. *Annu. Rev. Immunol.* **2011**, *29*, 493–525. [CrossRef] [PubMed]

12. Van de Wal, Y.; Kooy, Y.; van Veelen, P.; Peña, S.; Mearin, L.; Papadopoulos, G.; Koning, F. Cutting edge: Selective deamidation by tissue transglutaminase strongly enhances gliadin-specific t cell reactivity. *J. Immunol.* **1998**, *161*, 1585–1588.

13. Arentz-Hansen, H.; Körner, R.; Molberg, Ø.; Quarsten, H.; Vader, W.; Kooy, Y.M.C.; Lundin, K.E.A.; Koning, F.; Roepstorff, P.; Sollid, L.M.; *et al.* The intestinal T cell response to α-gliadin in adult celiac disease is focused on a single deamidated glutamine targeted by tissue transglutaminase. *J. Exp. Med.* **2000**, *191*, 603–612. [CrossRef] [PubMed]

14. Park, D.; Choi, S.; Ha, K.-S. Transglutaminase 2: A multi-functional protein in multiple subcellular compartments. *Amino Acids* **2010**, *39*, 619–631. [CrossRef] [PubMed]

15. Brusco, G.; Muzi, P.; Ciccocioppo, R.; Biagi, F.; Cifone, M.G.; Corazza, G.R. Transglutaminase and coeliac disease: Endomysial reactivity and small bowel expression. *Clin. Exp. Immunol.* **1999**, *118*, 371–375. [CrossRef] [PubMed]

16. Qiao, S.-W.; Iversen, R.; Ráki, M.; Sollid, L. The adaptive immune response in celiac disease. *Semin. Immunopathol.* **2012**, *34*, 523–540. [CrossRef] [PubMed]

17. Skovbjerg, H.; Koch, C.; Anthonsen, D.; Sjöström, H. Deamidation and cross-linking of gliadin peptides by transglutaminases and the relation to celiac disease. *Biochim. Biophys. Acta (BBA) Mol. Basis Dis.* **2004**, *1690*, 220–230. [CrossRef]

18. Sugimura, Y.; Hosono, M.; Wada, F.; Yoshimura, T.; Maki, M.; Hitomi, K. Screening for the preferred substrate sequence of transglutaminase using a phage-displayed peptide library: Identification of peptide substrates for tgase 2 and factor xiiia. *J. Biol. Chem.* **2006**, *281*, 17699–17706. [CrossRef] [PubMed]

19. Di Sabatino, A.; Vanoli, A.; Giuffrida, P.; Luinetti, O.; Solcia, E.; Corazza, G.R. The function of tissue transglutaminase in celiac disease. *Autoimmun. Rev.* **2012**, *11*, 746–753.

20. Di Cagno, R.; Barbato, M.; Di Camillo, C.; Rizzello, C.G.; De Angelis, M.; Giuliani, G.; De Vincenzi, M.; Gobbetti, M.; Cucchiara, S. Gluten-free sourdough wheat baked goods appear safe for young celiac patients: A pilot study. *J. Pediatric. Gastroenterol. Nutr.* **2010**, *51*, 777–783.

21. De Angelis, M.; Cassone, A.; Rizzello, C.G.; Gagliardi, F.; Minervini, F.; Calasso, M.; Di Cagno, R.; Francavilla, R.; Gobbetti, M. Mechanism of degradation of immunogenic gluten epitopes from triticum turgidum l. Var. Durum by sourdough lactobacilli and fungal proteases. *Appl. Environ. Microbiol.* **2010**, *76*, 508–518. [CrossRef] [PubMed]

22. Rizzello, C.G.; De Angelis, M.; Di Cagno, R.; Camarca, A.; Silano, M.; Losito, I.; De Vincenzi, M.; De Bari, M.D.; Palmisano, F.; Maurano, F.; *et al.* Highly efficient gluten degradation by lactobacilli and fungal proteases during food processing: New perspectives for celiac disease. *Appl. Environ. Microbiol.* **2007**, *73*, 4499–4507. [CrossRef] [PubMed]

23. Loponen, J.; Sontag-Strohm, T.; Venäläinen, J.; Salovaara, H. Prolamin hydrolysis in wheat sourdoughs with differing proteolytic activities. *J. Agric. Food Chem.* **2007**, *55*, 978–984. [CrossRef] [PubMed]

24. Gerez, C.L.; Dallagnol, A.; Rollán, G.; Font de Valdez, G. A combination of two lactic acid bacteria improves the hydrolysis of gliadin during wheat dough fermentation. *Food Microbiol.* **2012**, *32*, 427–430. [CrossRef] [PubMed]

25. Di Cagno, R.; De Angelis, M.; Auricchio, S.; Greco, L.; Clarke, C.; De Vincenzi, M.; Giovannini, C.; D'Archivio, M.; Landolfo, F.; Parrilli, G.; *et al.* Sourdough bread made from wheat and nontoxic flours and started with selected lactobacilli is tolerated in celiac sprue patients. *Appl. Environ. Microbiol.* **2004**, *70*, 1088–1096. [CrossRef] [PubMed]

26. Morón, B.; Bethune, M.T.; Comino, I.; Manyani, H.; Ferragud, M.; López, M.C.; Cebolla, Á.; Khosla, C.; Sousa, C. Toward the assessment of food toxicity for celiac patients: Characterization of monoclonal antibodies to a main immunogenic gluten peptide. *PLoS ONE* **2008**, *3*, e2294. [CrossRef] [PubMed]

27. Skovbjerg, H.; Norén, O.; Anthonsen, D.; Moller, J.; Sjöström, H. Coeliac disease gliadin is a good substrate of several transglutaminases: Possible implication in the pathogenesis of coeliac disease. *Scand. J. Gastroenterol.* **2002**, *37*, 812–817. [CrossRef] [PubMed]

28. Tye-Din, J.A.; Anderson, R.P.; Ffrench, R.A.; Brown, G.J.; Hodsman, P.; Siegel, M.; Botwick, W.; Shreeniwas, R. The effects of alv003 pre-digestion of gluten on immune response and symptoms in celiac disease *in vivo*. *Clin. Immunol.* **2010**, *134*, 289–295. [CrossRef] [PubMed]

29. Hartmann, G.; Koehler, P.; Wieser, H. Rapid degradation of gliadin peptides toxic for coeliac disease patients by proteases from germinating cereals. *J. Cereal Sci.* **2006**, *44*, 368–371. [CrossRef]

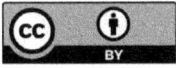

nutrients

MDPI

Article

Self-Reported Prevalence of Symptomatic Adverse Reactions to Gluten and Adherence to Gluten-Free Diet in an Adult Mexican Population

Noe Ontiveros [1], Jesús A. López-Gallardo [2], Marcela J. Vergara-Jiménez [2] and Francisco Cabrera-Chávez [2,*]

[1]   Regional Program for PhD in Biotechnology, FCQB, University of Sinaloa, Culiacán, Sinaloa 80019, México; noeontiveros@gmail.com
[2]   Nutrition Sciences Academic Unit, University of Sinaloa, Culiacán, Sinaloa 80019, México; aristeo.lopez37@hotmail.com (J.A.L.-G.); mjvergara@uas.edu.mx (M.J.V.-J.)
*   Correspondence: fcabrera@uas.edu.mx; Tel./Fax: +52-667-753-5454

Received: 31 May 2015; Accepted: 14 July 2015; Published: 21 July 2015

Abstract: The prevalence of symptomatic adverse reactions to gluten and adherence to gluten-free diet in Latin American countries is unknown. These measurements are strongly linked to gluten-related disorders. This work aimed to estimate the prevalence of adverse reactions to oral gluten and the adherence to gluten-free diet in the adult Mexican population. To reach this aim, a self-administered questionnaire was designed and tested for clarity/comprehension and reproducibility. Then, a self-administered questionnaire-based cross-sectional study was conducted in the Mexican population. The estimated prevalence rates were (95% CI): 11.9% (9.9–13.5) and 7.8 (6.4–9.4) for adverse and recurrent adverse reactions to gluten respectively; adherence to gluten-free diet 3.7% (2.7–4.8), wheat allergy 0.72% (0.38–1.37); celiac disease 0.08% (0.01–0.45), and NCGS 0.97% (0.55–1.68). Estimated pooled prevalence of self-reported physician-diagnosis of gluten-related disorders was 0.88% (0.49–1.5), and 93.3% respondents reported adherence to gluten-free diet without a physician-diagnosis of gluten-related disorders. Symptom comparisons between those who reported recurrent adverse reactions to gluten and other foods showed statistically significant differences for bloating, constipation, and tiredness ($p < 0.05$). Gluten-related disorders may be underdiagnosed in the Mexican population and most people adhering to a gluten-free diet are doing it without proper diagnostic work-up of these disorders, and probably without medical/dietician advice.

Keywords: prevalence; adverse reactions; gluten-free diet; gluten-related disorders

1. Introduction

Adverse reactions to foods can be mediated or not by immune mechanisms. Particularly, gluten related disorders such as wheat allergy and celiac disease are well known immune mediated conditions [1]. Another gluten related disorder is Non-Celiac gluten sensitivity (NCGS). These are cases where symptomatic adverse reactions to oral "gluten" occur, but in which neither allergic nor autoimmune mechanisms are involved [1,2]. However, other immune mechanisms related to the innate immune system could play a role in this condition, but the precise mechanisms underlying NCGS are not well understood yet [1,3]. Notably, all NCGS cases are symptomatic the hallmarks of this condition being gastrointestinal ornon-intestinal symptoms [4].

The existence of NCGS was supported a few years ago [5], but further studies carried out by the same group showed no gluten-specific symptomatic adverse reactions to gluten in a specific population [6]. This has led to the idea that other wheat components besides gluten could trigger the symptoms seen in NCGS cases. However, due to the lack of biomarkers for the diagnostic work-out of NCGS, a proper diagnosis of NCGS can be performed only after wheat allergy and celiac disease have been ruled-out, symptomatic relief is reached after gluten withdrawal, and gluten-specific symptoms are confirmed by a food challenge test [7,8].

Following a gluten-free diet is the only accepted treatment for those affected with celiac disease or NCGS. Wheat allergic patients do not necessary need to follow a gluten-free diet, but they have to avoid wheat in their diets. Although a gluten-free diet is costly and socially restrictive, it is possible that more people than those that truly benefit from it avoid gluten in their diets [9,10]. This could have some implications as adhering to a gluten-free diet could impact on the serum levels of some micronutrients such as iron and vitamin B [11,12]. Moreover, due to the reliability of celiac disease specific serology tests and pathology results are strongly influenced by gluten intake, adhering to a gluten-free diet without a proper diagnosis of celiac disease could complicate the diagnostic work-up of this condition [8].

Until now, it is been accepted that the prevalence of celiac disease is around 1% in the general population, but prevalence data about wheat allergy in adult population are scarce and data about NCGS highly differ. In fact, NCGS prevalence range from 1% to 13% according to studies carried out in the United States and Europe [1,13,14]. Furthermore, considering adherence to gluten-free diet in non-celiac population as a surrogate of NCGS, the prevalence of the latter condition in the United States is 0.55% [15], which is slightly lower than that of celiac disease (0.71%) [9]. Notably, although there are some prevalence data about celiac disease in Latin America, there is neither NCGS nor gluten-free diet adherence prevalence data in open populations within Latin American countries. Moreover, prevalence data related to other adverse reactions to foods such as food allergy are scarce. Identifying those cases that potentially develop symptomatic adverse reactions to foods is the first step to estimate with objective diagnostic criteria the prevalence of NCGS or other symptomatic adverse reactions to foods in population-based studies.

The main aim of this study was to estimate the prevalence of symptomatic adverse reactions to oral gluten and other foods as well as the adherence to gluten-free diet in the Mexican population aged 18 years or older. Moreover, due to the lack of a validated instrument to identify potential NCGS cases in a Latin population, an additional aim was to design and test a self-administered questionnaire to identify potential cases of symptomatic gluten-related disorders and other cases of adverse reactions to foods.

2. Experimental Section

2.1. Questionnaire Design

Based on two previously devised instruments and recognized NCGS symptoms published in scientific literature, a self-administered questionnaire was designed to identify people developing symptomatic adverse reactions to oral gluten and other foods. Gastrointestinal and extraintestinal symptoms were first recapitulated from an NCGS questionnaire devised by the Italian Celiac Disease Association and the Italian Celiac Foundation [14]. To ensure that most relevant NCGS-associated symptoms were included, additional scientific sources evaluating gluten-induced symptoms by oral gluten challenge test in NCGS population were consulted [5,16–18]. Thus, the NCGS-associated symptoms assessed in this study can be defined as literature-based NCGS symptoms and were chosen based on the frequencies of gastrointestinal and extraintestinal manifestations reported (material S3, questions 5 and 9).

Since the questionnaire devised by the Italian Celiac Disease Association/Foundation was designed for collecting clinical data by skilled investigators attending outpatient clinics, we took advantage of a previously validated Spanish version of an in-depth questionnaire intended to evaluate the prevalence of self-reported food allergy [19]. This instrument asks questions about typical symptoms of immediate hypersensitivity allergic reactions that have high sensitivity for positive specific food IgE [20,21]. Thus, the designed questionnaire includes not only items/questions related to NCGS, but also items/questions related to food allergy (Figure 1).

As expected, some items/questions of the in-depth Spanish questionnaire were adapted to ask questions about symptoms triggered by oral gluten or other foods, and to be self-administered. In this process a few words were changed from the original Chilean source to better fit the words for Mexican culture, but the ways to measure the variables of interest were not modified. To certify that the questions and responses were simple, clear, natural sounding, and the language used was at the level of understanding of the target population, we performed tests to evaluate comprehension, reproducibility, and wording of questions of the designed instrument.

2.2. Questionnaire Clarity/Comprehension and Wording of Questions Evaluation

Clarity/comprehension was evaluated as previously described [22]. This evaluation was performed by means of cognitive interviews in a sample of the target population (at least 20 subjects developing adverse reactions to gluten and 20 developing adverse reactions to other foods). The interviewees should evaluate each item/question in a three point scale; 1: Clear and comprehensible, 2: Difficult to understand, and 3: Incomprehensible (ordinal scale). Clarity/comprehension was also evaluated in a numerical scale from 0 to 10. For this evaluation 0 was considered very easy to understand and 10 very difficult to understand. The interviewees had to answer the question; how would you rate this item/question? Items/questions rated ≤3 were considered clear and comprehensible and, consequently, rewording was not required. We made sure that all possible answers were read/written immediately after the questions and the language used at the level of the target population. This can be helpful in cases of non-self-explanatory questions [23]. To verify the comprehension of the items and to evaluate the wording of questions, the interviewees should state with their own words the perceived meaning of each item and to answer the question: how would you write this item? These participants were identified in previous screening tests and were not included in the prevalence study.

2.3. Questionnaire Test-Retest Consistency

At least 20 subjects who reported adverse reactions to gluten and another 20 who reported adverse reactions to other foods answered the questionnaire twice. The time period interval between first and second application of the questionnaire was of at least two weeks (range: 2–4 weeks). These participants were identified in previous screening tests and were not included in the prevalence study. Intraclass or Lin's concordance correlation coefficients are commonly used for measuring test-retest consistency. These methods are useful to assess agreement in continuous variables, but most variables to be measured with the designed instrument were categorical. Thus, test-retest consistency analysis using the Kappa statistics was performed and results with 95% confidence intervals were reported. In addition, consistency was also reported as percentage of matched questions between first and second application of the questionnaire. A matched question was considered when the respondents reported the same gastrointestinal or extraintestinal symptoms in the first and second application of the questionnaire. The same approach was applied for other questions where more than one answer could be chosen. For the analysis, first and second applications of the questionnaire were considered as rater one and two respectively.

2.4. Population Survey

The survey was conducted outside mainstream shopping malls and urban parks of Culiacan, Sinaloa, Mexico. All data were collected during the period from January to April 2015. Inclusion criteria were as follows: subjects aged 18 years or older and able to read and answer the questionnaire by themselves. Exclusion criteria included subjects less than 18 years old or subjects that were not able to complete the questionnaire by themselves. Trained nutritional science students gave assistance on specific terms when it was requested. The first part of the questionnaire asked about demographics information including age, gender, and education. This part also includes contact information and a key question about adverse reactions to oral gluten (do you have some discomfort or adverse reaction when consuming wheat products?). Race/ethnicity was not considered as the city of Culiacan, Sinaloa is not characterized for being multicultural. The first section included 15 items/questions and was designed for those who reported adverse reactions to oral gluten. The first question in this section asked about the diagnostic work-up of gluten related disorders (have you ever been diagnosed with a disease related to the consumption of wheat or gluten?). The second section includes 14 items/questions and was designed for those who reported adverse reactions to other foods different from gluten. This section enables the estimation of general self-reported prevalence of adverse reactions to foods and, consequently, to estimate the magnitude of the symptomatic adverse reactions to gluten in the studied population. Additionally, prevalence rates of adverse reactions to individual foods including self-reported food allergy prevalence rates could be estimated (supplemental material). First and second section screened for gastrointestinal and extraintestinal symptoms, symptom frequency, time interval between the ingestion of food and symptom occurrence, and family history of celiac disease. In addition, first section screened for gluten-related disorders and the person who performed the diagnosis. All participants answered the question; do you keep a diet free of wheat or gluten?

A reported diagnosis of celiac disease was considered when the respondents were diagnosed by a physician or and were also following a gluten-free diet [13]. In addition to the previous criteria, self-reported wheat/food allergy was also considered when the respondents reported recurrent adverse reactions "convincing" of food allergy (Figure 1). This includes skin with hives and angio-edema, trouble breathing, wheezing or throat tightness, vomiting, and diarrhea, and the symptoms occurred within 2 h after food ingestion [19–21], or the respondents reported a previous diagnosis of food allergy (supplemental material S3, questions 13 or 26). Recurrent adverse reactions were considered when the respondents reported that the food-induced symptoms occurred always or most of the times.

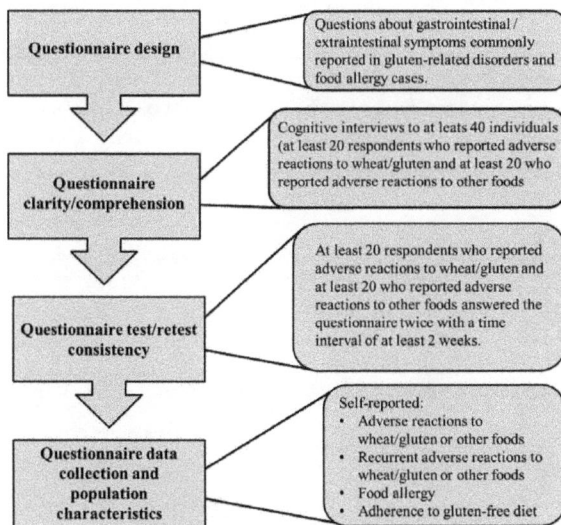

Figure 1. Flowchart of the study protocol.

2.5. Statistical and Ethical Issues

Statistical analysis was carried out using PASW statistics version 18.0 (SPSS Inc., Chicago, IL, USA). Categorical variables were summarized by descriptive statistics, including total numbers, percentages, odds ratio, 95% confidence interval, and associations were analyzed by two-tailed Fisher exact test. Odds ratio analysis was conducted to identify the symptoms preferentially associated to recurrent adverse reactions to gluten compared to other foods. Respondents that reported other allergies different from wheat allergy or dairy intolerance, but also reported recurrent adverse reactions to gluten were included in the analysis. Exposed and non-exposed cases were represented by those who reported and non-reported a specific symptom respectively, and cases and controls were represented by those who reported recurrent adverse reactions to gluten and recurrent adverse reactions to other foods respectively. Continuous variables were summarized by mean and range with differences between two groups calculated using the Student t-test. A p-value < 0.05 was considered statistically significant. Prevalence rates were calculated using OpenEpi software version 3.03 [24]. Rates were reported as rate (95% confidence intervals) per 100 inhabitants. Questionnaire completion and return was regarded as consent. An Ethics Review Board of the Autonomous University of Sinaloa approved the study protocol (ethic approval number CE-UACNYG-2014-AGO-001).

3. Results

3.1. Questionnaire Evaluation

Clarity/comprehension was evaluated in a population that reported recurrent-food-induced symptoms. For this purpose, twenty-two respondents had to answer Section 1 of the instrument designed (adverse reactions to gluten). Among these, eight respondents reported gluten-induced gastrointestinal and extraintestinal symptoms (36.4%). For Section 2 (adverse reactions to other foods), eight out of 20 respondents reported gastrointestinal and extraintestinal adverse reactions to foods different from gluten (40.0%). The school degree of the respondents in each section of the instrument ranged from elementary to postgraduate. Overall, clarity/comprehension evaluation was excellent with an ordinal scale score of clear and comprehensible, and numerical score of zero which means very easy to understand (Table 1). In line with this, when the respondents were asked a key question to verify comprehension and wording of items/questions (how would you write this item/question?), all of them answered that they would leave the items/questions as they were originally written. Consistency was evaluated in a separate group of respondents. This group shared characteristics with the clarity/comprehension group (as described above). Eight out of 20 respondents in Section 1 (40.0%) and 11 out of 24 in Section 2 (45.8%) reported a combination of recurrent-food-induced gastrointestinal and extraintestinal symptoms respectively. Percentages of matched questions between first and second application of the instrument were of 92.7% (range: 50%–100%) and 78.8% (range: 58.3%–100%) for Sections 1 and 2 respectively. The measure of agreement Kappa was found to be 0.92 (p < 0.001) and 0.77 (p < 0.001) for Sections 1 and 2 respectively (Table 1). These Kappa values can be interpreted as almost perfect agreement and moderate agreement respectively [25].

Table 1. Study population and test results of the designed questionnaire.

Assessment	Age Mean (Range)	*n* (Female/Male)	Adverse Reactions	Score
Clarity/comprehension	34.9 (20–66)	22 (5/17)	Gluten	Clear and comprehensible (0) *
	29.5 (18–50)	20 (12/8)	Other foods	Clear and comprehensible (0)
Consistency	33.2 (20–63)	20 (12/8)	Gluten	0.918 [#] (0.88–0.96) [##]
	22.1 (20–43)	24 (19/5)	Other foods	0.767 (0.71–0.82)

* Score in numeric scale. The Spanish version of the questionnaire was evaluated; [#] Measure of agreement Kappa; [##] 95% confidence interval.

3.2. Population Survey

A total of 1238 participants answered and returned the questionnaire (54.85% were female and 45.15% were male). The general prevalence of self-reported gluten-related disorders was 1.77% (n = 22) (95% CI: 1.2–2.7). Prevalence rates of self-reported NCGS, celiac disease, and wheat allergy were 0.97% (95% CI: 0.55–1.68), 0.08% (95% CI: 0.01–0.45), and 0.72% (95% CI: 0.38–1.37) respectively.

The characteristics of this population are given in Table 2. The prevalence rate of self-reported physician-diagnosed NCGS was 0.81% (95% CI: 0.41–1.53). Notably, only 27.3% (*n* = 6) of the self-reported gluten-related disorders group (*n* = 22) was following a gluten-free diet (Table 2). Overall, the prevalence rate of self-reported gluten-related disorders currently following a gluten-free diet was 0.48% (95% CI: 0.22–1.05).

Table 2. Characteristics of identified self-reported gluten-related disorder cases.

Gluten-Related Disorder	Mean Age in Years (Range)	Number of Cases (Female/Male)	Self-Reported	Self-Reported Physician-Diagnosed	Gluten-Free Diet (Yes/No)
Celiac disease *	45 (−)	1 (1/0)	0	1	1/0
Wheat allergy	30.5 (18–45)	9 (6/3)	9 [#]	0	3/6
NCGS **	37.2 (21–56)	12 (9/3)	2	10	2/10

* Diagnosed by gastroenterologist; ** Diagnosed by gastroenterologists (five cases) and general practitioners (five cases); [#] All cases were identified by means of self-reported convincing symptoms of acute allergic reactions.

Among those who reported recurrent adverse reactions to gluten (*n* = 96), we found 18 cases of self-reported gluten-related disorders (18.75%). In this group, eight respondents reported NCGS (six were physician-diagnosed), but only two of these were following a gluten-free diet (Table 2). Considering that the other four self-reported NCGS cases were not following a gluten-free diet, the general prevalence rate of self-reported NCGS currently following a gluten-free diet was 0.16% (95% CI: 0.04–0.58). On one hand, the general self-reported prevalence rate of wheat allergy currently following a gluten-free diet was 0.24% (95% CI: 0.08–0.71). Excluding the three physician-diagnosed gluten-related disorder cases adhering to a gluten-free diet (Table 2), six respondents who reported recurrent adverse reactions to gluten were following a gluten-free diet without proper diagnostic work-up of gluten-related disorders (6.25%), and thirty-five respondents reported that they were avoiding gluten in their diets (36.4%). On the other hand, nineteen respondents in this group had a physician diagnosis of colitis (19.8%) and they related the condition to gluten intake, but none of them were following a gluten-free diet.

Previous studies have used self-reported prevalence rates of adherence to a gluten-free diet among individuals without celiac disease as a surrogate marker for NCGS [15]. Consequently, the data were analyzed in this context. The estimated self-reported prevalence rate of adherence to gluten-free diet was 3.7% (95% CI: 2.7–4.8) (Table 3). Excluding the self-reported physician-diagnosed celiac disease case and three self-reported wheat allergy cases following a gluten-free diet (Table 2), the estimated prevalence of NCGS in the studied population would be 3.34% (95% CI: 2.47–4.49).

General prevalence estimations and prevalence comparisons by gender are given in Table 3. Except for the cases of dairy intolerance, all prevalence comparisons between genders were statistically significant (*p* < 0.05). Prevalence rate of recurrent adverse reactions to foods was 11.3% lower than the prevalence rate of general adverse reactions to foods, and this was statistically significant (*p* < 0.001) (Table 3). Similarly, the prevalence rate of recurrent adverse reactions to gluten was 4.1% lower than the prevalence rate of general adverse reactions to gluten, and this was also statistically significant (*p* < 0.05) (Table 3). Overall, recurrent adverse reactions to gluten represented more than 35% of the self-reported recurrent adverse reactions to any food.

The prevalence rate of recurrent adverse reactions to gluten was 7.8% (95% CI: 6.4–9.4) (Table 3). However, only 0.73% (*n* = 9) of the studied population reported both recurrent adverse reactions to gluten and adherence to a gluten-free diet. Consequently, most respondents (2.8% out of 3.7%) who were adhering to a gluten-free diet reported neither recurrent adverse reactions to gluten nor other foods. In fact, 93.3% of the respondents who reported adherence to a gluten-free diet had no self-reported physician-diagnosis of gluten-related disorders. Stratified by age, adherence to a gluten-free diet was more common in the group of respondents aged ≥39 years old than the group aged from 18 to 38 years old (6.3% *vs.* 3.0%), and this was statistically significant (*p* < 0.05).

Table 3. Study population and prevalence estimations.

Sample Size *	Assessment	(+) Cases **	Age [#] (Range)	Prevalence by Gender (95% CI)	*p* Value	General Prevalence (95% CI)
1238 M [##] = 559 F [##] = 679	Adverse reactions to foods	Total = 398 M = 141 F = 257	31.3 (18–85)	M 25.2 (21.8–29.0) F 37.8 (34.3–41.6)	<0.001	32.1 (29.6–34.8)
1230 M = 554 F = 676	Recurrent adverse reactions to foods	Total = 256 M = 81 F = 175	32.0 (18–84)	M 14.6 (11.9–17.8) F 22.7 (22.6–29.3)	<0.001	20.8 (18.6–23.2)
1221 M = 555 F = 666	Food allergy	Total = 67 M = 13 F = 54	27.4 (18–57)	M 2.3 (1.2–3.9) F 8.1 (6.3–10.4)	<0.001	5.5 (4.3–6.9)
1221 M = 555 F = 666	Dairy intolerance	Total = 43 M = 18 F = 25	30.8 (18–58)	M 3.2 (2.1–5.1) F 3.7 (2.6–5.5)	NS	3.5 (2.6–4.7)
1238 M = 559 F = 679	Adverse reactions to wheat/gluten	Total = 144 M = 45 F = 99	33.5 (18–71)	M 8.0 (6.0–10.6) F14.6 (12.1–17.4)	0.001	11.9 (9.9–13.5)
1237 M = 559 F = 678	Recurrent adverse reactions to wheat/gluten	Total = 96 M = 25 F = 71	34.2 (18–63)	M 4.5 (3.0–6.5) F 10.5 (8.4–13.0)	<0.001	7.8 (6.4–9.4)
1228 M = 556 F = 672	Adherence to gluten-free diet	Total = 45 M = 13 F = 32	32.0 (19–57)	M 2.3 (1.4–4.0) F 4.8 (3.4–6.6)	0.033	3.7 (2.7–4.8)

* The population school degree ranged from elementary to postgraduate; the sample size varies among assessments due to missed questions; ** Reported cases for the assessment; [#] Mean age (Years); [##] F: Female; M: Male.

Based on symptoms "convincing" of acute allergic reactions, general self-reported food allergy prevalence rate was 5.5% (95% CI: 4.3–6.9) (Table 3) and more than 40 foods were reported as the triggers of symptomatic adverse reactions (material S1). In addition, prevalence rates of self-reported food allergy to individual foods were also reported (material S2).

Recurrent-food-induced gastrointestinal symptoms were reported for 90 out of 96 (93.7%) respondents from the adverse reactions to gluten group, and 140 out of 160 (87.5%) from the adverse reaction to other foods group ($p > 0.05$) (Table 4). More frequently reported gastrointestinal symptoms were bloating and abdominal pain in both groups. After odds ratio analyses, bloating and constipation were the symptoms more frequently reported by the recurrent adverse reactions to gluten group compared to the opposite group (Table 4). However, a high proportion of those who reported recurrent adverse reactions to foods different from gluten experienced bloating (59.3%) and constipation was reported for less than 35% of the respondents who reported recurrent adverse reactions to gluten (Table 4). Age when gastrointestinal or extraintestinal symptoms appeared did not differ between the groups that reported adverse reactions to gluten and adverse reactions to other foods ($p > 0.05$). Diarrhea was far more common in those cases that reported adverse reactions to other foods different from gluten (19.3% *vs.* 10.0%), but this was not statistically significant ($p > 0.05$) (Table 4). There were more cases of family history of celiac disease in the group of adverse reactions to gluten ($n = 7$; 14.9%) than the group of adverse reactions to other foods ($n = 5$; 4.9%). Although this difference was not statistically significant ($p > 0.05$), risk analysis of family history of celiac disease showed an odds ratio of 3.4 (95% CI: 1.02–11.3).

Extraintestinal symptoms were less common in the recurrent adverse reactions to gluten group ($n = 31$; 32.3%) than the recurrent adverse reactions to other foods group ($n = 79$; 49.4%) ($p < 0.05$). More frequently reported extraintestinal symptoms in the recurrent adverse reactions to gluten group were tiredness (38.7%), headache (35.5%), and anxiety (35.5%) (Figure 2). In the opposite group, these symptoms were skin with hives (30.4%), headache (26.6%), trouble breathing (25.3%), and anxiety (25.3%). A statistically significant difference was found for tiredness ($p < 0.05$) this symptom being more frequent in the recurrent adverse reactions to gluten group (Figure 2). Risk analysis of this extraintestinal symptom showed an odds ratio of 2.93 (95% CI: 1.16–7.39). However, this symptom was reported for less than 40% and more than 15% of the recurrent adverse reactions to gluten group and the opposite group respectively (Figure 2). In the adverse reactions to gluten and adverse reactions to other foods groups the mean age when extraintestinal symptoms appeared was of 26.9 (Range: 5–56; $n = 22$) and 19.6 (Range: 3–50; $n = 57$) years respectively, and this was statistically significant ($p < 0.05$).

Table 4. Comparison between identified self-reported recurrent adverse reactions to gluten and recurrent adverse reactions to other foods cases.

Variable	Adverse Reactions to				Odds Ratio (95% CI)
	Wheat/Gluten ($N = 90$)		Other Foods ($N = 140$)		
	—	n	—	n	
Mean age in years (range) [#]	34.1 (18–63)	—	30.5 (18-84)	—	—
Gender (female/male) (%)	73.3/26.7	66/24	63.6/36.4	89/51	1.57 (0.88–2.9)
Bloating (%)	83.3	75	59.3	83	3.4 (1.8–6.6)
Abdominal pain (%)	44.4	40	48.6	68	0.85 (0.49–1.4)
Abdominal discomfort (%)	37.8	34	30.7	43	1.4 (0.78–2.4)
Constipation (%)	34.3	31	10.0	14	4.7 (2.3–9.5)
Flatulence (%)	30.0	27	24.3	34	1.3 (0.74–2.4)
Reflux (%)	24.4	22	22.1	31	1.1 (0.61–2.1)
Acidity (%)	22.2	20	23.6	33	0.93 (0.49–1.7)
Nausea (%)	16.7	15	14.3	20	1.2 (0.58–2.5)
Diarrhea (%)	10.0	9	19.3	27	0.46 (0.21–1.0)
Vomit (%)	5.5	5	8.6	12	0.63 (0.21–1.8)
Dairy intolerance (%)	17.7	16	14.8	21	1.4 (0.72–2.9)
IBS (%)	12.5	12	8.6	12	1.5 (0.67–3.4)

[#] Age comparison by Student t test ($p > 0.05$).

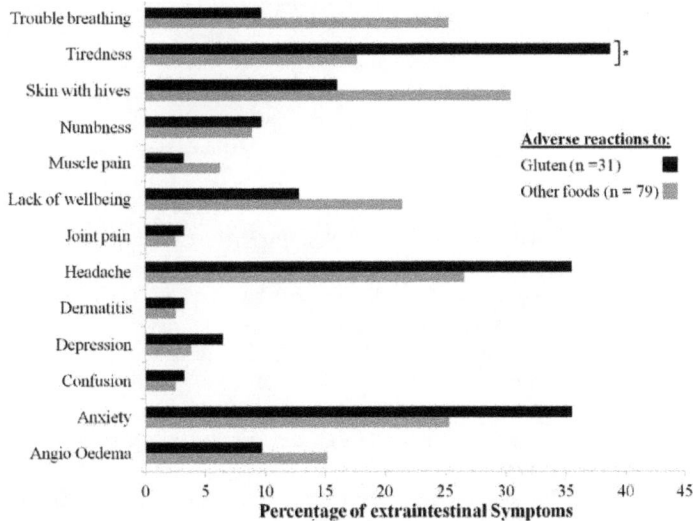

Figure 2. Recurrent self-reported extraintestinal symptoms. [*] $p < 0.05$.

4. Discussion

A self-administered questionnaire for the assessment of adverse reactions to gluten and other foods was designed as a part of this study. This instrument was not reworded in its entirety, but it had to be culturally adapted to be administered in the Mexican population [26]. Previous studies have utilized questionnaires to estimate the prevalence of adverse reactions to gluten or food allergy in open populations [13,14,19,20]. However, there is not instrument designed to estimate the self-reported symptomatic adverse reactions to gluten including wheat allergy and other foods in Latin American countries. Notably, the prevalence estimation of adverse reactions to other foods different from gluten enables the measurement of the magnitude of symptomatic adverse reactions to gluten in a specific population. On one hand, the evaluation of "convincing" symptoms of food allergy not only enables the prevalence estimation of wheat allergy. On the other hand, it could also be a helpful tool to make decisions when particular cases are to be confirmed with objective diagnostic criteria. The instrument designed in this study can be reliably applied in the Mexican population and other Latin American countries after cultural adaptation. Furthermore, it measures not only variables associated to wheat allergy, but also variables associated to other gluten-related disorders.

A recent study carried out in adult Mexican population has estimated the self-reported prevalence of food hypersensitivity, defined as those adverse reactions to foods mediated or not by immunological mechanism [27,28]. Notably, no wheat hypersensitivity cases were reported. Contrary, in our study 11.9% and 7.8% of the respondents reported adverse reactions or recurrent adverse reactions to gluten respectively, highlighting that these reactions could be common in Mexican population. It should be noted that different instruments were utilized for the assessment of adverse reactions to foods, and this could partially explain the discrepancy between the two studies. Certainly, our results are in line with previous studies carried out in the United Kingdom where the estimated prevalence of gluten-sensitivity was 13% [13]. Furthermore, the estimated prevalence of self-reported wheat allergy in our study (0.72%) is in line with studies carried out in other countries where self-reported wheat allergy prevalence rates ranged from 0.5% to 1.17% [29–31].

A previous study carried out in Mexico reported that the prevalence of celiac disease was 0.6% (1/166) [32]. In the present study just one respondent reported a physician diagnosis of celiac disease (0.08%; 1/1238). This could be influenced in part by the fact that the frequency of classical celiac disease (symptomatic) has dropped substantially and more commonly cases are identified as non-classical celiac disease (asymptomatic) [8,33,34]. Certainly, these results suggest that celiac disease either classical or non-classical is a condition commonly underdiagnosed in the Mexican population. Therefore, screening studies of the condition in populations at risk of developing celiac disease could be helpful to avoid long-term complications.

Prevalence of NCGS largely varies among studies. Reported NCGS prevalence rates typically fluctuate between 0.55% and 18.5% [1,13–15]. Although most patients complaining of gluten-related symptoms did not experience symptomatic relief after gluten withdrawal [35], wheat allergy and celiac disease have to be excluded in the diagnostic work-up of NCGS [1,8]. The estimated self-reported prevalence rates of NCGS in our study ranged from 0.16% to 3.34% depending on how the analyses were conducted. Certainly, a proper diagnosis of NCGS requires not only the exclusion of other gluten-related disorders and informed symptomatic relief after gluten withdrawal, but also the gluten-attributed symptoms should be confirmed by a food challenge test [7,8]. Overall, our study highlights that prevalence estimations of NCGS should be interpreted with caution and special attention should be paid to study designs.

The self-reported prevalence of adhering to a gluten-free diet in the studied population was 3.7%. This is 6.7 fold higher than that reported in a recent study carried out in the USA where the self-reported adherence to gluten-free diet was 0.55% [15]. Unfortunately, a clear explanation of this discrepancy between studies is beyond the scope of our work. Certainly, this is probably not due to differences in the studied populations as most of the cases that reported adherence to a gluten-free diet in the USA study were over 18 years old [15]. Furthermore, in line with the USA study, we found that the prevalence of adherence to a gluten-free diet increased more than two fold among those aged ≥39 years old.

Most respondents (93.3%) who were adhering to a gluten-free diet in our study had no self-reported physician-diagnosis of gluten related disorders. Patients that benefit from a gluten-free or a wheat-free diet should be referred to a dietitian to receive dietary counseling for the diet [36]. Adhering to a gluten-free diet without proper dietary counseling could lead to iron and vitamin B deficiencies [11,12]. Furthermore, adhering to the diet without proper diagnostic work-up of celiac disease makes the practice of a six week gluten challenge in those with genetic predisposition for this condition necessary [8,37]. The main concern in this practice is that symptomatic relapse commonly precedes serology and/or histology relapse making six weeks gluten challenge intolerable for many patients [18]. Under these conditions, celiac disease could not be excluded and a proper diagnosis of NCGS would not be possible.

Previous studies have evaluated the self-reported intestinal and extraintestinal manifestations in suspected NCGS [13,14]. In this study there were evaluated the self-reported symptomatic adverse reactions to oral gluten in open population. Notably, the more commonly gluten-associated symptoms reported, either intestinal or extraintestinal, were reproducible among the studies despite different approaches or instruments were utilized to assess the manifestations. However, our results also showed that the symptoms preferentially associated with adverse reactions to gluten were not truly representative of this type of reactions as they were also frequent or unusual manifestations in those who reported recurrent adverse reactions to other foods different from gluten. These results show that symptom evaluation *per se* is not enough to confidently attribute the manifestations reported to gluten intake, and further evaluations with objective diagnostic criteria are required before making definitive conclusions.

It should be acknowledged that our study has some limitations. Firstly; this study was self-administered and questionnaire-based and the adverse reactions to foods reported, either recurrent or not, could be intoxications or other gastrointestinal conditions different from gluten-related disorders. Secondly; the use of self-reporting to estimate prevalence rates has been found to overestimate the real prevalence rates and our data were not confirmed by more specific diagnostic studies [38]. Thirdly; the instrument utilized in this study was mainly designed to estimate the prevalence of adverse reactions to gluten and consequently the manifestations evaluated were all associated to gluten-related disorders. Other variables that could be relevant to better interpretation of parts of the results were not included because of the length of the instrument. For instance, questionnaires intended to evaluate the self-reported prevalence of food allergy normally inquire about atopic diseases such as rhinitis, asthma, and eczema, and a list of potential allergens is given to improve the survey's accuracy. Undoubtedly, the best way to evaluate prevalence of food allergy and NCGS is by designing studies that include the use of an oral food challenge, ideally double-blinded and placebo-controlled [7,8,18,39]. Thus, the main utility of self-reported questionnaire-based studies is to serve as a groundwork for further objective studies.

5. Conclusions

It was designed a self-administered instrument to estimate the prevalence rates of self-reported adverse reactions to gluten and other foods and adherence to a gluten-free diet. The instrument can be reliably applied in adult populations. Using this instrument, it was found that recurrent-symptomatic adverse reactions to gluten are common in Mexican population, but gluten-related disorders could be underdiagnosed. Consequently, most people adhering to a gluten-free diet had no physician-diagnosis of gluten-related disorders and this makes it highly possible that most people adhering to the diet are doing it without medical/dietary advice. To our knowledge, this is the first population-based study conducted to evaluate the prevalence of symptomatic adverse reactions to oral gluten and adherence to gluten-free diet in Latin American countries.

Acknowledgments: Authors are grateful to Eduardo E. Valdez-Meza, Jesús A. Ibarra-Duarte, Giovanni I. Ramírez-Torres, Ivan R. Chiquete-Elizalde, Anna P. Islas-Zamorano and Saraí Moreno-Munguía for assistance in data collection. Thanks to PROFAPI 2013/026 grant for financial support. We thank Melinda Hardy for assistance in preparing this manuscript.

Author Contributions: Noe Ontiveros: Study concept and design, analysis and interpretation of the data, statistical analysis, and manuscript preparation; Jesús A. López-Gallardo: Responsible for substantial acquisition of the data, statistical analysis, and manuscript preparation; Marcela J. Vergara-Jiménez: Study design, acquisition of the data, and analysis of the data; Francisco Cabrera-Chávez: Study concept and design, analysis and interpretation of the data, statistical analysis, and manuscript preparation. Noe Ontiveros and Francisco Cabrera-Chávez designed the questionnaire utilized in this study.

Conflicts of Interest: All authors declare no conflict of interest.

References

1. Sapone, A.; Bai, J.C.; Ciacci, C.; Dolinsek, J.; Green, P.H.; Hadjivassiliou, M.; Kaukinen, K.; Rostami, K.; Sanders, D.S.; Schumann, M.; *et al.* Spectrum of gluten-related disorders: Consensus on new nomenclature and classification. *BMC Med.* **2012**, *10*, 13. [CrossRef] [PubMed]
2. Ludvigsson, J.F.; Leffler, D.A.; Bai, J.C.; Biaqi, F.; Fasano, A.; Green, P.H.; Hadjivassiliou, M.; Kaukiken, K.; Kelly, C.P.; Leonard, J.N.; *et al.* The Oslo definitions for coeliac disease and related terms. *Gut* **2012**, *62*, 43–52. [CrossRef] [PubMed]
3. Sapone, A.; Lammers, K.M.; Casolaro, V.; Cammarota, M.; Giuliano, M.T.; de Rosa, M.; Stefanile, R.; Mazzarella, G.; Tolone, C.; Russo, M.I.; *et al.* Divergence of gut permeability and mucosal immune gene expression in two gluten-associated conditions: Celiac disease and gluten sensitivity. *BMC Med.* **2011**, *9*, 23. [CrossRef] [PubMed]
4. Pietzak, M. Celiac disease, wheat allergy, and gluten sensivity: When gluten free is not a fad. *JPEN J. Parenter. Enteral Nutr.* **2012**, *36*, 68S–75S. [CrossRef] [PubMed]
5. Biesiekierski, J.R.; Newnham, E.D.; Irving, P.M.; Barrett, J.S.; Haines, M.; Doecke, J.D.; Shepherd, S.J.; Muir, J.G.; Gibson, P.R. Gluten causes gastrointestinal symptoms in subjects without celiac disease: A double-blind randomized placebo-controlled trial. *Am. J Gastroenterol.* **2011**, *106*, 508–514. [CrossRef] [PubMed]
6. Biesiekierski, J.R.; Peters, S.L.; Newnham, E.D.; Rosella, O.; Muir, J.G.; Gibson, P.R. No effects of gluten in patients with self-reported non-celiac gluten sensitivity after dietary reduction of fermentable, poorly absorbed, short-chain carbohydrates. *Gastroenterology* **2013**, *145*, 320–328. [CrossRef] [PubMed]
7. Catassi, C.; Elli, L.; Bonaz, B.; Bouma, G.; Carroccio, A.; Castillejo, G.; Cellier, C.; Cristofori, F.; de Magistris, L.; Dolinsek, J.; *et al.* Diagnosis of Non-Celiac Gluten Sensitivity (NCGS): The Salerno Experts' Criteria. *Nutrients* **2015**, *7*, 4966–4977. [CrossRef] [PubMed]
8. Ontiveros, N.; Hardy, M.Y.; Cabrera-Chavez, F. Assessing of Celiac Disease and Nonceliac Gluten Sensitivity. *Gastroenterol. Res. Pract.* **2015**. [CrossRef]
9. Rubio-Tapia, A.; Ludvigsson, J.F.; Brantner, T.L.; Murray, J.A.; Everhart, J.E. The prevalence of celiac disease in the United States. *Am. J. Gastroenterol.* **2012**, *107*, 1538–1544. [CrossRef] [PubMed]
10. Tanpowpong, P.; Ingham, T.R.; Lampshire, P.K.; Kirchberg, F.F.; Epton, M.J.; Crane, J.; Camargo, C.A., Jr.; New Zealand Asthma and Allergy Cohort Study Group. Coeliac disease and gluten avoidance in New Zealand children. *Arch. Dis. Child.* **2012**, *97*, 2–6. [CrossRef] [PubMed]
11. Hallert, C.; Svensson, M.; Tholstrup, J.; Hultberg, B. Clinical trial: B vitamins improve health in patients with coeliac disease living on a gluten-free diet. *Aliment. Pharmacol. Ther.* **2009**, *29*, 811–816. [CrossRef] [PubMed]
12. Wild, D.; Robins, G.G.; Burly, V.J.; Howdle, P.D. Evidence of high sugar intake, and low fibre and mineral intake, in the gluten-free diet. *Aliment. Pharmacol. Ther.* **2010**, *32*, 573–581. [CrossRef] [PubMed]
13. Aziz, I.; Lewis, N.R.; Hadjivassiliou, M.; Winfiled, S.N.; Rugg, N.; Kelsall, A.; Newrick, L.; Sanders, D.S. A UK study assessing the population prevalence of self-reported gluten sensivity and referral characteristics to secondary care. *Eur. J. Gastroenterol. Hepatol.* **2014**, *26*, 33–39. [CrossRef] [PubMed]
14. Volta, U.; Bardella, M.T.; Calabró, A.; Tranconne, R.; Corazza, G.R. An Italian prospective multicenter survey on patients suspected of having non-celiac-gluten sensitivity. *BMC Med.* **2014**. [CrossRef] [PubMed]

15. DiGiacomo, D.V.; Terryson, C.A.; Green, P.H.; Demmert, R.T. Prevalence of gluten-free diet adherence among individuals without celiac disease in the USA: Results from the Continuous National Health and Nutrition Examination Survey 2009–2010. *Scand. J. Gastroenterol.* **2013**, *48*, 921–925. [CrossRef] [PubMed]

16. Carroccio, A.; Mansueto, P.; Iacono, G.; Soresi, M.; D'Alcamo, A.; Cavataio, F.; Brusca, I.; Florena, A.M.; Ambrosiano, G.; Seidita, A.; et al. Non-celiac wheat sensitivity diagnosed by double-blind placebo-controlled challenge: Exploring a new clinical entity. *Am. J. Gastroenterol.* **2012**, *107*, 1898–1906. [CrossRef] [PubMed]

17. Peters, S.L.; Biesiekierski, J.R.; Yelland, G.W.; Muir, G.J.; Gibson, P.R. Randomised clinical trial: Gluten may cause depression in subjects with non-coeliac gluten sensitivity—An exploratory clinical study. *Aliment. Pharmacol. Ther.* **2014**, *39*, 1104–1112. [CrossRef] [PubMed]

18. Ontiveros, N.; Tye-Din, J.A.; Hardy, M.Y.; Anderson, R.P. Ex-vivo whole blood secretion of interferon (IFN)-γ and IFN-γ-inducible protein-10 measured by enzyme-linked immunosorbent assay are as sensitive as IFN-γ enzyme-linked immunospot for the detection of gluten-reactive T cells in human leucocyte antigen (HLA)-DQ2-5(+) -associated coeliac disease. *Clin. Exp. Immunol.* **2014**, *175*, 305–315. [PubMed]

19. Hoyos-Bachiloglu, R.; Ivanovic-Zuvic, D.; Alvarez, J.; Linn, K.; Thöne, K.; de los Ángeles, P.M.; Borzutzky, A. Prevalence of parent-reported immediate hypersensitivity food allergy in Chilean school-aged children. *Allergol. Immnunopathol.* **2014**, *42*, 527–532. [CrossRef] [PubMed]

20. Sicherer, S.H.; Burks, A.W.; Sampson, H.A. Clinical features of acute allergic reactions to peanut and tree nuts in children. *Pediatrics* **1998**, *102*, e6. [CrossRef] [PubMed]

21. Sicherer, S.H.; Muñoz-Furlong, A.; Godbold, J.H.; Sampson, H.A. US prevalence of selft-reported peanut, tree nut, and sesame allergy: 11-year follow-up. *J. Allergy Clin. Immunol.* **2010**, *125*, 1322–1326. [CrossRef] [PubMed]

22. Gusi, N.; Badia, X.; Herdman, M.; Olivares, P. Translation and cultural adaptation of the Spanish version of EQ-5D-Y questionnaire for children and adolescents. *Aten Primaria* **2009**, *41*, 19–23. [CrossRef] [PubMed]

23. Kazi, A.M.; Khalid, W. Questionnaire designing and validation. *J. Pak. Med. Assoc.* **2012**, *62*, 514–516. [PubMed]

24. OpenEpi Open Source Epidemiologic Statistics for Public Health. Available online: http://www.openepi.com/ (accessed on 25 April 2015).

25. Landis, J.R.; Koch, G.G. An application of hierarchical kappa-type statistics in the assessment of majority agreement among multiple observers. *Biometrics* **1977**, *33*, 363–374. [CrossRef] [PubMed]

26. Beaton, D.E.; Bombardier, C.; Guillemin, F.; Ferraz, M.B. Guidelines for the process of cross-cultural adaptation of self-report measures. *SPINE* **2000**, *25*, 3186–3191. [CrossRef] [PubMed]

27. Bedolla-Barajas, M.; Bedolla-Pulido, T.R.; Camacho-Peña, A.S.; González-García, E.; Morales-Romero, J. Food hypersensitivity in Mexican adults at 18 to 50 years of age: A questionnaire survey. *Allergy Asthma Immunol. Res.* **2014**, *6*, 511–516. [CrossRef] [PubMed]

28. Johansson, S.G.; Hourihane, J.O.; Bousquet, J.; Bruijnzeel-Koomen, C.; Dreborg, S.; Haahtela, T.; Kowalski, M.L.; Mygind, N.; Ring, J.; van Cauwenberge, P.; et al. A revised nomenclature for allergy. An EAACI position statement from the EAACI nomenclature task force. *Allergy* **2011**, *56*, 813–824.

29. Vierk, K.A.; Koehler, K.M.; Fein, S.B.; Street, D.A. Prevalence of self-reported food allergy in American adults and use of food labels. *J. Allergy Clin. Immunol.* **2007**, *119*, 1504–1510. [CrossRef] [PubMed]

30. Zuidmeer, L.; Goldhahn, K.; Rona, R.J.; Gislason, D.; Madsen, C.; Summers, C.; Sodergren, E.; Dahistrom, J.; Lindner, T.; Siqurdardottir, S.T.; et al. The prevalence of plant food allergies: A systematic review. *J. Allery Clin. Immunol.* **2008**, *121*, 1210–1218. [CrossRef] [PubMed]

31. Morita, E.; Chinuki, Y.; Takahashi, H.; Nabika, T.; Yamasaki, M.; Shiwaku, K. Prevalence of wheat allergy in Japanese adults. *Allergol Int.* **2012**, *61*, 101–105. [CrossRef] [PubMed]

32. Remes-Troche, J.M.; Nuñez-Alvarez, C.; Uscanga-Dominguez, L.F. Celiac Disease in Mexican population: An update. *Am. J. Gastroenterol.* **2013**, *108*, 283–284. [CrossRef] [PubMed]

33. Balamtekin, N.; Uslu, N.; Baysoy, G.; Usta, Y.; Demir, H.; Saltik-Temize, I.N.; Ozen, H.; Gürakan, F.; Yüce, A. The presentation of celiac disease in 220 Turkish children. *Turk. J. Pediatr.* **2010**, *52*, 239–244. [PubMed]

34. Admou, B.; Essaadouni, L.; Krati, K.; Zaher, K.; Sbihi, M.; Chabaa, L.; Belaabidia, B.; Alaoui-Yazidi, A. Atypical celiac disease: From recognizing to managing. *Gastroenterol. Res. Pract.* **2012**. [CrossRef] [PubMed]

35. Capannolo, A.; Viscido, A.; Barkad, M.A.; Valerii, G.; Ciccone, F.; Melideo, D.; Frieri, G.; Latella, G. Non-Celiac gluten sensitivity among patients perceiving gluten-related symptoms. *Digestion* **2015**, *92*, 8–13. [CrossRef] [PubMed]

36. Rubio-Tapia, A.; Hill, I.D.; Kelly, C.P.; Calderwood, A.H.; Murray, J.A. ACG clinical guidelines: Diagnosis and management of celiac disease. *Am. J. Gastroenterol.* **2013**, *108*, 656–676. [CrossRef] [PubMed]

37. Rostom, A.; Murray, J.A.; Kagnoff, M.F. American Gastroenterological Association (AGA) Institute technical review on the diagnosis and management of celiac disease. *Gastroenterology.* **2006**, *131*, 1981–2002. [CrossRef] [PubMed]

38. Rona, R.J.; Keil, T.; Summers, C.; Gislason, D.; Zuidmeer, L.; Sodergren, E.; Siqurdardottir, S.T.; Lindner, T.; Goldhahn, K.; Dahistrom, J.; *et al.* The prevalence of food allergy: A meta-analysis. *Allergy Clin. Immunol.* **2007**, *120*, 638–646. [CrossRef] [PubMed]

39. Ontiveros, N.; Flores-Mendoza, L.K.; Canizalez-Román, V.A.; Cabrera-Chavez, F. Food allergy: Prevalence and food technology approaches for the Control of IgE-mediated food allergy. *Austin J Nutr. Food Sci.* **2014**, *2*, 1029.

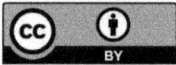

nutrients

MDPI

Review

Bones of Contention: Bone Mineral Density Recovery in Celiac Disease—A Systematic Review

Patricia Grace-Farfaglia [1,2,*]

1 Department of Nutritional Sciences, The University of Connecticut, Waterbury, CT 06702, USA
2 Health and Wellness Promotion, Rocky Mountain University of Health Professions, Provo, UT 84606, USA

Received: 19 January 2015; Accepted: 26 March 2015; Published: 7 May 2015

Abstract: Metabolic bone disease is a frequent co-morbidity in newly diagnosed adults with celiac disease (CD), an autoimmune disorder triggered by the ingestion of dietary gluten. This systematic review of studies looked at the efficacy of the gluten-free diet, physical activity, nutrient supplementation, and bisphosphonates for low bone density treatment. Case control and cohort designs were identified from PubMed and other academic databases (from 1996 to 2015) that observed newly diagnosed adults with CD for at least one year after diet treatment using the dual-energy x-ray absorptiometry (DXA) scan. Only 20 out of 207 studies met the inclusion criteria. Methodological quality was assessed using the Strengthening of the Reporting of Observational Studies in Epidemiology (STROBE) statement checklist. Gluten-free diet adherence resulted in partial recovery of bone density by one year in all studies, and full recovery by the fifth year. No treatment differences were observed between the gluten-free diet alone and diet plus bisphosphonates in one study. For malnourished patients, supplementation with vitamin D and calcium resulted in significant improvement. Evidence for the impact of physical activity on bone density was limited. Therapeutic strategies aimed at modifying lifestyle factors throughout the lifespan should be studied.

Keywords: celiac disease; gluten; osteoporosis; diet; physical activity; bone density; nutrient deficiency

1. Introduction

Celiac disease (CD) is triggered in genetically susceptible individuals by dietary gluten that results in intestinal damage and occurs in 1% of the population in Europe and the United States [1]. Approximately 75% of newly diagnosed patients with celiac disease have low bone mineral density (BMD). And when matched by age and gender to a non-affected population, celiac patients have a 40% greater risk for bone fracture [2]. Even with a silent or extra-intestinal presentation such as dermatitis herpetiformis or dementia, low bone mass is frequently found [3–5]. One-third of newly diagnosed cases are over 60 years of age which coincides with a period of an increased risk of falls only worsened by the presence of co-morbidities [6,7]. Women with celiac disease have a much higher rate of fractures during the 10 year period prior to diagnosis and 5 years afterward [8]. The cumulative effects of gluten-induced inflammation, treatment delay, and malabsorption result in lower bone density and bone fragility.

The most effective treatment for celiac disease and related co-morbidities, the gluten-free diet (GFD), is without dispute in the literature. Yet, improvements in BMD after treatment can take as long as two to five years after mucosal recovery [9–12] Nutritional deficiencies are common during the initial year of treatment for celiac disease, but little data exists on adult micronutrient status and bone mineral density in this population beyond calcium and vitamin D status [13–16].

The objective of this systematic review is to examine whether a GFD, alone or in combination with other interventions, leads to bone mineral recovery in newly diagnosed adults with celiac disease. A second objective is to identify gaps in the literature that would inform the design of future clinical trials and health intervention studies.

2. Methods

2.1. Criteria for Considering Studies for this Review

The literature search was limited to English-language articles on untreated and treated adults with celiac disease observed for one year or more. Studies that were exclusively silent or asymptomatic were included if they were part of the sample due to their known bone mineral status. The types of studies considered were cohort, case-control, and randomized controlled designs. Case report and case series were excluded from the analysis. Studies that included co-morbid conditions, such as diabetes or primary hyperparathyroidism, were excluded. Randomized controlled trials and interventions that identified the dose, frequency, type of nutrition supplementation, and physical activity were sought.

2.2. Search Strategy for Identification of Studies

A keyword search was accomplished in PubMed (January 1996 to April 2015); Embase; CINAHL plus full text; EBSCO; Scopus; ProQuest Dissertations and Theses, and University of Connecticut library resources (HOMER). The MEDLINE search strategy keywords were "celiac disease" [MeSH]) AND ("bone mineral density" OR "osteoporosis" OR "bone density") AND ("exercise" OR "physical activity") AND ("nutrition" OR "gluten-free") in publication title, abstract, or full-text. The inclusion criteria for this effort were studies with a focus on the treatment of newly diagnosed adults with celiac disease that reported the dependent variable as bone mineral density (BMD) as a dual-energy X-ray absorptiometry (DXA) T-score at baseline and at the annual assessment. Treatment modalities sought included gluten-free diet, physical activity, or vitamin and mineral supplementation. Case studies and papers that did not report DXA data at baseline were excluded.

Key article reference lists were hand searched from the Cochrane database of systematic reviews, meta-analyses, and review articles, as well as papers in (Bone, Gut, Osteoporosis International, and American Journal of Gastroenterology). Finally, journal review articles, and meta-analyses for non-celiac studies of low BMD were reviewed.

2.3. Quality Assessments

The clinical trials meeting the criteria are listed in Table 1. Methodological quality was assessed using the STROBE (Strengthening the Reporting of Observational Studies in Epidemiology Statement) recommendations using separate checklists for conference abstracts, case control studies, cohort studies, and cross-sectional studies [17]. The use of a qualitative assessment using a percentage system to categorize the studies as proposed by other authors proved to be unreasonable because of the age of some of the papers, published years before the STROBE recommendations [18]. The final system used was a combination of STROBE (50%–80% fulfilled) and whether missing items left the reader questioning eligibility criteria or bias in the results reported. After 2008, most of the papers fell into the "A" quality category.

2.4. Overview of Studies

Three categories of study were identified: GFD; GFD and nutritional supplement; GFD and bisphosphonates; and a combination of GFD, supplement and exercise. The outcome measures in selected articles included: DXA (femoral neck, trochanter and lumbar spine), ligand of receptor activator of NFκB (RANKL) /osteoprotegerin (OPG) ratio, adherence to a GFD, and physical activity level. The clinical trials meeting the criteria are listed in Table 1.

Table 1. Studies meeting search criteria.

Author Publication Year	Summary Title	Design	Treatment	Participants	Results	Quality
Corazza (1996) [22]	Reversal of osteopenia with diet in adult coeliac disease	Prospective, case-control	GFD	Gender (M/F) Classical CD 9/10, Mdn age = 26.5 years, Subclinical untreated 11/14, Mdn age = 28.5 years, Control 13/15 (Mdn age = 28)	GFD normalizes BMD in subclinical, but not classical CD.	B
Valdimarsson (1996) [23]	Influence of pattern of clinical presentation and of gluten-free diet on bone mass and metabolism in adult coeliac disease	Prospective, case-control	GFD	n = 63, Age range = 17–79 years, M/F = 28/35	After one year taking a GFD bone mineral density increased at all sites ($p < 0.01$). Seven patients with dermatitis herpetiformis had normal BMD, vitamin D & PTH status	B
McFarlane (1996) [24]	Effect of a gluten free diet on osteopenia in adults with newly diagnosed coeliac disease	Prospective, cohort	GFD	n = 21 M/F = 14/7, Mean age = 49.7 years (31.0 to 66.1)	Almost half of subjects had osteoporosis. After 1 year of treatment there was significant improvement in BMD	B
Ciacci (1997) [25]	Effects of dietary treatment on bone mineral density in adults with celiac disease: factors predicting response	Prospective, case-control	GFD & calcium	Gender (M/F) 11/30 n = 41, M/F = 11/30, Mean age = 34.3	Mean BMD (g cm^{-2}) significantly improved by one year after GFD treatment in most, but not all subjects.	B
Mautalen (1997) [26]	Effect of treatment on bone mass, mineral metabolism, and body composition in untreated celiac disease patients.	Prospective, RCT	GFD or GFD plus calcium (1 g day^{-1}) & vitamin D (32,000 IU week^{-1})	n = 41, M/F = 11/30, Mean age = 34.3 years	Mean BMD (g cm^{-2}) significantly improved by one year in most but not all subjects.	B
Kempainen (1999) [27]	Bone recovery after a gluten-free diet: a 5-year follow-up study	Prospective, cohort	GFD	n = 28 newly diagnosed CD patients (9 men, 19 women) recruited from 1990 to 1991. 6 patients withdrew. Women Age = 44.1 ± 13.6 and Men Age = 48.6 ± 12.3 Compliance with the GFD was good: 96% at 1 year and 82% at 5 years.	Bone disease "cured" by 5 years; with most of improvement in the first 12 months.	A
Valdimarsson (1999) [28]	Low circulating insulin-like growth factor 1 in coeliac disease and its relation to bone mineral density	Prospective, case-control, longitudinal	GFD	n = 29 CD, Mean age = 41 years, (range 21–66), M/F 8/21, n = 29 controls, age and gender matched	BMD and circulating IGF-1 levels are low in adults with untreated CD.	A
Sategna-Guidetti (2000) [29]	The effects of 1-year gluten withdrawal on bone mass, bone metabolism and nutritional status in newly-diagnosed adult coeliac disease patients	Prospective, cohort	GFD	n = 86 newly diagnosed CD, M/F = 22/64, mean age M/F = 29/29	GFD leads to significant increase in BMD and IGF-1 levels in postmenopausal women and in patients with incomplete mucosal recovery. Folic acid, albumin and pre-albumin serum levels low for those with incomplete recovery.	A
Taranta (2004) [30]	Imbalance of osteoclastogenesis-regulating factors in patients with celiac disease	Prospective, case-control, longitudinal	GFD	n = 25 treated, n = 17 untreated, n = 17 controls, Treated group mean age = 35.7 ± 7.9 years, Untreated mean age = 43 ± 9.9	Results suggest that bone loss in CD caused by a cytokine imbalance directly affecting osteoclastogenesis. RANKL/osteoprotegerin ratio was increased in patients not on the GFD.	A

Table 1. *Cont.*

Author Publication Year	Summary Title	Design	Treatment	Participants	Results	Quality
Bucci (2008) [31]	PO.7 Physical activity does not influence bone mass density in celiac adult patients	Prospective cohort	Unrestricted and GFD	n = 57 adults, age range = 18–45, CD enrolled, 38 completed the study protocol after a 24 months of GFD. High rate of dropout (33%).	GFD induced increase of BMD at femur independently of the amount of reported physical activity, but difference was not significant from baseline to follow-up in the low BMD group. PA was did not differ from baseline at 24 months.	B
Kurppa (2010) [32]	Gastrointestinal symptoms, quality of life and bone mineral density in mild enteropathic coeliac disease: A prospective clinical trial.	Prospective, cohort study	GFD	n = 27 (mild enteropathy), mean age (16–70); n = 46 (celiac), mean age 46 (16–70); BMD measured in n = 19 (normal villi), n = 39 (villus atrophy); n = 110 non-celiac controls mean age 49 (24–87)	Osteoporosis or osteopenia was detected in 58% of subjects in the mild enteropathy group and there was a trend towards improved bone mineral density after the treatment.	B
Papamichael (2010) [33]	S2044 effect of a gluten free diet on bone mineral density in patients with celiac disease.	Prospective cohort	GFD/Vitamin D and calcium	n = 22 CD patients, M/F = 7/15, mean age = 33 (21–69) years	Women diagnosed with CD because of overt malabsorption had osteoporosis despite supplementation with calcium and vitamin D. At baseline 10 female and all male patients had osteopenia. After 1 year 3 osteoporotic women had osteopenia, while the remaining 19 patients had a normal BMD.	B
Duerksen & Leslie (2011) [34]	Longitudinal evaluation of bone mineral density and body composition in patients with positive celiac serology	Retrospective cohort, database	GFD	Age > 40 years at baseline and testing for CD within 6 mo of baseline DXA test Groups: 37 (seropositive)/214 (controls)	Increase in BMD, BMI, and abdominal fat on GFD. Seropositive versus seronegative individuals had greater increases in mean spine BMD (4.6%/year vs. 0.7% spine, p < 0.0001), hip BMD (3.0%/year vs. 0.2% year−1 hip, p < 0.0001).	A
Vilppula (2011) [35]	Clinical benefit of gluten-free diet in screen-detected older celiac disease patients.	Prospective, cohort study	GFD	n = 35, Median age = 61 years (range 52–76), M/F = 15/20	Screen detected older celiac may suffer from subclinical malnutrition, GI symptoms or bone disease. Significant difference between pre & post-treatment femoral and lumbar spine Z scores.	A
Casella (2012) [36]	Celiac disease in elderly adults: clinical, serological, and histological characteristics and the effect of a gluten-free diet	Retrospective, cohorts grouped by age	GFD	M: n = 16(A), n = 306(B) F: n = 43(A), n = 860(B) Mean Age at diagnosis, μ ± SD: 70.1 ± 4.3 (65–83 years), 35.2 ± 10.6 (18–64 years)	Prevalence of osteoporosis was 67% in older and 14% in younger male participants and 70% in older and 9% in younger female participants (p < 0.001). Lumbar-sacral and femoral T-scores increased significantly during GFD in pooled results of 48 older and younger participants studied before and during GFD.	A

Table 1. *Cont.*

Author Publication Year	Summary Title	Design	Treatment	Participants	Results	Quality
Passananti (2012) [37]	Bone mass in women with celiac disease: role of exercise and gluten-free diet	Prospective, cohort, longitudinal	GFD	48 women of 2-year FU group (Mean age = 35.1 ± 8.7 years) and 47 women of 5-year FU group (Mean age = 35.1 ± 11.3 years)	Improvement in BMD on GFD was significant after 2 years; physical activity was frequently low. No significant relationship was observed between the BMD for 2-year FU and 5-year FU and level of physical activity at diagnosis ($p > 0.05$) for the lumbar spine and for the proximal femur).	B
Szymczak (2012) [38]	Low bone mineral density in adult patients with coeliac disease	Prospective, case-control, longitudinal	GFD plus calcium & alfacalcidol (vitamin D)	$n = 19$ treated, $n = 16$ untreated and 36 controls, second study of supplementation and GFD $n = 35$ CD group M/F = 6/29, Mean age 41.5 ± 13.6 years	Adult CD subjects treated with GFD for one year. They were deficient in calcium, vitamin D, and had lower BMD than controls. Then treated and untreated subjects given diet and supplements for one year. GFD compliant subjects taking supplements had a 35% increase in BMD, but gain was less in non-adherent subjects.	B
Kumar (2013) [39]	Effect of zoledronic acid on bone mineral density in patients of celiac disease: a prospective, randomized, pilot study	Randomized, prospective	GFD group A; and GFD & 4 mg zoledronic acid, calcium (1000 mg) and cholecalciferol (0.6 million units) if serum vitamin D was low, group B	$n = 13$ (11 completes), and $n = 15M/F = 7/6$ and 7/8, Mean age 28.2 ± 12.8 years; 25.3 ± 9.1 years	Significant improvement in clinical, biochemical parameters in both groups; GFD with Zoledronic acid was not found to be better than GFD alone after one year.	A
Kurppa (2014) [40]	Benefits of a gluten-free diet for asymptomatic patients with serologic markers of celiac disease.	Prospective, cohort, RCT	Unrestricted and GFD	$n = 40$ randomized to GFD group or unrestricted group, $n = 20$ (M/F = 15/5), $n = 20$ (11/9), Mean age: 42 (21–74) years GFD, Mean age: 42 (21–74) years, unrestricted diet	There were no differences between groups in laboratory test results, BMD (lumbar spine and femur neck), or body composition. Most measured parameters (GI symptoms, psych well-being, and SF-36 QOL) improved when patients in the gluten-containing diet group were placed on GFDs.	A
Pantaleoni (2014) [4]	Bone mineral density at diagnosis of celiac disease and after 1 year of gluten-free diet.	Prospective cohort	GFD	(M/F) $n = 146/23$ Mean age: 38.9 ± 12.6 years, pre/post-menopausal = 104/42	Stratification of patients according to sex and age showed a higher prevalence of low bone mineral density in men older than 30 years and in women of all ages. GFD led to a significant improvement in lumbar spine and femoral neck mean T-score value	A

CD: celiac disease; F: female, M: male; BMD: bone mineral density; GFD: gluten-free diet; PA: physical activity; DXA: dual-energy X-ray absorptiometry; BMI: body mass index; FU: follow-up; SF-36 QOL: standard quality of life index; yr: year; Quality assessment was performed by the author according to STROBE recommendations. RANKL: receptor activator of nuclear factor-κB ligand; PTH: parathyroid hormone; IGF-1: Insulin-like growth factor 1; PA: Physical activity.

3. Results

After the initial screening of articles and abstracts from the initial search strategy, a total of 180 articles were retrieved. The systematic process yielded 20 reports (Figure 1). During the period of this review there was an evolution in diagnosis and classification of CD with greater acceptance of serology test results for screening and monitoring in adults, combined with biopsy for diagnosis [19–21]. These developments made study comparisons more difficult because of the clinical heterogeneity between subjects with little or no villous atrophy.

Various tests are used to measure bone density, including the DXA, quantitative computed tomography (QTC), photon absorptiometry, and ultrasound. Adult bone mineral loss is categorized into osteopenia and osteoporosis. The World Health Organization (WHO) has established DXA as the best densitometry technique for the measurement of bone density in postmenopausal women, but the sensitivity of the DXA is lower compared to QTC in individuals with celiac disease [41]. A T-score between −1 and −2.5 and ≤2.5 indicates bone mineral loss with a greater than average risk of fracture [12]. Multiple risk factors and the results of the DXA scan are good predictors of relative fracture risk, and prediction is enhanced when co-morbidities, such as celiac disease, are added to the FRAX (WHO Fracture Risk Assessment Tool) index [42].

3.1. Diet Therapy

The studies reviewed that reported a dietary compliance measure demonstrated that adherence to the GFD has a positive effect on bone mineral density [4,36,38,43]. The greatest diet treatment gain occurs in the first year of in longitudinal studies that followed individuals for more than 12 months [27,34,37]. But full recovery for adults was mainly achieved after 5 years [27]. Newly diagnosed older adults benefit from the GFD with significant gains in femoral and lumbar spine being reported in the first year of treatment [35,36]. Malabsorption associated malnutrition delayed restoration of BMD in a vitamin D and calcium supplemented high risk group, while less nutritionally compromised individuals in the same study progressed from osteoporosis to osteopenia by one year of treatment [33]. Bone turnover markers Interleukin-18 (IL-18), Interleukin-6 (IL-6), and *N*-terminal telopeptide of procollagen type I were measured in treated ($n = 25$), untreated individuals ($n = 17$), and controls ($n = 21$) [30]. The GFD group had reduced levels of IL-18 and a lower RANKL/osteoprotegerin (OPG) ratio compared to untreated subjects, while the *N*-terminal telopeptide of procollagen type I was comparable to controls. Another study looked at the regulation of osteoclastogenesis and bone turnover in celiac disease in a cohort study of healthy premenopausal female subjects and diet compliant individuals with celiac disease who had no evidence of hypoparathyroidism [44]. The authors reported that the OPG/RANKL ratio was significantly lower in CD patients than in controls (14.8 ± 6.9 *vs.* 19.4 ± 9.2; $p < 0.05$).

Overall, the studies have shown that a GFD for the majority of patients is an effective therapy for long-term bone mineral recovery. The use of intermediate measures such as BMD, quality of life, and bone turnover, is more practical than fracture reduction estimates because these studies followed patients for one to five years. The incidence of fractures in a group of diet compliant participants ($n = 265$, M/F = 422/223) before and 5 years after diagnosis was compared to a cohort of patients with functional gastrointestinal disorders ($n = 530$, M/F = 84/446) [45]. The incidence of fractures declined after treatment (Incidence Rate (IR) = −1.22 events per 1000 patients year^{-1}) and Health Risk (HR) of fracture was comparable to controls (HR: 1.28, 95% CI: 0.74–2.21, p = ns), thus confirming the long-term benefit of the GFD.

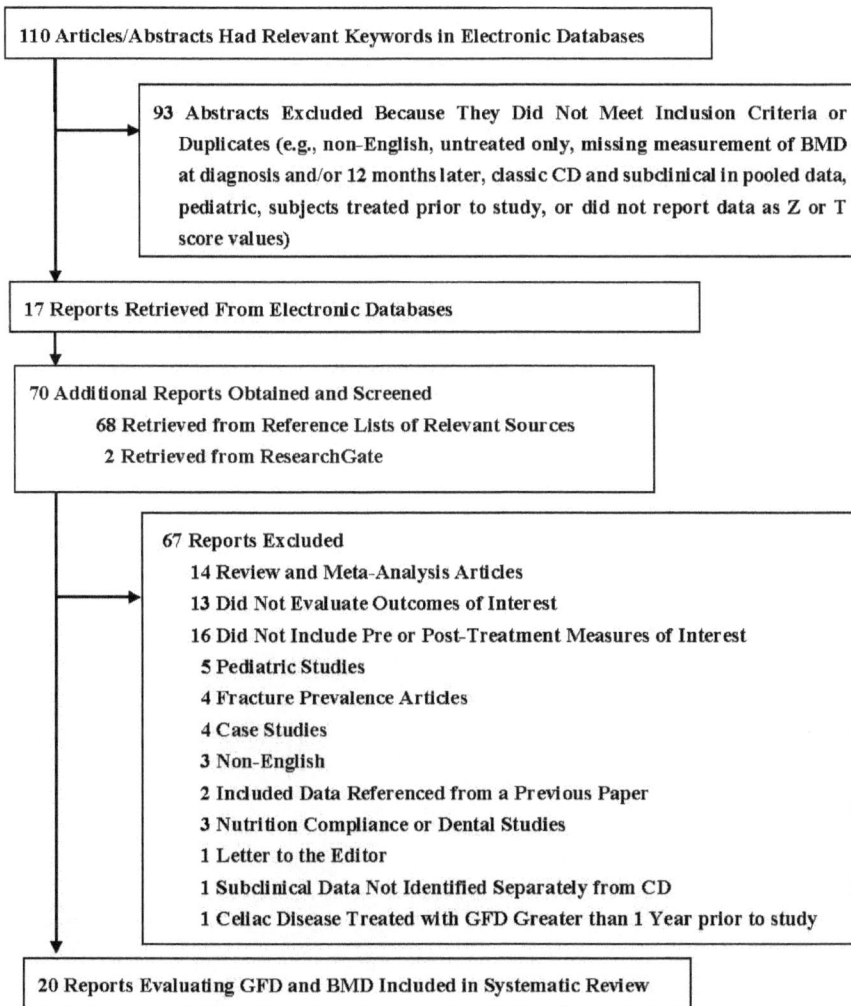

Figure 1. Selection process for studies included in the systematic review.

3.1.1. GFD and Nutrient Supplementation

The review identified 3 articles that addressed the treatment effects of vitamin and mineral supplementation on BMD [25,26,33]. The approach of Ciacci, *et al.* was a constant dietary calcium level of 1250 mg daily with diet alone or the addition of a supplement for those who were intolerant to lactose [25]. There was no significant change in vitamin D, urinary calcium increased, and a significant increase in BMD in the lumbar spine, femoral neck, and Ward's triangle in this study. Non-responders were more likely to be older and menopausal. Mautalen and associates randomized participants to a gluten-free diet condition ($n = 7$) or diet plus calcium (1.0 g day^{-1}) and vitamin D ($32,000$ IU week^{-1}) ($n = 7$) [26]. This trial's results were compromised by non-compliance. Adherent subjects had significant gains in BMD compared to patients that with frequent lapses, and improvement favored the axial compared to the peripheral skeleton. Lastly, Papamichael, *et al.* observed serum $25(OH)D_3$, parathyroid hormone (PTH), and calcium before and after treatment [33]. Only women with severe malabsorption were given supplements, the rest of the study group relied on the GFD and sunshine. In summary, the effect of supplementation depends on the disease severity at diagnosis and environmental exposure to UV radiation. The BMD of the majority of patients improved significantly to adequate vitamin D and calcium in the first year.

Satenga-Guidetti, *et al.* evaluated the pre- and post-treatment nutrient status of subjects ($n = 86$) on a GFD with no supplementation with serum folate, 25OH-D, hemoglobin, transferrin, and albumin measurement, as well as urinary calcium [29]. The researchers observed after a one-year follow-up that 34% of 86 newly diagnosed CD patients had a normal bone mineral density, while 40% had osteopenia and 26% osteoporosis with dietary treatment. There were no differences between gender in bone metabolism markers or most nutritional indices. The only difference was between pre- and post-menopausal women, where BMD and several bone metabolic markers were significantly different. This is in contrast to another study where reduced BMD was found after complete healing of duodenal lesions in one half of their patient sample [46]. The researchers concluded that additional measures beyond dietary compliance and counseling should be taken into account in order to increase BMD.

Treatment failure may actually be the result of a highly processed GFD as it is associated with small bowel bacterial overgrowth (SIBO) [47]. A highly processed GFD has been shown to alter the gut microbiome and increase GI symptoms which leads to an increased permeability of the epithelial barrier in patients with CD [48–50]. The health of the gut microbiota and the symptoms related to SIBO impact normalization of bone metabolism. The GFD does not reduce the risk of serious co-morbidities such as small bowel adenocarcinoma, Enteropathy-Associated T-cell Lymphoma (EATL), abortions, myocardial infarction, colonic adenocarcinoma, gastric MALT-lymphoma, ulcerative jejuno-ileitis, Cholangitis, severe non-alcoholicsteato-hepatitis, and autoimmune thrombocytopenia [51].

Nutritional status at time of diagnosis, age, menopausal status, environment, and dietary compliance moderate the effect of dietary supplements on BMD. Controversy exists regarding the amount of supplementation required to reverse malnutrition for key nutrients. A large clinical trial comparing the constant vitamin D and calcium dietary approach to a GFD without supplementation is needed. Because the maintenance of serum vitamin D is improved in the presence of adequate calcium intakes and high levels of physical activity, the study should collect direct measures of total UV radiation exposure and physical activity [52].

3.1.2. GFD and Bisphosphonates

The use of hormone replacement therapy or bisphosphonates, has been shown in healthy pre- and post-menopausal women to be effective in restoring bone mass; and the data suggests that combining these therapies with weight-bearing exercise may have additive effects [53,54]. A small pilot study ($n = 28$) treating CD patients with either GFD and zoledronic acid, or a calcium and cholecalciferol supplemented GFD reported that there were no significant difference in effectiveness [39]. Replication of this study with a larger sample size that includes older adults may be more representative of the adult CD population.

3.1.3. GFD and Physical Activity

Few researchers have studied the effect of physical activity on bone density in this population. Passananti and associates studied two groups of women (20–60 years), and compared baseline measures for the International Physical Activity Questionnaire (IPAQ), fatigue visual analogue scale (VAS), dietary compliance, gastrointestinal symptoms, serum vitamin D, anti-transglutaminase antibodies (U mL^{-1}), and BMD in 2 or 5 year follow-up cohorts [37]. Women who were taking oral contraceptives or hormone replacement therapy were excluded. A total of 110 participants were enrolled into the study, but 15 were either lost to follow-up or did not adhere to the GFD. The final sample size of the two cohorts were $n = 48$, $n = 47$, for the 2 and 5 year follow-up cohorts respectively. BMD measurements were taken at the right femur and lumbar spine. Chi-square tests were used for categorical data and ANOVA for continuous measures. Baseline and follow-up (FU) BMD was analyzed by two-sample and pairwise t-tests with a confidence interval set at 95%. Health measures also included BMI, small intestine pathology using Marsh categories for lesion comparisons and age of menarche and menopause. In the 2-year FU group 53.7% of participants reported low physical activity, and 10.6% were highly active (IPAQ = 3). Compared to baseline fatigue in this group, there was no statistical difference. The 5-year FU group was more active, with 46.3% reporting low levels and 14.6% highly active. Yet, the active subjects in in this group were more likely to report fatigue ($p = 0.039$ *post hoc*). The mean IPAQ score for both groups were not significantly different (1.60 ± 0.67 *vs.* 1.87 ± 0.88; $p > 0.05$). There was no significant difference between groups at FU for BMD and no relationship between BMD and intensity of Physical activity (PA) ($p > 0.05$ at the lumbar spine and proximal femur). The researchers concluded that physical activity has a minor role in supporting the bone mineral recovery in celiac patients. It is important to note that the study participants had normal vitamin D levels, but did not meet their dietary needs for calcium.

Di Stefano (2000) observed lifestyle factors in untreated patients with CD and BMD [55]. The participants ($n = 39$) were drawn from a consecutive patient pool with a spectrum of gluten-sensitive disorders: classical celiac, herpetiformis dermatitis, subclinical, or refractory (non-responsive) sprue. The independent variables were gender, smoking status, symptom severity, symptom duration, sunlight exposure, and level of physical activity. PA level was determined by self-report of occupational, recreational (cycling and brisk walking), and activities of daily living on a 0–4 scale of frequency [56]. Predictors of BMD were gender, malnutrition, severity, and PA. Symptom severity predicted low BMD in lumbar and femoral neck (-2.5 ± 0.8, $p < 0.001$). PA was correlated with BMD at the lumbar ($r = 0.57$, $p < 0.004$) and femoral ($r = -0.71$, $p < 0.004$); and bone mineral content (BMC) was correlated with lumbar BMC ($r = 0.59$, $p < 0.001$) and femoral BMC ($r = 0.58$, $p < 0.001$).

Studies concur that fatigue and celiac symptoms impact the frequency and intensity of exercise. The outcome measures, whether biochemical or radiologic, do not take muscle strength or flexibility into account. No direct measure of fitness level or every-day movement has been published. Aside from a study by Gonzalez *et al.* [57], few papers have identified overall body composition changes in spite of observations that treatment results in obesity in some patients [58,59]. In the elderly the impact of exercise on biochemical pathways involved in bone remodeling, such as receptor activator of nuclear factor-κB (RANK) /RANKL/OPG, is positive and particularly responsive to specific types of exercise (e.g., high or low impact exercise and resistance training) [60]. It has been observed that individuals with CD have an altered osteoprotegerin/RANKL ratio, which may also predispose patients to cardiovascular disease [44,61] Future health intervention research in celiac disease should focus on improving wellness, strength, and functional capacity in this population.

A randomized, double-blinded *vs.* placebo parallel study of the effectiveness of L-carnitine on fatigue in patients with celiac disease [62]. Participants were given a placebo or 2 g L-carnitine daily for 180 days. L-carnitine plays an important role in muscle contraction and energy production. The experimental group experienced an increase in organic cation transporter 2 (OCTN2), a sodium-dependent transporter for carnitine that facilitates carnitine absorption, as well as amines, some vitamins. The L-carnitine treatment group reported significant improvement in fatigue, as evaluated by the VAS scale. The rise in OCTN2 might explain this change. Ultimately, low levels of physical activity in persons with CD may be improved through L-carnitine treatment, which may aid in stimulation of bone mineral deposition.

The specific type of exercise may be a critical factor for improving bone health. Marques and associates studied the effect of resistance and moderate-impact aerobics training protocols on proximal femur BMD, muscle strength, balance, body composition, serum OPG, and RANKL levels in older women ($n = 71$). After eight months of the intervention, only the resistance training group experienced positive changes in BMD and muscle strength [63]. Both protocols had significant effects on functional balance control, a key factor in fall prevention. A later study by this author observed the effect of combined impact training for balance and lower-extremity muscle strength in men and women; the researchers reported improvement in dynamic balance (6.4%), muscle strength (11.0%) and trochanter

(0.7%), intertrochanter (0.7%), total hip (0.6%), and lumbar spine BMD (1.7%), while osteocalcin, OPG and RANKL levels remained unchanged [64]. Exercise performed with adequate dose and intensity addresses multiple risk factors for osteoporosis and fractures. Further research on celiac disease lifestyle intervention should begin with known barriers to PA and motivational therapies in other populations [65].

3.1.4. Nutritional Deficiencies, Dietary Sodium, Dysbiosis, and Inflammation

Folate supplementation is an effective treatment for elevated homocysteine in CD [66]. B12 and iron deficiency is a common symptom in untreated CD and in one study it was discovered in 41% of participants [67]. Dahele and Ghosh reported that after oral and parenteral administration of B12, all patients (n = 39) had normal serum levels of B12 at one year follow-up. A new role for B12 in bone health has been demonstrated in a mouse model of B12 deficiency demonstrating that deficiency impairs taurine synthesis and enhances Growth hormone-dependent IGF-1 synthesis in the liver; this subsequently increases osteoblast function (Figure 1) [68]. Research in humans should focus on reevaluating vitamin B12 requirements in CD to determine its role in bone remineralization.

Intestinal microbiota has been implicated in the development of CD which may not be corrected after treatment. Due to the low level of phylum *Bacteroides* and abundance of *Firmicutes* in the stools of people with CD, this imbalance has a pro-inflammatory effect by increasing IL-10 cytokine [69]. The GFD did not normalize gut bacteria in one two-year follow-up study of children with CD, and has been shown to induce dysbiosis in healthy adults fed a gluten-free diet for one month [50,70]. Vitamin D metabolite $25(OH)_2D_3$ has been shown in one vitro study to prime dendritic cells to induce regulatory T (Treg) cells [71]. In that study, the results showed that Dermal dendritic cell-derived IL-10 induce IL-10+ TR1 cells. Gut microbiota also affects T cell differentiation and host susceptibility to autoimmune disease [72]. *Bifidobacterium* genus is low in the stools of celiac patients on a GFD compared to healthy controls consuming a regular diet. This genus has been shown to protect against inflammation and mucosal damage caused by gliadin peptides *in vitro* [73].

A change in diet can bring about long-term improvement in chronic inflammation and malabsorption of nutrients due to alterations in the gut microbiome [74]. Enhanced barrier function due to diet and physical activity was shown in a study of professional elite rugby players eating a diet high in whey protein, fruits, and vegetables during training camp [75]. The DNA from fecal samples showed a rich diversity of organism such as phylum Firmicutes, genus Akkermansia, and fewer Bacteroides than in two less active controls groups comprised of normal weight and obese individuals.

The conclusion of a multivariate analysis of factors predicting recovery in 30 women and 11 men w with CD as that gender (women), pretreatment age, and pretreatment BMD independently predict bone mineralization, especially in the lumbar spine [25]. The regression coefficient for lumbar spine BMD (+0.060 to +0.160 g cm^{-2}) did not overlap the 95% confidence interval. The authors identified in their discussion that vitamin D_3 supplementation may be an important factor that was not addressed in their study. In a double blind placebo controlled study, Fickling and associates (2001) administered 300,000 units of choiecalciferol (vitamin D) by intramuscular injection or saline placebo to newly diagnosed CD patients [76]. Data was collected at 6, 12, and 24 months. Both groups saw improvements in BMD, but no significant difference was found between groups.

A case report of a woman with severe bone mineral loss illustrates the need for individualized treatment of CD [14]. A 37-year-old, sedentary woman diagnosed with CD initially had a low BMD and was prescribed calcium (1000 mg day^{-1}) and vitamin D (400 IU day^{-1}). After one year a Registered Dietitian-Nutritionist verified diet compliance, serum vitamin D remained low (33 nmol L^{-1}), and the dose was subsequently increased to 1000 IU day^{-1}. After an 81% increase in the spine and 60% change in the hip at year 3, her bone mass plateaued by year 4. This demonstrates the need to evaluate lifestyle, nutrition, and bone status throughout treatment.

A 10-year study of individuals with CD reported that more than half suffered from vitamin deficiencies in folate, B12 and B6, as evidenced by elevated homocysteine levels, low plasma folate, and B6 [77]. In a Dutch study of newly diagnosed adults ($n = 80$), researchers observed deficiencies in vitamin A, B6, folic acid, B12, and zinc in 67% of participants [78]. B12 and iron deficiency are common in untreated CD and in one study it was discovered in 41% of participants [67]. Dahele and Ghosh reported that after oral and parenteral administration of B12, all patients ($n = 39$) had normal serum levels of B12 at one year follow-up [67]. A new role for B12 in bone health has been shown in a mouse model of B12 deficiency demonstrating that deficiency impairs taurine synthesis and enhances growth hormone-dependent IGF-1 synthesis in the liver; this subsequently increases osteoblast function [68]. Research in humans should focus on reevaluating vitamin B12 requirements in celiac disease to determine its role in bone remineralization.

4. Discussion

Our understanding of bone mineral metabolism and the impact of diet and exercise in the treatment of bone mineral loss for people with celiac disease is incomplete. For this review, the author identified published works and most of these were small, non-randomised clinical trials. Because most participants were recruited from University hospitals and specialty treatment centers, the results may be subject to sampling bias. In spite of an exhaustive search only two studies were found using randomised control, and these did not use an intention-to-treat analysis in spite of subject attrition. Studies also lacked uniformity in dietary intake and compliance assessment measures. It is critical to develop a database of individual raw data from studies on bone density and celiac disease so that a meta-analysis of individual participant data can be published [79]. This type of analysis can differentiate treatment effects for different sub-groups, such as non-responders. The incidence of CD continues to rise in all ages groups, creating need for better management of low BMD in adults and elderly [80].

Nutrient malabsorption due to chronic inflammation and villus atrophy are thought to be the major causes of low BMD (Figure 2). In bone, calcium is regulated by parathyroid hormone (PTH), 1,25-dihydroxyvitamin D (Vitamin D3), and calcitonin [81]. Hyperparathyroidism is common in untreated celiac disease and is characterized by high bone turnover and cortical bone loss [82]. In addition, alterations in gallbladder function, exocrine pancreatic insufficiency, and gut permeability reduce the absorption of essential nutrients [83]. BMD is directly related to the extent of villus atrophy which results in malabsorption of calcium, iron, vitamin D, and folic acid [84]. Even after long after the initiation of diet treatment calcium absorption may be reduced [85]. When administered with vitamin D, Vitamin K has been shown to increase BMD in osteoporosis and reduce fracture rates due to its role in calcium balance [86].

Bone is dynamic tissue that is continuously going through resorption and absorption of calcium from blood to bone in a process called remodeling (Figure 3). The loss of bone density in CD is caused by an imbalance in osteoclastogenesis and osteoblast activity as reported from a study on newly diagnosed patients compared to individuals on a GFD [30]. The authors reported that proinflammatory factors, N-terminal telopeptide of procollagen type I and IL-6, were higher in the untreated CD group, thus suggesting that bone-turnover regulating factors contributed to the reduced bone mass. Other inflammatory factors involved in the pathogenesis of bone metabolism are osteoprotegerin (OPG), a member of the tumor necrosis factor receptor family, and RANKL. RANKL is a cytokine that stimulates osteoclast formation and activation in bone, while OPG acts as a decoy receptor for RANKL, thereby controlling its function. The OPG/RANKL ratio was significantly lower in CD patients in a controlled study of premenopausal women than age matched controls, and the OPG/RANKL ratio was correlated with loss of BMD at the spine [44]. Demographic and lifestyle factors such as age, gender, eating disorders, alcohol abuse, low physical activity, and smoking are also associated with low BMD in CD [55,80,87].

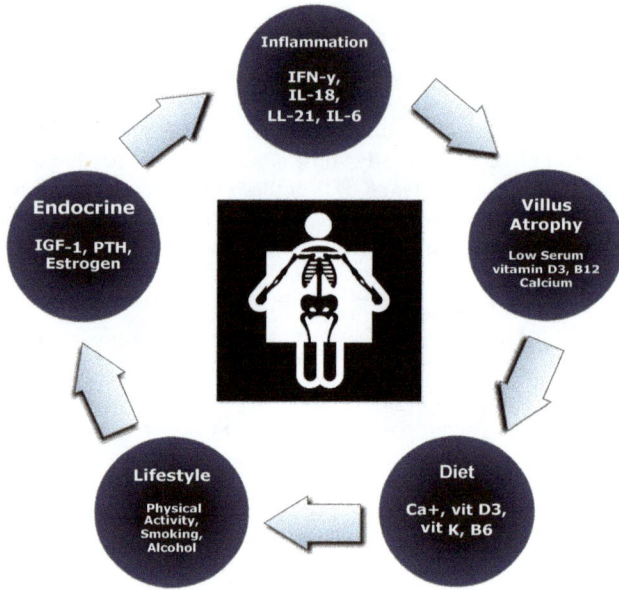

Figure 2. Dysfunctional bone metabolism in celiac disease.

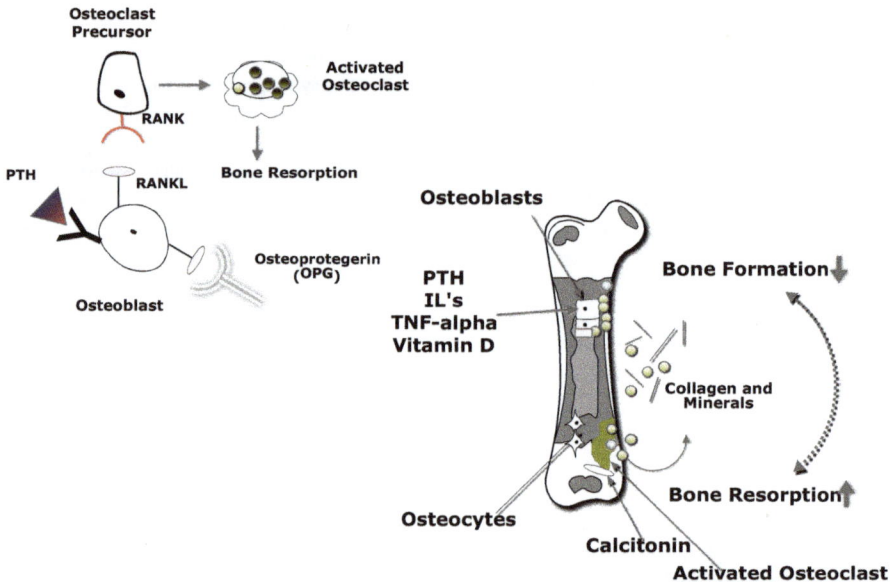

Figure 3. Bone Remodeling. As PTH levels rise, osteoblasts up-regulate the expression of RANKL, which binds to RANK, activating signaling pathways that promote osteoclast differentiation. Osteoblasts secrete osteoprotegerin which protects bone from resorption. Osteoprotegerin binds to RANKL and prevents binding to RANK, therefore the rate stimulation of osteoclastogenesis is reduced. PTH: parathyroid hormone; RANK: receptor activator of nuclear factor-κB; RANKL: receptor activator of nuclear factor-κB ligand.

Nutrients 2015, *7*, 3347–3369

5. Conclusions

The most important behavior impacting bone density in celiac disease is diet adherence. The psychological determinants of GFD adherence, such as self-discipline, values, depression, anxiety, and presence of other food intolerances may have an effect on bone rehabilitation [88]. Patients who struggle with personality and psychological barriers to diet compliance may benefit from motivational interviewing techniques early in treatment [89]. Adults diagnosed with celiac disease may have malabsorption of long-standing, therefore may benefit from iron, folate, B12, vitamin D3, vitamin K, calcium, magnesium and docosahexaenoic acid (DHA) therapy [66,77,90]. The nutrient density shortcomings of the gluten-free diet call for the early and individualized services of a registered dietitian-nutritionist with celiac disease expertise in both medical nutrition therapy and lifestyle coaching [91].

Acknowledgments: The author wants to thank the colleagues in her Health Promotion and Wellness cohort at Rocky Mountain University of Health Professions, experts in the fields of nutrition, physical therapy, occupational therapy, or athletic training, for providing me with constructive criticism that influenced the initial drafts of this manuscript. The author is grateful for the assistance of Teresa E. Araas who critically reviewed subsequent revisions.

Conflicts of Interest: The author declares no conflict of interest.

References

1. Lohi, S.; Mustalahti, K.; Kaukinen, K.; Laurila, K.; Collin, P.; Rissanen, H.; Lohi, O.; Bravi, E.; Gasparin, M.; Reunanen, A.; *et al.* Increasing prevalence of coeliac disease over time. *Aliment. Pharmacol. Ther.* **2007**, *26*, 1217–1225. [CrossRef] [PubMed]
2. Lucendo, A.J.; Garcia-Manzanares, A. Bone mineral density in adult coeliac disease: An updated review. *Rev. Esp. Enferm. Dig.* **2013**, *105*, 154–162. [CrossRef] [PubMed]
3. Tursi, A.; Giorgetti, G.; Brandimarte, G.; Rubino, E.; Lombardi, D.; Gasbarrini, G. Prevalence and clinical presentation of subclinical/silent celiac disease in adults: An analysis on a 12-year observation. *Hepato-Gastroenterol.* **2001**, *48*, 462–464.
4. Pantaleoni, S.; Luchino, M.; Adriani, A.; Pellicano, R.; Stradella, D.; Ribaldone, D.G.; Sapone, N.; Isaia, G.C.; Di Stefano, M.; Astegiano, M. Bone mineral density at diagnosis of celiac disease and after 1 year of gluten-free diet. *Sci. World J.* **2014**, *2014*, 173082. [CrossRef]
5. Lorinczy, K.; Juhász, M.; Csontos, Á.; Fekete, B.; Terjék, O.; Lakatos, P.L.; Miheller, P.; Kocsis, D.; Kárpáti, S.; Tulassay, Z.; *et al.* Does dermatitis herpetiformis result in bone loss as coeliac disease does? A cross sectional study. *Rev. Esp. Enferm. Dig.* **2013**, *105*, 187. [CrossRef] [PubMed]
6. Johnson, M.W.; Ellis, H.J.; Asante, M.A.; Ciclitira, P.J. Celiac disease in the elderly. *Nat. Clin. Pract. Gastroenterol. Hepatol.* **2008**, *5*, 697–706. [CrossRef] [PubMed]
7. Finlayson, M.L.; Peterson, E.W. Falls, aging, and disability. *Phys. Med. Rehabil. Clin. N. Am.* **2010**, *21*, 357–373. [CrossRef] [PubMed]
8. Davie, M.W.; Gaywood, I.; George, E.; Jones, P.W.; Masud, T.; Price, T.; Summers, G.D. Excess non-spine fractures in women over 50 years with celiac disease: A cross-sectional, questionnaire-based study. *Osteoporos. Int.* **2005**, *16*, 1150–1155. [CrossRef] [PubMed]
9. Hjelle, A.M.; Apalset, E.; Mielnik, P.; Bollerslev, J.; Lundin, K.E.; Tell, G.S. Celiac disease and risk of fracture in adults—A review. *Osteoporos. Int.* **2014**, *25*, 1667–1676. [CrossRef] [PubMed]
10. Ludvigsson, J.F.; Michaelsson, K.; Ekbom, A.; Montgomery, S.M. Coeliac disease and the risk of fractures–A general population-based cohort study. *Aliment. Pharm. Ther.* **2007**, *25*, 273–285. [CrossRef]
11. Capriles, V.D.; Martini, L.A.; Areas, J.A. Metabolic osteopathy in celiac disease: Importance of a gluten-free diet. *Nutr. Rev.* **2009**, *67*, 599–606. [CrossRef] [PubMed]
12. Larussa, T.; Suraci, E.; Nazionale, I.; Abenavoli, L.; Imeneo, M.; Luzza, F. Bone mineralization in celiac disease. *Gastroenterol. Res. Pract.* **2012**, *2012*, 198025. [CrossRef] [PubMed]
13. Albulova, E.A.; Drozdov, V.N.; Parfenov, A.I.; Viazhevich Iu, V.; Petrakov, A.V.; Varvanina, G.G. Bone mineral density in patients with gluten-sensitivity celiac disease. *Ter. Arkh.* **2010**, *82*, 43–48. [PubMed]

14. Duerksen, D.R.; Ali, M.; Leslie, W.D. Dramatic effect of vitamin d supplementation and a gluten-free diet on bone mineral density in a patient with celiac disease. *J. Clin. Densitometr.* **2012**, *15*, 120–123. [CrossRef]

15. Caraceni, M.P.; Molteni, N.; Bardella, M.T.; Ortolani, S.; Nogara, A.; Bianchi, P.A. Bone and mineral metabolism in adult celiac disease. *Am. J. Gastroenterol.* **1988**, *83*, 274–277. [PubMed]

16. Caruso, R.; Pallone, F.; Stasi, E.; Romeo, S.; Monteleone, G. Appropriate nutrient supplementation in celiac disease. *Ann. Med.* **2013**, *45*, 522–531. [CrossRef] [PubMed]

17. Sanderson, S.; Tatt, I.D.; Higgins, J.P.T. Tools for assessing quality and susceptibility to bias in observational studies in epidemiology: A systematic review and annotated bibliography. *Int. J. Epidemiol.* **2007**, *36*, 666–676. [CrossRef] [PubMed]

18. Olmos, M.; Antelo, M.; Vazquez, H.; Smecuol, E.; Maurino, E.; Bai, J.C. Systematic review and meta-analysis of observational studies on the prevalence of fractures in coeliac disease. *Dig. Liver Dis.* **2008**, *40*, 46–53. [CrossRef] [PubMed]

19. Wakim-Fleming, J.; Pagadala, M.R.; Lemyre, M.S.; Lopez, R.; Kumaravel, A.; Carey, W.D.; Zein, N.N. Diagnosis of celiac disease in adults based on serology test results, without small-bowel biopsy. *Clin. Gastroenterol. Hepatol.* **2013**, *11*, 511–516. [CrossRef] [PubMed]

20. Rubio-Tapia, A.; Hill, I.D.; Kelly, C.P.; Calderwood, A.H.; Murray, J.A.; American College of, G. Acg clinical guidelines: Diagnosis and management of celiac disease. *Am. J. Gastroenterol.* **2013**, *108*, 656–676. [CrossRef] [PubMed]

21. Kelly, C.P.; Bai, J.C.; Liu, E.; Leffler, D.A. Advances in diagnosis and management of celiac disease. *Gastroenterology* **2015**, *148*, 1175–1186. [CrossRef] [PubMed]

22. Corazza, G.R.; Di Sario, A.; Cecchetti, L.; Jorizzo, R.A.; Di Stefano, M.; Minguzzi, L.; Brusco, G.; Bernardi, M.; Gasbarrini, G. Influence of pattern of clinical presentation and of gluten-free diet on bone mass and metabolism in adult coeliac disease. *Bone* **1996**, *18*, 525–530. [CrossRef] [PubMed]

23. Valdimarsson, T.; Lofman, O.; Toss, G.; Strom, M. Reversal of osteopenia with diet in adult coeliac disease. *Gut* **1996**, *38*, 322–327. [CrossRef] [PubMed]

24. McFarlane, X.A.; Bhalla, A.K.; Robertson, D.A. Effect of a gluten free diet on osteopenia in adults with newly diagnosed coeliac disease. *Gut* **1996**, *39*, 180–184. [CrossRef] [PubMed]

25. Ciacci, C.; Maurelli, L.; Klain, M.; Savino, G.; Salvatore, M.; Mazzacca, G.; Cirillo, M. Effects of dietary treatment on bone mineral density in adults with celiac disease: Factors predicting response. *Am. J. Gastroenterol.* **1997**, *92*, 992–996. [PubMed]

26. Mautalen, C.; Gonzalez, D.; Mazure, R.; Vazquez, H.; Lorenzetti, M.P.; Maurino, E.; Niveloni, S.; Pedreira, S.; Smecuol, E.; Boerr, L.A.; *et al.* Effect of treatment on bone mass, mineral metabolism, and body composition in untreated celiac disease patients. *Am. J. Gastroenterol.* **1997**, *92*, 313–318. [PubMed]

27. Kemppainen, T.; Kroger, H.; Janatuinen, E.; Arnala, I.; Lamberg-Allardt, C.; Karkkainen, M.; Kosma, V.M.; Julkunen, R.; Jurvelin, J.; Alhava, E.; *et al.* Bone recovery after a gluten-free diet: A 5-year follow-up study. *Bone* **1999**, *25*, 355–360. [CrossRef] [PubMed]

28. Valdimarsson, T.; Arnqvist, H.J.; Toss, G.; Jarnerot, G.; Nystrom, F.; Strom, M. Low circulating insulin-like growth factor I in coeliac disease and its relation to bone mineral density. *Scand. J. Gastroenterol.* **1999**, *34*, 904–908. [CrossRef] [PubMed]

29. Sategna-Guidetti, C.; Grosso, S.B.; Grosso, S.; Mengozzi, G.; Aimo, G.; Zaccaria, T.; Di Stefano, M.; Isaia, G.C. The effects of 1-year gluten withdrawal on bone mass, bone metabolism and nutritional status in newly-diagnosed adult coeliac disease patients. *Aliment. Pharmcol. Ther.* **2000**, *14*, 35–43. [CrossRef]

30. Taranta, A.; Fortunati, D.; Longo, M.; Rucci, N.; Iacomino, E.; Aliberti, F.; Facciuto, E.; Migliaccio, S.; Bardella, M.T.; Dubini, A.; *et al.* Imbalance of osteoclastogenesis-regulating factors in patients with celiac disease. *J. Miner. Res.* **2004**, *19*, 1112–1121. [CrossRef]

31. Bucci, C.; Iovino, P.; Tortora, R.; Zingone, F.; Franzese, M.D.; Cappello, C.; Passananti, V.; Ciacci, C. S1264 the lazy celiac adults and their bone density. *Gastroenterology* **2008**, *134*, A213–A214. [CrossRef]

32. Kurppa, K.; Collin, P.; Sievanen, H.; Huhtala, H.; Maki, M.; Kaukinen, K. Gastrointestinal symptoms, quality of life and bone mineral density in mild enteropathic coeliac disease: A prospective clinical trial. *Scand. J. Gastroenterol.* **2010**, *45*, 305–314. [CrossRef] [PubMed]

33. Papamichael, K.; Kokkinakis, E.; Archavlis, E.J.; Theodoropoulos, I.; Tzivras, D.; Karakoidas, C.; Papaioannou, F.; Tsironikos, D.; Karga, H.; Mantzaris, G.J. S2044 effect of a gluten free diet on bone mineral density in patients with celiac disease. *Gastroenterology* **2010**, *138*, S308. [CrossRef]

34. Duerksen, D.R.; Leslie, W.D. Longitudinal evaluation of bone mineral density and body composition in patients with positive celiac serology. *J. Clin. Densitometr.* **2011**, *14*, 478–483. [CrossRef]

35. Vilppula, A.; Kaukinen, K.; Luostarinen, L.; Krekela, I.; Patrikainen, H.; Valve, R.; Luostarinen, M.; Laurila, K.; Maki, M.; Collin, P. Clinical benefit of gluten-free diet in screen-detected older celiac disease patients. *BMC Gastroenterol.* **2011**, *11*, 136. [CrossRef] [PubMed]

36. Casella, S.; Zanini, B.; Lanzarotto, F.; Villanacci, V.; Ricci, C.; Lanzini, A. Celiac disease in elderly adults: Clinical, serological, and histological characteristics and the effect of a gluten-free diet. *J. Am. Geriatr. Soc.* **2012**, *60*, 1064–1069. [CrossRef] [PubMed]

37. Passananti, V.; Santonicola, A.; Bucci, C.; Andreozzi, P.; Ranaudo, A.; Di Giacomo, D.V.; Ciacci, C. Bone mass in women with celiac disease: Role of exercise and gluten-free diet. *Dig. Liver Dis.* **2012**, *44*, 379–383. [CrossRef] [PubMed]

38. Szymczak, J.; Bohdanowicz-Pawlak, A.; Waszczuk, E.; Jakubowska, J. Low bone mineral density in adult patients with coeliac disease. *Endokrynol. Pol.* **2012**, *63*, 270–276. [PubMed]

39. Kumar, M.; Rastogi, A.; Bhadada, S.K.; Bhansali, A.; Vaiphei, K.; Kochhar, R. Effect of zoledronic acid on bone mineral density in patients of celiac disease: A prospective, randomized, pilot study. *Indian J. Med. Res.* **2013**, *138*, 882–887. [PubMed]

40. Kurppa, K.; Paavola, A.; Collin, P.; Sievanen, H.; Laurila, K.; Huhtala, H.; Saavalainen, P.; Maki, M.; Kaukinen, K. Benefits of a gluten-free diet for asymptomatic patients with serologic markers of celiac disease. *Gastroenterology* **2014**, *147*, 610–617. [CrossRef] [PubMed]

41. Masala, S.; Annibale, B.; Fiori, R.; Capurso, G.; Marinetti, A.; Simonetti, G. Dxa *vs.* qct for subclinical celiac disease patients. *Acta Diabetol.* **2003**, *40*, S174–S176. [CrossRef] [PubMed]

42. Dennison, E.M.; Compston, J.E.; Flahive, J.; Siris, E.S.; Gehlbach, S.H.; Adachi, J.D.; Boonen, S.; Chapurlat, R.; Diez-Perez, A.; Anderson, F.A.; *et al.* Effect of co-morbidities on fracture risk: Findings from the global longitudinal study of osteoporosis in women (glow). *Bone* **2012**, *50*, 1288–1293. [CrossRef] [PubMed]

43. Di Stefano, M.; Mengoli, C.; Tomarchio, O.; Bergonzi, M.; De Amici, M.; Ilardo, D.; Vattiato, C.; Biagi, F.; Zanaboni, A.M.; Miceli, E.; *et al.* P.05.6 high levels of osteoprotegerin and low levels of cooh-terminal propeptide of type I procollagen characterize the persisting bone derangement in celiac disease patients on long-term gluten-free diet. *Dig. Dis.* **2013**, *45*, S120–S121.

44. Fiore, C.E.; Pennisi, P.; Ferro, G.; Ximenes, B.; Privitelli, L.; Mangiafico, R.A.; Santoro, F.; Parisi, N.; Lombardo, T. Altered osteoprotegerin/rankl ratio and low bone mineral density in celiac patients on long-term treatment with gluten-free diet. *Horm. Metab. Res.* **2006**, *38*, 417–422. [CrossRef] [PubMed]

45. Sanchez, M.I.; Mohaidle, A.; Baistrocchi, A.; Matoso, D.; Vazquez, H.; Gonzalez, A.; Mazure, R.; Maffei, E.; Ferrari, G.; Smecuol, E.; *et al.* Risk of fracture in celiac disease: Gender, dietary compliance, or both? *World J. Gastroenterol.* **2011**, *17*, 3035–3042. [CrossRef] [PubMed]

46. Larussa, T.; Suraci, E.; Montalcini, T.; Nazionale, I.; Abenavoli, L.; Imeneo, M.; Luzza, F. P.41 reduced bone mineral density is frequent in treated adult coeliac disease notwithstanding complete normalization of duodenal lesions. *Dig. Liver Dis.* **2010**, *42*, S117. [CrossRef]

47. Tursi, A.; Brandimarte, G.; Giorgetti, G. High prevalence of small intestinal bacterial overgrowth in celiac patients with persistence of gastrointestinal symptoms after gluten withdrawal. *Am. J. Gastroenterol.* **2003**, *98*, 839–843. [CrossRef] [PubMed]

48. Brown, K.; DeCoffe, D.; Molcan, E.; Gibson, D.L. Diet-induced dysbiosis of the intestinal microbiota and the effects on immunity and disease. *Nutrients* **2012**, *4*, 1095–1119. [CrossRef] [PubMed]

49. Sanz, Y.; De Pama, G.; Laparra, M. Unraveling the ties between celiac disease and intestinal microbiota. *Int. Rev. Immunol.* **2011**, *30*, 207–218. [CrossRef] [PubMed]

50. Sanz, Y. Effects of a gluten-free diet on gut microbiota and immune function in healthy adult humans. *Gut Microb.* **2010**, *1*, 135–137. [CrossRef]

51. Tursi, A.; Giorgetti, G.M.; Elisei, W.; Brandimarte, G.; Aiello, F. Pa.47 complications in coeliac disease under gluten-free diet. *Dig. Liver Dis.* **2008**, *40*, S92–S93. [CrossRef]

52. Mason, R.S.; Sequeira, V.B.; Gordon-Thomson, C. Vitamin D: The light side of sunshine. *Eur. J. Clin. Nutr.* **2011**, *65*, 986–993. [CrossRef] [PubMed]

53. Going, S.; Lohman, T.; Houtkooper, L.; Metcalfe, L.; Flint-Wagner, H.; Blew, R.; Stanford, V.; Cussler, E.; Martin, J.; Teixeira, P.; *et al.* Effects of exercise on bone mineral density in calcium-replete postmenopausal women with and without hormone replacement therapy. *Osteoporos. Int.* **2003**, *14*, 637–643. [CrossRef] [PubMed]

54. Zhao, R.; Zhao, M.; Zhang, L. Efficiency of jumping exercise in improving bone mineral density among premenopausal women: A meta-analysis. *Sports Med.* **2014**, *44*, 1393–1402. [CrossRef] [PubMed]

55. Di Stefano, M.; Veneto, G.; Corrao, G.; Corazza, G.R. Role of lifestyle factors in the pathogenesis of osteopenia in adult coeliac disease: A multivariate analysis. *Eur. J. Gastroenterol. Hepatol.* **2000**, *12*, 1195–1199.

56. Elders, P.J.; Netelenbos, J.C.; Lips, P.; Khoe, E.; van Ginkel, F.C.; Hulshof, K.F.; van der Stelt, P.F. Perimenopausal bone mass and risk factors. *Bone Miner.* **1989**, *7*, 289–299. [CrossRef] [PubMed]

57. González, D.; Mazure, R.; Mautalen, C.; Vazquez, H.; Bai, J. Body composition and bone mineral density in untreated and treated patients with celiac disease. *Bone* **1995**, *16*, 231–234. [CrossRef] [PubMed]

58. Kabbani, T.A.; Goldberg, A.; Kelly, C.P.; Pallav, K.; Tariq, S.; Peer, A.; Hansen, J.; Dennis, M.; Leffler, D.A. Body mass index and the risk of obesity in coeliac disease treated with the gluten-free diet. *Aliment. Pharmacol. Ther.* **2012**, *35*, 723–729. [CrossRef] [PubMed]

59. Sonti, R.; Green, P.H. Celiac disease: Obesity in celiac disease. *Nat. Rev. Gastroenterol. Hepatol.* **2012**, *9*, 247–248. [CrossRef] [PubMed]

60. Keramaris, N.; Malliaropoulos, N.; Padhiar, N.; King, J.; Maffulli, N. The effect of physical exercise on musculo-skeletal metabolism: A systematic review of the role of rank/rankl/opg pathway. *Br. J. Sports Med.* **2013**, *47*, e3. [CrossRef]

61. Whitney, C.; Warburton, D.E.; Frohlich, J.; Chan, S.Y.; McKay, H.; Khan, K. Are cardiovascular disease and osteoporosis directly linked? *Sports Med.* **2004**, *34*, 779–807. [CrossRef] [PubMed]

62. Ciacci, C.; Peluso, G.; Iannoni, E.; Siniscalchi, M.; Iovino, P.; Rispo, A.; Tortora, R.; Bucci, C.; Zingone, F.; Margarucci, S.; *et al.* L-carnitine in the treatment of fatigue in adult celiac disease patients: A pilot study. *Dig. Liver Dis.* **2007**, *39*, 922–928. [CrossRef] [PubMed]

63. Marques, E.A.; Wanderley, F.; Machado, L.; Sousa, F.; Viana, J.L.; Moreira-Goncalves, D.; Moreira, P.; Mota, J.; Carvalho, J. Effects of resistance and aerobic exercise on physical function, bone mineral density, opg and rankl in older women. *Exp. Gerontol.* **2011**, *46*, 524–532. [CrossRef] [PubMed]

64. Marques, E.A.; Mota, J.; Carvalho, J. Exercise effects on bone mineral density in older adults: A meta-analysis of randomized controlled trials. *Age* **2012**, *34*, 1493–1515. [CrossRef] [PubMed]

65. Baert, V.; Gorus, E.; Mets, T.; Bautmans, I. Motivators and barriers for physical activity in older adults with osteoporosis. *J. Geriatr. Phys. Ther.* **2015**. [CrossRef]

66. Hadithi, M.; Mulder, C.J.; Stam, F.; Azizi, J.; Crusius, J.B.; Pena, A.S.; Stehouwer, C.D.; Smulders, Y.M. Effect of B vitamin supplementation on plasma homocysteine levels in celiac disease. *World J. Gastroenterol.* **2009**, *15*, 955–960. [CrossRef] [PubMed]

67. Dahele, A.; Ghosh, S. Vitamin B12 deficiency in untreated celiac disease. *Am. J. Gastroenterol.* **2001**, *96*, 745–750. [CrossRef] [PubMed]

68. Roman-Garcia, P.; Quiros-Gonzalez, I.; Mottram, L.; Lieben, L.; Sharan, K.; Wangwiwatsin, A.; Tubio, J.; Lewis, K.; Wilkinson, D.; Santhanam, B.; *et al.* Vitamin B-12-dependent taurine synthesis regulates growth and bone mass. *J. Clin. Investig.* **2014**, *124*, 2988–3002. [CrossRef] [PubMed]

69. Calabro, A.; Gralka, E.; Luchinat, C.; Saccenti, E.; Tenori, L. A metabolomic perspective on coeliac disease. *Autoimmun. Dis.* **2014**, *2014*, 756138.

70. Di Cagno, R.; De Angelis, M.; De Pasquale, I.; Ndagijimana, M.; Vernocchi, P.; Ricciuti, P.; Gagliardi, F.; Laghi, L.; Crecchio, C.; Guerzoni, M.E.; *et al.* Duodenal and faecal microbiota of celiac children: Molecular, phenotype and metabolome characterization. *BMC Microbiol.* **2011**, *11*, 219.

71. Van der Aar, A.M.; Sibiryak, D.S.; Bakdash, G.; van Capel, T.M.; van der Kleij, H.P.; Opstelten, D.J.; Teunissen, M.B.; Kapsenberg, M.L.; de Jong, E.C. Vitamin D3 targets epidermal and dermal dendritic cells for induction of distinct regulatory T cells. *J. Allergy Clin. Immunol.* **2011**, *127*, 1532–1540.

72. Atarashi, K.; Honda, K. Microbiota in autoimmunity and tolerance. *Curr. Opin. Immunol.* **2011**, *23*, 761–768. [CrossRef] [PubMed]

73. Golfetto, L.; Senna, F.D.; Hermes, J.; Beserra, B.T.; Franca Fda, S.; Martinello, F. Lower bifidobacteria counts in adult patients with celiac disease on a gluten-free diet. *Arquivos Gastroenterol.* **2014**, *51*, 139–143. [CrossRef]

74. Krajmalnik-Brown, R.; Ilhan, Z.E.; Kang, D.W.; DiBaise, J.K. Effects of gut microbes on nutrient absorption and energy regulation. *Nutr. Clin. Pract.* **2012**, *27*, 201–214. [CrossRef]

75. Clarke, S.F.; Murphy, E.F.; O'Sullivan, O.; Lucey, A.J.; Humphreys, M.; Hogan, A.; Hayes, P.; O'Reilly, M.; Jeffery, I.B.; Wood-Martin, R.; *et al.* Exercise and associated dietary extremes impact on gut microbial diversity. *Gut* **2014**, *63*, 1913–1920. [CrossRef] [PubMed]

76. Fickling, W.E.; Gupta, R.; Speden, D.; Bhalla, A.K.; Ring, F.J.; Robertson, D.A. Parenteral vitamin D in newly diagnosed coeliac disese—Prelimineary analysis of double blind placebo controlled study. *Gastroenterology* **2001**, *120*, A394. [CrossRef]

77. Hallert, C.; Grant, C.; Grehn, S.; Granno, C.; Hulten, S.; Midhagen, G.; Strom, M.; Svensson, H.; Valdimarsson, T. Evidence of poor vitamin status in coeliac patients on a gluten-free diet for 10 years. *Aliment. Pharmacolo. Ther.* **2002**, *16*, 1333–1339. [CrossRef]

78. Wierdsma, N.J.; van Bokhorst-de van der Schueren, M.A.; Berkenpas, M.; Mulder, C.J.; van Bodegraven, A.A. Vitamin and mineral deficiencies are highly prevalent in newly diagnosed celiac disease patients. *Nutrients* **2013**, *5*, 3975–3992. [CrossRef] [PubMed]

79. Riley, R.D.; Lambert, P.C.; Abo-Zaid, G. Meta-analysis of individual participant data: Rationale, conduct, and reporting. *Res. Methods Rep.* **2010**, *340*. [CrossRef]

80. Rashtak, S.; Murray, J.A. Celiac disease in the elderly. *Gastroenterol. Clin. N. Am.* **2009**, *38*, 433–446. [CrossRef]

81. Krupa-Kozak, U. Pathologic bone alterations in celiac disease: Etiology, epidemiology, and treatment. *Nutrition* **2014**, *30*, 16–24. [CrossRef] [PubMed]

82. Zanchi, C.; Di Leo, G.; Ronfani, L.; Martelossi, S.; Not, T.; Ventura, A. Bone metabolism in celiac disease. *J. Pediatr.* **2008**, *153*, 262–265. [CrossRef] [PubMed]

83. Farnetti, S.; Zocco, M.A.; Garcovich, M.; Gasbarrini, A.; Capristo, E. Functional and metabolic disorders in celiac disease: New implications for nutritional treatment. *J. Med. Food* **2014**, *17*, 1159–1164. [CrossRef] [PubMed]

84. Garcia-Manzanares, A.; Tenias, J.M.; Lucendo, A.J. Bone mineral density directly correlates with duodenal marsh stage in newly diagnosed adult celiac patients. *Scand. J. Gastroenterol.* **2012**, *47*, 927–936. [CrossRef] [PubMed]

85. Pazianas, M.; Butcher, G.P.; Subhani, J.M.; Finch, P.J.; Ang, L.; Collins, C.; Heaney, R.P.; Zaidi, M.; Maxwell, J.D. Calcium absorption and bone mineral density in celiacs after long term treatment with gluten-free diet and adequate calcium intake. *Osteoporos. Int.* **2005**, *16*, 56–63. [CrossRef] [PubMed]

86. Weber, P. Vitamin K and bone health. *Nutrition* **2001**, *17*, 880–887. [CrossRef] [PubMed]

87. Molteni, N.; Caraceni, M.P.; Bardella, M.T.; Ortolani, S.; Gandolini, G.G.; Bianchi, P. Bone mineral density in adult celiac patients and the effect of gluten-free diet from childhood. *Am. J. Gastroenterol.* **1990**, *85*, 51–53. [PubMed]

88. Edwards George, J.B.; Leffler, D.A.; Dennis, M.D.; Franko, D.L.; Blom-Hoffman, J.; Kelly, C.P. Psychological correlates of gluten-free diet adherence in adults with celiac disease. *J. Clin. Gastroenterol.* **2009**, *43*, 301.

89. Thorpe, M. Motivational interviewing and dietary behavior change. *J. Am. Diet. Assoc.* **2003**, *103*, 150–151. [CrossRef] [PubMed]

90. Genuis, S.J.; Bouchard, T.P. Combination of micronutrients for bone (comb) study: Bone density after micronutrient intervention. *J. Environ. Public Health* **2012**, *2012*, 354151. [PubMed]

91. Grace-Farfaglia, P. Celiac & gluten intolerance: A wellness perspective. *J. Nutr. Health Food Eng.* **2014**, *1*, 14.

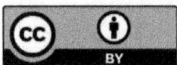

nutrients

MDPI

Article

Analysis of Body Composition and Food Habits of Spanish Celiac Women

Itziar Churruca, Jonatan Miranda, Arrate Lasa, María Á. Bustamante, Idoia Larretxi and Edurne Simon *

Gluten Analysis Laboratory of University of the Basque Country, Department of Nutrition and Food Science, University of the Basque Country (UPV/EHU), Vitoria-Gasteiz 01006, Spain; itziar.txurruka@ehu.es (I.C.); jonatan.miranda@ehu.es (J.M.); arrate.lasa@ehu.es (A.L.); marian.bustamante@ehu.es (M.A.B.); idoia.larrechi@ehu.es (I.L.)

* Correspondence: edurne.simon@ehu.es; Tel.: +34-945-013-069; Fax: +34-945-013-014

Received: 28 May 2015; Accepted: 1 July 2015; Published: 8 July 2015

Abstract: The purpose of the present work was both to analyze composition of Spanish celiac women and to study the food habits and gluten-free diet of these celiac patients, in order to determine whether they achieve a balanced and healthy diet as well as to highlight nutritional qualitative and/or quantitative differences. 54 adult celiac women (34 ± 13 years) took part in the six-month study. Height, weight and body composition were measured. An analysis of energy consumption and of the macronutrient distribution of their diet was carried out. Their fulfillment of micronutrient intake recommendations was verified. Participants showed a Body Mass Index of 21.6 ± 2.4 kg/m^2. Energy Intake was slightly lower than the Dietary Reference Intakes. Excessive protein apart from over-consumption of fat was observed. More than three quarters of participants consumed meat in excess. Carbohydrate consumption along with that of fiber was below recommended levels. Vitamin D, iron, and iodine had a low percentage of recommendation compliance. In general, participants followed the recommendations of dairy products and fruit intake whereas vegetable consumption was not enough for the vast majority. We conclude that although the diet of celiac women does not differ much from the diet of general population, some considerations, such as reducing fat and protein consumption and increasing fiber intake, must be taken into account.

Keywords: celiac disease; gluten-free diet; diary recommended intake; food habit; body composition

---

1. Introduction

Celiac disease (CD) is one of the most common chronic intestinal diseases in Europe and is defined as a permanent intolerance to gluten proteins. This intolerance is maintained throughout a lifetime and is presented in genetically predisposed subjects. Its aetiology is unknown but genetic, environmental (gluten) and immunological factors contribute to its development [1]. Its estimated prevalence in Europeans and their descendants is 1%, this being more frequent in women in a 2:1 ratio [2]. Moreover, there is a significant percentage of patients who remain undiagnosed [2].

The only effective treatment for celiac disease is a strict lifelong gluten-free diet (GFD). To meet this challenge, it is essential to control the production of foods and dishes for celiac people, in order to guarantee the absence of these proteins in them. Catassi *et al.* [3] demonstrated that the ingestion of small amounts of gluten, as little as 50 mg of gluten per day over three months, can cause important damage in the intestinal mucosa. In this context a GFD with the threshold of 20 mg/kg ensures an intake of less than 50 mg/day of gluten and provides a sufficient safety margin [4,5].

Apart from gluten control, the correct suitable GFD must be nutritionally balanced too; it must fulfil all the energy and nutrient requirements and be sufficient to meet the nutritional needs of each person and prevent deficiencies. The possibility that excessively restricted cereal consumption as a solution to avoid gluten intake becomes a low carbohydrate (CHO) intake with an excess of fat and protein cannot be discarded. Additionally, the American Dietetic Association mentions in its guide for celiac patients [6] the possible consequences of complying with a GFD. According to this guide, following this diet could imply a low intake of carbohydrates, iron, folate, niacin, zinc, and fiber. Other authors also indicate that consumption of refined grains, processed as gluten-free products, entails a lower intake of vitamin B group, vitamin D, and calcium [7].

It must be taken into account that the prevalence of some diseases such as cardiovascular diseases is associated with low fiber and high saturated fat intake. Similarly, anaemia, related to a lack of iron and folic acid, and osteoporosis, associated with a lack of calcium and vitamin D, are closely linked with common symptoms of celiac patients [8,9].

As far as we know no data exist concerning the nutritional adequacy of a GFD for celiac women in Spain. In this context, the main aim of the present work was to evaluate body composition and the nutritional composition of the GFD followed by adult celiac women, as well as to compare it with the international recommendations, in order to highlight qualitative and quantitative nutritional differences. Furthermore, we found it relevant to describe the food intake and habits of celiac women in comparison with Spanish women in the general population.

2. Experimental Section

2.1. Participants and Procedure

Gluten and Food Safety is a prospective SUSFOOD study conducted in the Basque Country (Spain). The present study makes use of data from the celiac women cohort recruited in 2011 from three regions in the north of Spain (Alava, Gipuzkoa, and Bizkaia). All celiac patients were members of the Basque Country Celiac Society, with a confirmation of CD diagnosis (intestinal biopsy and/or serological test). Participants had all been compliant with the GFD for at least one year (mean length in years $\pm$ SD: 23 $\pm$ 11) and were followed up on for this analysis until April 2012 (for six months). 54 celiac women and older than 16 years took part in the study (mean age $\pm$ SD: 34 $\pm$ 13). All women claimed to be in remission from clinical symptoms. Exclusion criteria included a history of cardiovascular disease or diabetes, pregnancy, hyperthyroidism/hypothyroidism, total cholesterol levels > 300 mg/dL, levels of triglyceride > 300 mg/dL and blood pressure level > 140/90 mm Hg. All participants received verbal and written information about the nature and purpose of the survey, and all gave their written consent for their involvement in the study. This study was approved by the Ethical Committee of the University of The Basque Country (CEISH/76/2011).

Each subject underwent anthropometric parameters and dietary habits record for nutritional status assessment.

2.2. Anthropometric Measurements

Body weight ($\pm$10 g) was measured after voiding using a digital integrating scale (SECA 760, SECA, Hamburg, Germany). Height was measured to the nearest 5 mm using a stadiometer (SECA 220, SECA, Hamburg, Germany).

For each subject body mass index (BMI) was calculated as weight (kg)/height (m)^2. The BMI values were categorized according to the World Health Organization (WHO) criteria as follows: Below 18.5 kg/m^2 as underweight, 18.5–24.9 kg/m^2 as normal weight, 25–29.9 kg/m^2 as overweight and $\geq$30 kg/m^2 as obese [10].

2.3. Body Composition and Energy Expenditure

Body composition (fat mass and fat-free mass) was estimated with a direct segmental multiple-frequency bioelectrical impedance analysis method (Inbody 230; Biospace, Seoul, Korea). Two skin electrodes were placed on the feet and two electrodes on the hands. According to the standard procedure, whole-body resistance and reactance were measured. For all subjects, fat mass and fat-free mass were evaluated from total-body impedance (Z). Energy expenditure was calculated using Harris-Benedict formula and applying 1.5 factor for mild/light physical activity.

Regarding the percentage of body fat, the guidelines of Gallagher *et al.* were used as reference [11].

2.4. Dietary Assessment

24 h food recall (24HR) of three days and a food frequency questionnaire (FFQ), previously described [12], were kept for each patient with food portions and amounts determined by using photographs of rations and sizes described in Photo Album food [13]. Trained nutritionist-dieticians carried out the 24HRs, two on weekdays and one at the weekend. Nutrient intake was calculated by using a computerized program system (AyS, Software, Tandem Innova, Inc., Huesca, Spain). The nutrient content data of the specific gluten-free products manufactured for celiac people were collected from the manufacturers and added into the food composition database of the program before calculations. As gluten-free product labels did not indicate micronutrient content (vitamins and minerals), an estimation with homologous gluten-containing products was carried out [12]. Dietary reference intakes (DRI) for Spanish population issued by the Spanish Societies of Nutrition, Feeding and Dietetics (FESNAD) in 2010 were taken as references for the interpretation of the 24HR [14]. Other Recommended Dietary Values such as Institute of Medicine (IoM) were taken into consideration [15].

In the case of FFQ, Spanish Society of Community Nutrition (SENC) recommendations were used for the correct interpretation of the results [16]. The energy, nutrient and food intakes of celiac women were compared to nutritional data obtained from a Spanish reference women population in ENIDE [17], a nutritional survey carried out in 2011, at the same period of time as the present work.

ENIDE study is representative at national level of the adult population. It was based on a random selection of more than 3323 individuals, providing a level of confidence of 95% and an accuracy of ±1.8%. The survey was conducted on 1589 men and 1734 women aged between 18 and 65 years old. The methodology used 24 h recall, daily food over three random days, and a food frequency questionnaire [17].

2.5. Mediterranean-Diet Score

Adherence to the Mediterranean diet was measured by the Mediterranean-Diet Score (MDS) [18]. The diet score varied from 0 (low quality diet) to 9 (high quality diet). With regard to fruits and nuts, vegetables/potatoes, legumes, fish, and cereals as well as the component ratio between monounsaturated fatty acids and saturated fatty acids, a value of 1 was assigned to celiac women whose consumption was equal to or higher than the median value, and 0 to the others. For meat and meat products and dairy products, a value 1 was assigned to celiac women whose consumption was less than the median, and 0 to the others. Although seven participants were under 18 years, taking into account that they consume alcohol, these criteria were also computed for MDS.

2.6. Statistical Analysis

Statistical analyses of our results were performed by using the IBM SPSS statistical program 19 (IBM Inc., Armonk, NY, USA). The results for continuous variables are given as the arithmetic mean ± SD and the range. The results for non-continuous variables are given as the frequency and the percentage. Statistical analyses were performed with Student's or Welch's *t* test and *F*-Snedecor test. *p* values < 0.05 were accepted as significant.

3. Results

3.1. Anthropometric and Body Composition Measurements

Main anagraphic data and anthropometric/body composition measurements of CD women are shown in Table 1. The BMI were within normal in 81.5% of cases, and there were only six people with low weight and four cases of overweight women. None of them were obese. Accordingly, the majority of adult women had a normal fat percentage [11].

Table 1. Characteristic of celiac participants included in survey.

Characteristic	Women
n	54
Age (year)	34.4 ± 12.9
Mean duration of GFD (year)	10.9 ± 8.5
Height (cm)	164 ± 6
Weight (kg)	57.9 ± 7.3
Body Fat %	27.1 ± 6.9
Body-mass index	
Mean (kg/m^2)	21.4 ± 27
Underweight <18.5—no. (%)	6 (11.1)
Normal 18.5–24.9—no. (%)	44 (81.5)
Overweight 25–30—no. (%)	4 (7.4)

Notes: Values are means ± SD; SD, standard deviation; no, number of subjects; GFD, gluten free diet.

3.2. Dietary Intakes

3.2.1. Energy, Macronutrients and Fiber

The average energy intake of celiac women (Table 2) was in good accordance with their estimated energy expenditure (1904 ± 161 kcal) but below that of the DRI's [14]. Although this was also observed in women from the ENIDE study, the energy intake of celiac patients was significantly lower (Table 2). When comparing energy sources among groups, similar macronutrient intakes were found between celiac and Spanish women—control women groups (Figure 1).

Regarding proteins, this nutrient intake represented 17.3% of total energy intake, which was similar to the data observed in the Spanish survey (Figure 1), therefore it was consumed in excess in both celiac and general women—control women populations. Animal protein intakes were the main contributor (69%) to the total protein consumption. Dairy products provided nearly 20% of total protein intake whereas meat and meat products, fish and eggs provided nearly 50%.

Carbohydrate consumption was enough to cover the minimum established as DRI (130 g/day) by FESNAD (Table 2). With regard to lipids, the percentage of this macronutrient markedly exceeded the recommendations (Figure 1). In fact, almost all the celiac women reached a fat consumption which represented over 30% of total energy. In order to evaluate the dietary fat quality, the lipid profile was calculated. In general terms, saturated and unsaturated fatty acids related ratios were reached, as was the case in the ENIDE survey (Table 2) [19].

Celiac women consume small amounts of dietary fiber. Indeed, 43% of celiac women did not reach 15 grams per day (Table 2). Compared to Spanish women—control women from the ENIDE survey, the celiac group consumed a significantly lower daily amount of fiber (Table 2). Low fiber intake was more frequent in young adult celiac women; the mean fiber consumption in the 16–44 years celiac women (*n* = 41) was 15.6 ± 5.5 g/day, women older than 45 years (*n* = 13) consumed on average 19.0 ± 5.1 g/day (*p* = 0.005).

Table 2. Energy and nutrient distribution in celiac and Spanish women.

	Celiac Women ($n = 54$)	Spanish Women—Control Women ($n = 1734$)	p
Energy (kcal)	1847 ± 362	2038 ± 655	0.003
Protein (g)	79.2 ± 16.6	88.0 ± 37.8	< 0.001
Carbohydrate (g)	192.3 ± 40.7	199.7 ± 75.9	0.002
Fat (g)	84.6 ± 23.0	93.2 ± 35.6	0.022
(PUFA+MUFA)/SFA	2.1	2.0	-
PUFA/SFA	0.49	0.49	-
Cholesterol (mg)	324 ± 137	336 ± 151	0.544
Fiber (g)	16.4 ± 5.6	18.9 ± 10.1	0.002

Notes: Values are means ± SD; Spanish Adult women data were taken from the Spanish dietary nutritional assessment (ENIDE study, representative of the adult population at national level); SD, standard deviation; PUFA, polyunsaturated fatty acids; MUFA, monounsaturated fatty acids; SFA, saturated fatty acids.

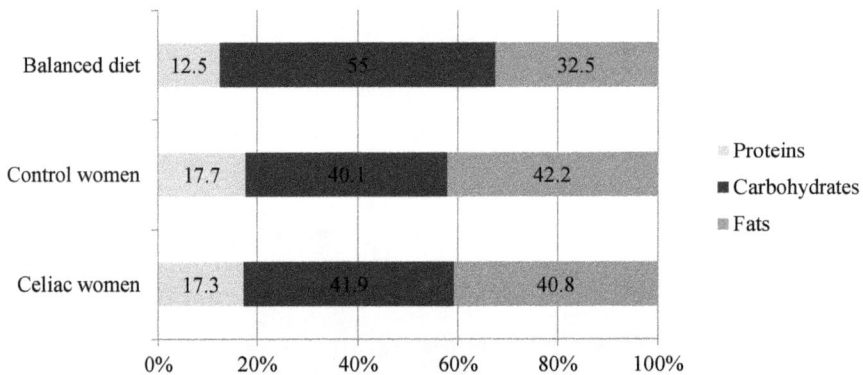

Figure 1. Energy percentage from each macronutrient in celiac ($n = 54$) and Spanish women—control women ($n = 1734$) (ENIDE study, representative at national level of the adult population) compared to the recommended percentage in a balanced diet proposed by the Federation of Spanish Societies of Nutrition and Dietetics (FESNAD).

3.2.2. Micronutrients

Of the 19 micronutrients analyzed, vitamin D, vitamin E, folate, iodine, iron, calcium, and selenium had an especially marked low compliance and these deficiencies were also similar to those found in general population (Table 3). None of the celiac women showed low intakes of vitamin B12 (Table 3). According to FESNAD recommendations, iodine, vitamin D, and vitamin E deficiencies were highly presented because 80%, 48% and 39%, respectively, of the celiac women did not accomplish 2/3 of DRI of these nutrients (Figure 2). Also, nearly 1 in 3 women did not achieve 2/3 of the iron and selenium DRIs (Figure 2). With respect to folate, calcium and vitamin A, around 18%, 13% and 11% of celiac were below 2/3 of recommended levels (Figure 2).

Comparing these with the Spanish general population survey—control women, micronutrient deficiencies follow a very similar scheme/ pattern (Table 3). Statistical differences were found in some of them, such as vitamin E and niacin as well as magnesium and selenium minerals, which were lower in celiacs (Table 3). On the other hand, riboflavin, vitamin B6, and folate were noticeably higher in the celiac group (Table 3).

Table 3. Micronutrient intake in celiac and Spanish women compared to the FESNAD' and IoM' recommendations.

	Celiac Women (*n* = 54)	Spanish Women—Control Women (*n* = 1734)	*p*	DRI FESNAD (2010) [14]	DRI: RDA and AI IoM (2011) [15]
Vitamin A (µg)	819 ± 556	723 ± 323	0.001	600	700
Thiamin (mg)	2.1 ± 3.5	1.8 ± 4.9	0.056	1	1.1 [k]
Riboflavin (mg)	2.1 ± 1.5	1.4 ± 3.2	0.001	1.3 [a]	1.1 [k]
Vitamin B6 (mg)	2.1 ± 0.8	1.7 ± 3.7	< 0.001	1.2 [b]	1.3 [b]
Vitamin B12 (µg)	8.1 ± 5.6	6.1 ± 4.9	0.230	2	2.4
Vitamin C (mg)	153 ± 65	133 ± 80	0.180	60 [c]	75
Vitamin D (µg)	4.9 ± 4.0	3.7 ± 3.7	0.331	5	15
Vitamin E (mg)	11.2 ± 3.8	13.4 ± 7.0	0.003	15	15
Niacin (mg)	26.4 ± 11.4	39.4 ± 39.7	< 0.001	14	14
Folate (µg)	373 ± 556	266 ± 113	< 0.001	300	400 [j]
Calcium (mg)	897 ± 264	835 ± 293	0.274	900 [d]	1000 [d]
Iron (mg)	14.5 ± 5.0	13.7 ± 6.2	0.162	18 [e]	18 [e]
Magnesium (mg)	297 ± 92	354 ± 126	0.011	300 [f]	320 [f]
Iodine (µg)	78.7 ± 38.7	84.8 ± 47.3	0.187	150	150
Phosphorus (mg)	1223 ± 314	1295 ± 380	0.191	700 [g]	700 [g]
Zinc (mg)	9.2 ± 4.0	8.7 ± 3.3	0.156	7 [g]	8
Sodium (mg)	1916 ± 802	2349 ± 810	0.505	1500	1500 [l]
Potassium (mg)	2950 ± 806	2858 ± 827	0.485	3100 [h]	4700
Selenium (µg)	48.2 ± 19.3	53.7 ± 28.9	0.031	55 [i]	55

Notes: Values are means ± SD; Spanish Adult women data were taken from the Spanish dietary nutritional assessment (ENIDE study, representative of the adult population at national level); SD, standard deviation; DRI, dietary reference intake; RDA, recommended dietary allowances; AI, adequate intake; FESNAD, Federation of Spanish Societies of Nutrition and Dietetics; IoM, Institute of Medicine; [a] Riboflavin, 1.2 mg for 16–19 range and >60 years women; [b] Vitamin B6, 1.3 mg for 16–19 years old women (FESNAD), 1.2 mg for 16–18 years and 1.5 mg for >50 (IoM); [c] Vitamin C, 65 mg for 16–18 years (IoM) and 70 mg for >60 years (FESNAD); [d] Calcium 1000 mg (FESNAD) or 1300 mg (IoM) for 16–19 years range and 1000 mg >50 years women (FESNAD) or 1200 mg (ioM) for >50 years; [e] Iron, 15 mg for 16–19 years, 50–59 years and 10 mg for >60 years (FESNAD) or15 mg for 16–18 years and 8 mg for >51 years (IoM); [f] Magnesium 360 mg for 16–18 years, 310 mg for 18–30 years, 320 mg for >60 years (IoM); [g] Phosphorus and Zinc, 800 and 8 for 16–19years (FESNAD) or 1250 mg and 9 for 16–18 years (IoM); [h] Sodium, 1300 mg for >50 years women; [i] Selenium, 45 µg for 16–19 years (FESNAD); [k] Thiamin and Riboflavin: 1.0 mg for 16–18 years; [l] Sodium, 1300 mg for 51–70 years and 1200 mg for >70 years (IoM).

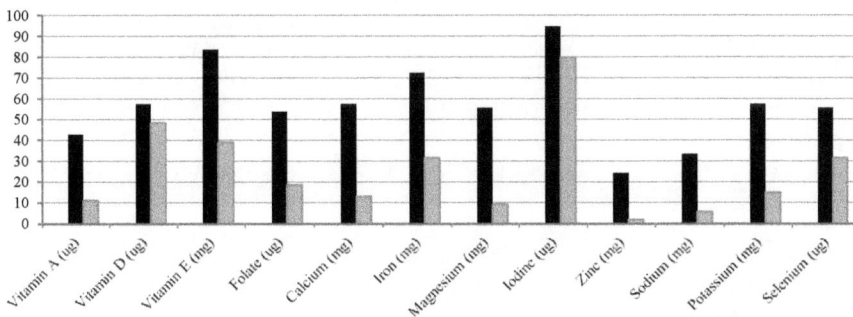

Figure 2. Percentage of celiac women who do not achieve dietary reference intake of the vitamins and minerals proposed by the Federation of Spanish Societies of Nutrition and Dietetics (FESNAD). ■ Do not fulfilled completely (100%) dietary reference intakes; ■ with a fulfillment of dietary reference intakes in the range of 99%–67%.

3.3. Food Consumption Frequency

Main food group consumption is summarized in Figure 3. The cereal consumption data indicated that only one out of ten celiac people ate the minimum of four recommended servings per day. Moreover, nearly half the celiac women (48%) consumed a very small amount of cereals (fewer than two servings) per day. Nevertheless, three day 24HR questionnaires showed that grains and cereal derivatives provided 23% of total energy intake and that these were the main source of CHO (37.9%). Cereal derivatives consumed usually took the form of naturally gluten-free grains and the incorporation of gluten free rendered cereals (GFP) into GFD was quite low. Specifically gluten-free products formed only 3% of total energy intake and contained only about 11 g of the 73 carbohydrate g provided by the cereal group.

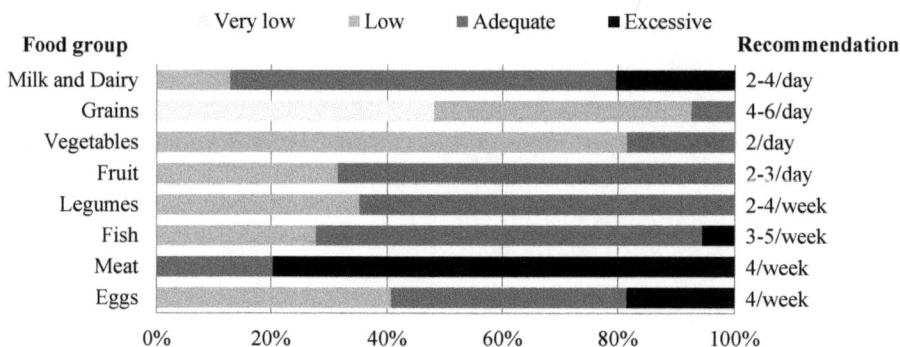

Figure 3. Compliance of food frequency consumption of celiac women by servings per day or week, according to Spanish Society of Community Nutrition (SENC).

One third of celiac women did not consume the minimum recommended two servings of fruit daily. In relation to the intake of vegetables, only 18.5% of celiacs consumed the daily minimum of two servings. Even weekly, the vast majority of participants, 70%, did not reach vegetable consumption recommendations (10 portions/week) [16].

As far as food of animal origin is concerned, 87% of celiac patients consumed two or more serving daily of milk or dairy products. Almost 40% of celiac patients reached the weekly recommended egg consumption by SENC. More than three quarters of participants had an excessive consumption of meat and meat products. Additionally, half this amount was fatty meat/red meat (pork, beef, lamb for instance). In the case of fish, its consumption was sufficient in two out of three adult celiacs and very few consumed it in excess. This food group (meat, fish and eggs) supplied 18% of total energy, and nearly 50% of total protein intake, whereas milk derivatives contributed 14% of total energy and 20% of total protein.

65% of celiac women usually included two or more portions of legumes and, on average, daily intake was about 20 g. Chickpeas, beans and lentils were the preferred pulses, making up 3% of the total daily energy intake.

With respect to other energy sources such as vegetable oils, sugar, chocolate, alcohol and/or pastries, most participants consumed them fairly correctly (data not shown). In general, this population chose olive oil as its fat source, a positive aspect that contributed to maintaining the high proportion of monounsaturated fatty acid in the diet.

3.4. Score for Adherence to Mediterranean Diet

The MDS showed that diet followed by celiac women was intermediate in quality, in terms of adherence to the Mediterranean pattern. The mean MDS for all studied participants was 4.6 ± 1.8.

4. Discussion

Dietary treatment of celiac disease involves certain dietary restrictions that can limit the nutritional status of celiac people and make the implementation of the recommendations for a balanced diet difficult. In a previous study carried out by our research group, females and males were collected in order to analyze their GFD and to carry out a nutritional comparison between gluten-free diets and diets containing equivalent products with gluten [14]. Surprisingly, women and men showed different patterns of eating habits. Following a GF diet in women resulted in a lower protein intake and in a higher fat intake when comparing the same diet with equivalent products containing gluten. However in men these differences were not observed. Taking these results into account, a more in-depth study should be carried out in order to analyze the nutritional status of celiac women following a GFD. Thus, in the present research, we evaluated this situation in 54 celiac women from the Basque Country (from Alava, Gipuzkoa, and Bizkaia regions in the north of Spain), in order to point out any differences between celiac women and women in the general population.

The anthropometric study conducted with celiac women indicated that only less than 6.5% were overweight and that there were no cases of obesity. In good accordance with these results, Bardella *et al.* found a lower BMI index in celiac people than in the general population [20]. Our results were also lower than those corresponding to Spanish women—control women overall [21]. There are several reasons that could justify this fact: (1) the celiac disease pathological situation could provoke a low bioavailability of nutrients as was reported by others in newly diagnosed celiacs [22]; (2) these patients were more concerned about their dietary habits than the general population and therefore there is a lower percentage or incidence of overweight and obesity.

With regard to the first issue, it is hard to believe that malabsorption related to celiac disease could be an explanation, considering that participants in our study had followed a long-term GFD (10.9 years). However, it is true that in the case of the adult celiac population complete normalization of duodenal lesions is rare [23], leading to additional nutrient deficiencies. One of the weaknesses of the present research is that no intestinal biopsy was performed prior to the study, therefore there was no possibility of ensuring the histological remission of celiac disease, which makes it difficult to discount if any of the celiacs studied might have more deficiencies or not. Nevertheless, the purpose of the study was to define whether GFD itself could provoke nutrient deficiencies or not, regardless of histological remission. Despite its limitations, the information extracted from the present research could answer why celiac patients in biopsy-proven remission and who adhered to a strict gluten-free diet for years were prone to the development of various vitamin deficiency states [24].

The second reason itself could also be considered as one possible limitation of this work, due to the fact that research study participants usually show more interest in the topic of nutrition. Taking into account that the present study was voluntary and was not done randomly, the self-selection bias was inevitable. However, it is noteworthy that our results were consistent with those obtained in a study conducted with an American celiac population. Zipser *et al.* [25] found a prevalence of overweight and obesity of 14% and 4% respectively in American Celiac population, percentages which were a long way from the prevalence of overweight and obesity in the United States. Other recent research carried out in Finland also showed that although the mean BMI is significantly increasing in Western countries and a similar trend is described for celiac patients, a more favourable BMI [26] is found in the latter population.

Another important aspect in assessing the nutritional status of celiac was the dietary intake evaluation. Nowadays there are no databases that include specific composition of GFP. Furthermore, gluten-free product labels do not indicate micronutrient (vitamin and mineral) content. As stated before, in the present study an estimation using homologous gluten-containing products was carried out. This strategy has also been used by other authors, publishing some results in good accordance to ours [27].

According to data obtained from the three day records, the macronutrient imbalance in the celiac population was quite predictable considering that it also exists in the general population. In fact, the national survey of dietary intake of Spain (ENIDE) showed that a similar percentage of energy intake comes from protein, and a slightly larger one from fats (42.2%) in the Spanish population—control women [17]. These similarities between GFD energy distribution and that of the general population have been reported in other studies conducted in Europe [28,29].

It is important to remark that the low consumption of CHO detected in celiac women by our study, was accentuated in general Spanish population—control women. Furthermore, it must be considered that the percentage contribution of carbohydrates to total energy has steadily decreased in recent years. This fact is due at least in part to reductions in cereal and grain intake. The ENIDE survey indicated that 39% of total energy from CHO came from cereal, and that this food group contributed 17% (394 kcal) of total energy, which is comparable to the data reached by our celiac group (37,9% of total carbohydrate and 23% of total energy; 417 kcal) [17]. Both sets of data, the ENIDE survey and our study, showed cereal and grain consumption below Spanish data registered in 2006 and in previous years [30].

With the outcomes obtained from celiac women *vs.* general women population—control women it could be hypothesized that the dietary habits of celiac women were healthier than those of the general population. Zuccotti *et al.* [29] compared dietary intake of celiac children to a control group, suggesting a similar conclusion. Food frequency questionnaires of that study revealed a difference in eating habits. Indeed, celiac children consumed more bread and rice, accompanied by greater gluten-free product consumption than controls [29]. Nevertheless, it is necessary to point out that celiac women from our research did not consume such a large amount of commercially available gluten-free foods as those children did.

As suggested by Subar *et al.* [31], in the general United States population grain foods contribute a large percentage to the adult daily intake of several nutrients including thiamine, riboflavin, niacin, folate, iron, and fiber [31]. Therefore, non-consumption of the recommended amount of whole grain products could have important implications for dietary intakes of B-vitamins, iron, and fiber.

With regard to our results, the intake of dietary fiber in a GFD was a long way from the recommended amount and it was even much lower than Spanish women's consumption—control women. This fact was not surprising, taking into account that GFD and GFP are often formulated and produced in low fiber forms to avoid the risk of gluten cross-contamination [32]. Unlike our results, in a recent study conducted with the German celiac population, dietary fiber intake was very similar to that of the general German population [33], which suggests that perhaps commercial gluten-free food contains added fiber in that country. However, another study conducted with Spanish families [34] indicated that the average fiber consumption is about 16.4 g/day, which would be a similar amount to that found in the celiac women population. Therefore it could be postulated that adult celiac women share nutritional goals with the rest of the Spanish population, at least for this component of the diet.

As micronutrients are concerned, if we compare the results of the celiac population with Spanish general population—control women, the data are similar to those reported in the ENIDE study [17]. Vitamin D and iodine represent the most important deficiencies in the celiac women of this study [14].

The compliance rate for recommended vitamin D consumption, both for the celiac as well as for the general population, is around 70%–80% of RDI. The lack of vitamin D can alter the normal metabolism of the bone, which can lead to rickets in children or osteoporosis or osteomalacia in adults [35]. In fact, numerous studies indicate that a suitable intake of calcium is crucial in the celiac group [36,37]. In this sense, the data showed that 57% of celiacs do not obey the FESNAD DRI for calcium [14]. A review of the topic suggested that up to 75% of celiac people exhibit low bone density and increased risk of fractures [38]. What is more, a study of persistent mucosal damage and the risk of fracture in celiac disease concluded that the association between persistent villous atrophy and hip fractures implies thinner subcutaneous tissue [39]. Taking into account that our result showed that 6% of participants were underweight and deficient in vitamin D intake, the risk of fractures in our cohort is more than probable.

Similarly, as in the Spanish general population—control women, there was a deficiency of iodine in the celiac participants (94% of them demonstrated iodine deficiency according to FESNAD's recommendations) [14]. In good accordance with the result obtained, remarkably low iodine intake was also found in Europe in 2010 for the general population [40]. Nevertheless, it is important to point out that celiac disease is accompanied by other pathologies related to thyroid function, where adequate iodine consumption is a limiting factor to avoid clinical consequences [41].

In the case of vitamin A, this micronutrient had a low rate of compliance in celiac women, even though the average intake was greater than in the Spanish general population—control women (ENIDE study) [17]. For the rest of the minerals and vitamins analyzed, recommended intakes were reached (Table 3) [14]. Although, riboflavin results show that the celiac population had doubled RDI [14], there is no evidence of adverse effects due to excessive intake of riboflavin, possibly due to a limited extent of absorption in the intestine and its rapid excretion in urine.

Vitamin 6, folate, and vitamin B12 deficiencies commonly lead to moderate elevations in total plasma homocysteine levels which, in turn, may increase the tendency to develop occlusive venous and arterial disease in both celiac people and the general population [42]. In our research, the recommendations for vitamin B6, folate, and vitamin B12 were amply fulfilled by celiac women. Taking into account that it has been demonstrated that most bread, pastas, and cold cereals are not fortified with folate for instance [43], the intake of this vitamin, like that of B12 and B6, must have been compensated by other sources.

The frequency consumption questionnaire conducted revealed the daily or weekly consumed rations of different food groups. Although macronutrient distribution of the diet was similar to the rest of the Spanish population [16], this questionnaire highlighted that the food source of these nutrients was different. CHO in the general population should come from cereals, fruits and pulses/legumes, respectively. As represented in Figure 3, celiac women consumed a very low amount of cereals, consequently in the case of celiac people the pulses and legumes group had greater importance as sources of CHO. Thus, if we compare the consumption of legumes of celiac people in our research with Spanish general population [30], it is possible to point out the great difference between groups (19.3 g/day *vs.* 11.9 g/day). The strategy followed by celiac people consists in focussing on avoiding gluten in the diet, promoting the consumption of legumes instead of cereals [44].

In relation to the intake of vegetables, although only 19% of celiac adults consume the daily minimum of two servings these data are in good accordance with the rest of the Spanish adult population—control women [17]. More than three quarters of participants reported excessive (more than three servings) consumption of meat and meat products per week. Additionally, rather than celiac people consuming one serving per week of fatty meat/red meat, the data obtained revealed that half of their meat consumption was pork, beef, or lamb. Nevertheless, the daily consumption of meat by celiac patients was lower than that of the general Spanish population (110 g/day *vs.* 179 g/day) [30].

The PREDIMED trial among others, has demonstrated that following a Mediterranean Diet can be considered a sustainable ideal model for cardiovascular disease prevention [45]. According to data published in the ENIDE study, celiac women demonstrated better adhesion to the Mediterranean diet than did the general Spanish women population—control women. The percentage of celiac women with low adherence to the Mediterranean dietary pattern (less than index 4) was 30%, while in the Spanish women population—control women this reached 62%. Consequently, celiac women showed higher percentages of intermediate (indexes 4–6) and high (>6) Mediterranean-Diet Score; 56 *vs.* 31 and 13 *vs.* 7 respectively. In good accordance with the results obtained in the present work, a recent study conducted with Spanish women—control women established a relationship between higher adhesion to the Mediterranean diet and decreased risk of overweight or obesity [46].

In summary, as far as our result is concerned there are marked differences between the body composition of adult celiac and non-celiac women. Furthermore it could be postulated that energy and macronutrient intake of celiac women follows trends similar to those found in Spanish women—control women as a whole, with an imbalanced distribution of macronutrients and an inadequate consumption of certain micronutrients and fiber (Table 4).

Table 4. Summary of Spanish societies recommendations' compliance concerning energy intake, obese and overweight percentage, nutrients, fiber and food consumption frequency by celiac women and Spanish women.

	Compliance/Suggestion	
	Celiac Women	Spanish Women—Control Women
Energy intake (kcal)		√
Obese and overweight (%)	√	×/↓
Macronutrient distribution		
Protein (%)		×/↓
Carbohydrate (%)		×/↑
Fat (%)		×/↓
Fiber (g)	×/↑↑	×/↑
Micronutrient intake		
Vitamin D (μg)		×/↑
Vitamin E (mg)		×/↑
Folate (μg)		×/↑
Calcium (mg)		×/↑
Iron (mg)		×/↑
Iodine (μg)		×/↑
Selenium (μg)		×/↑
Food consumption frequency		
Grains	×/↑	√/=
Legumes	√/=	×/↑
Vegetables		×/↑

Notes: ×, values do not achieve Spanish societies (FESNAD and SENC) recommendations; √ values do achieve Spanish societies (FESNAD and SENC) recommendations; ↑ it is suggested an intake increase; ↓ it is suggested an intake reduction; FESNAD, Federation of Spanish Societies of Nutrition and Dietetics; SENC, Spanish Society of Community Nutrition.

5. Conclusions

Even though specific nutritional education is not necessary for celiac people some specific consideration must be provided in order to improve eating habits and nutritional status among adult celiac women.

Acknowledgments: This research was supported by a grant from the University of the Basque Country, Vitoria-Gasteiz, Spain (UPV/EHU) (University-Society US12/10). We thank the collaboration of "Federación Española de Asociaciones de Celiacos (FACE), Madrid, Spain", specifically that of Mireia Apraiz, and the efforts of dieticians Beatriz Zulueta, Nerea Segura and Estibaliz Olabarri.

Author Contributions: Itziar Churruca and Edurne Simon conceived and designed the experiments; Arrate Lasa and Idoia Larretxi performed the experiments; Jonatan Miranda analyzed the data; María Á. Bustamante contributed materials/analysis tools; Itziar Churruca wrote the paper.

Conflicts of Interest: The authors declare no conflict of interest.

References

1. Ludvigsson, J.F.; Green, P.H. Clinical management of coeliac disease. *J. Int. Med.* **2011**, *269*, 560–571. [CrossRef] [PubMed]
2. Catassi, C.; Gatti, S.; Fasano, A. The new epidemiology of celiac disease. *J Pediatr. Gastroenterol. Nutr.* **2014**, *59*, S7–S9. [CrossRef] [PubMed]
3. Catassi, C.; Fabiani, E.; Iacono, G.; D'Agate, C.; Francavilla, R.; Biagi, F.; Volta, U.; Accomando, S.; Picarelli, A.; de Vitis, I.; *et al.* A prospective, double-blind, placebo-controlled trial to establish a safe gluten threshold for patients with celiac disease. *Am. J. Clin. Nutr.* **2007**, *85*, 160–166. [PubMed]
4. Rajpoot, P.; Makharia, G.K. Problems and challenges to adaptation of gluten free diet by Indian patients with celiac disease. *Nutrients* **2013**, *5*, 4869–4879. [CrossRef] [PubMed]

5. Gibert, A.; Kruizinga, A.G.; Neuhold, S.; Houben, G.F.; Canela, M.A.; Fasano, A.; Catassi, C. Might gluten traces in wheat substitutes pose a risk in patients with celiac disease? A population-based probabilistic approach to risk estimation. *Am. J. Clin. Nutr.* **2013**, *97*, 109–116. [CrossRef] [PubMed]

6. American-Dietetic-Association. Celiac disease. In *Evidence Based Nutrition Practice Guideline*; American-Dietetic-Association: Chicago, IL, USA, 2009.

7. Saturni, L.; Ferretti, G.; Bacchetti, T. The gluten-free diet: Safety and nutritional quality. *Nutrients* **2010**, *2*, 16–34. [CrossRef] [PubMed]

8. Pietzak, M.M. Follow-up of patients with celiac disease: Achieving compliance with treatment. *Gastroenterology* **2005**, *128*, S135–S141. [CrossRef] [PubMed]

9. Valdimarsson, T.; Toss, G.; Löfman, O.; Ström, M. Three years' follow-up of bone density in adult coeliac disease: Significance of secondary hyperparathyroidism. *Scand. J. Gastroenterol.* **2000**, *35*, 274–280. [CrossRef] [PubMed]

10. World Health Organization (WHO). Obesity: Preventing and managing the global epidemic. In *Report of a WHO Consultation on Obesity*; World Health Organization: Geneva, Switzerland, 1997; p. 276.

11. Gallagher, D.; Heymsfield, S.B.; Heo, M.; Jebb, S.A.; Murgatroyd, P.R.; Sakamoto, Y. Healthy percentage body fat ranges: An approach for developing guidelines based on body mass index. *Am. J. Clin. Nutr.* **2000**, *72*, 694–701. [PubMed]

12. Miranda, J.; Lasa, A.; Bustamante, M.A.; Churruca, I.; Simon, E. Nutritional differences between a gluten-free diet and a diet containing equivalent products with gluten. *Plant. Foods. Hum. Nutr.* **2014**, *69*, 182–187. [CrossRef] [PubMed]

13. Russolillo, G.; Marques, I. *Food Portion Sizes Album*; Imagen Comunicación Multimedia: Madrid, Spain, 2008; p. 186.

14. Federation of Spanish Societies of Nutrition and Dietetics (FESNAD). Dietary reference intakes (DRI) for spanish population, 2010. *Act Diet.* **2010**, *14*, 196–197.

15. Ross, C.; Taylor, C.; Yaktine, A.; del Valle, H. *Dietary Reference Intakes for Calcium and Vitamin D*; The National Academies Press: Washington, DC, USA, 2011; p. 1132.

16. Aranceta, J.; Serra-Majem, L. Dietary guidelines for the Spanish population. *Public. Health. Nutr.* **2001**, *4*, 1403–1408. [CrossRef] [PubMed]

17. Nutritional Assessment Studies: Spanish Population Dietary Intakes. National Health Survey. ENIDE. Available online: http://aesan.msssi.gob.es/AESAN/web/evaluacion_riesgos/seccion/estudios_evaluacion_nutricional.shtml (accessed on 25 May 2015).

18. Trichopoulou, A.; Costacou, T.; Bamia, C.; Trichopoulos, D. Adherence to a Mediterranean diet and survival in a Greek population. *N. Engl. J. Med.* **2003**, *348*, 2599–2608. [CrossRef] [PubMed]

19. Serra-Majem, L.; Aranceta, J. Nutritional objectives for the Spanish population: Consensus from the Spanish Society of Community Nutrition. *Public Health Nutr.* **2001**, *4*, 1409–1413. [CrossRef] [PubMed]

20. Bardella, M.T.; Fredella, C.; Prampolini, L.; Molteni, N.; Giunta, A.M.; Bianchi, P.A. Body composition and dietary intakes in adult celiac disease patients consuming a strict gluten-free diet. *Am. J. Clin. Nutr.* **2000**, *72*, 937–939. [PubMed]

21. Pedrera-Zamorano, J.D.; Roncero-Martin, R.; Lavado-Garcia, J.M.; Calderon-Garcia, J.F.; Rey-Sanchez, P.; Vera, V.; Martinez, M.; Moran, J.M. Segmental fat-free and fat mass measurements by bioelectrical impedance analysis in 2224 healthy Spanish women aged 18–85 years. *Am. J. Hum. Biol.* **2014**. [CrossRef]

22. Wierdsma, N.J.; van Bokhorst-de van der Schueren, M.A.; Berkenpas, M.; Mulder, C.J.; van Bodegraven, A.A. Vitamin and mineral deficiencies are highly prevalent in newly diagnosed celiac disease patients. *Nutrients* **2013**, *5*, 3975–3992. [CrossRef] [PubMed]

23. Lanzini, A.; Lanzarotto, F.; Villanacci, V.; Mora, A.; Bertolazzi, S.; Turini, D.; Carella, G.; Malagoli, A.; Ferrante, G.; Cesana, B.M.; *et al.* Complete recovery of intestinal mucosa occurs very rarely in adult coeliac patients despite adherence to gluten-free diet. *Aliment. Pharmacol. Ther.* **2009**, *29*, 1299–1308. [CrossRef] [PubMed]

24. Hallert, C.; Grant, C.; Grehn, S.; Grännö, C.; Hultén, S.; Midhagen, G.; Ström, M.; Svensson, H.; Valdimarsson, T. Evidence of poor vitamin status in coeliac patients on a gluten-free diet for 10 years. *Aliment. Pharmacol. Ther.* **2002**, *16*, 1333–1339. [CrossRef] [PubMed]

25. Zipser, R.D.; Patel, S.; Yahya, K.Z.; Baisch, D.W.; Monarch, E. Presentations of adult celiac disease in a nationwide patient support group. *Dig. Dis. Sci.* **2003**, *48*, 761–764. [CrossRef] [PubMed]

26. Ukkola, A.; Mäki, M.; Kurppa, K.; Collin, P.; Huhtala, H.; Kekkonen, L.; Kaukinen, K. Changes in body mass index on a gluten-free diet in coeliac disease: A nationwide study. *Eur. J. Int. Med.* **2012**, *23*, 384–388. [CrossRef] [PubMed]

27. Pellegrini, N.; Agostoni, C. Nutritional aspects of gluten-free products. *J. Sci Food. Agric.* **2015**, in press.

28. Martin, J.; Geisel, T.; Maresch, C.; Krieger, K.; Stein, J. Inadequate nutrient intake in patients with celiac disease: Results from a German dietary survey. *Digestion* **2013**, *87*, 240–246. [CrossRef] [PubMed]

29. Zuccotti, G.; Fabiano, V.; Dilillo, D.; Picca, M.; Cravidi, C.; Brambilla, P. Intakes of nutrients in Italian children with celiac disease and the role of commercially available gluten-free products. *J. Hum. Nutr. Diet.* **2013**, *26*, 436–444. [CrossRef] [PubMed]

30. Varela-Moreiras, G.; Avila, J.M.; Cuadrado, C.; del Pozo, S.; Ruiz, E.; Moreiras, O. Evaluation of food consumption and dietary patterns in Spain by the Food Consumption Survey: Updated information. *Eur. J. Clin. Nutr.* **2010**, *64*, S37–S43. [CrossRef] [PubMed]

31. Subar, A.F.; Krebs-Smith, S.M.; Cook, A.; Kahle, L.L. Dietary sources of nutrients among US adults, 1989 to 1991. *J. Am. Diet. Assoc.* **1998**, *98*, 537–547. [CrossRef]

32. Gallagher, E.; Gormley, T.R.; Arendt, E.K. Recent advances in the formulation of gluten-free cereal-based products. *Trends Food. Sci. Technol.* **2004**, *15*, 143–152. [CrossRef]

33. Martin, U.; Mercer, S.W. A comparison of general practitioners prescribing of gluten-free foods for the treatment of coeliac disease with national prescribing guidelines. *J. Hum. Nutr. Diet.* **2014**, *27*, 96–104. [CrossRef] [PubMed]

34. Ruiz-Roso Calvo de Mora, B.; Perez-Olleros Conde, L. Preliminary results on dietary fibre intake in Spain and health benefits associated to soluble fiber intake. *Res. Esp Nutr. Comunitaria* **2010**, *16*, 147–153. [CrossRef]

35. Yoshida, T.; Stern, P.H. How vitamin D works on bone. *Endocrinol. Metab. Clin. North. Am.* **2012**, *41*, 557–569. [CrossRef] [PubMed]

36. Cellier, C.; Flobert, C.; Cormier, C.; Roux, C.; Schmitz, J. Severe osteopenia in symptom-free adults with a childhood diagnosis of coeliac disease. *Lancet* **2000**. [CrossRef]

37. Kalayci, A.G.; Kansu, A.; Girgin, N.; Kucuk, O.; Aras, G. Bone mineral density and importance of a gluten-free diet in patients with celiac disease in childhood. *Pediatrics* **2001**, *108*, E89. [CrossRef] [PubMed]

38. Lucendo, A.J.; García-Manzanares, A. Bone mineral density in adult coeliac disease: An updated review. *Rev. Esp. Enferm. Dig.* **2013**, *105*, 154–162. [CrossRef] [PubMed]

39. Lebwohl, B.; Michaëlsson, K.; Green, P.H.; Ludvigsson, J.F. Persistent mucosal damage and risk of fracture in celiac disease. *J. Clin. Endocrinol. Metab.* **2014**, *99*, 609–616. [CrossRef] [PubMed]

40. Zimmermann, M.B.; Andersson, M. Prevalence of iodine deficiency in Europe in 2010. *Ann. Endocrinol.* **2011**, *72*, 164–166. [CrossRef] [PubMed]

41. Kalyoncu, D.; Urganci, N. Antithyroid antibodies and thyroid function in pediatric patients with celiac disease. *Int. J. Endocrinol.* **2015**. [CrossRef] [PubMed]

42. Hadithi, M.; Mulder, C.J.; Stam, F.; Azizi, J.; Crusius, J.B.; Peña, A.S.; Stehouwer, C.D.; Smulders, Y.M. Effect of B vitamin supplementation on plasma homocysteine levels in celiac disease. *World. J. Gastroenterol.* **2009**, *15*, 955–960. [CrossRef] [PubMed]

43. Thompson, T. Folate, iron, and dietary fiber contents of the gluten-free diet. *J. Am. Diet. Assoc.* **2000**, *100*, 1389–1396. [CrossRef]

44. Mlynekov, Z.; Chrenkov, Mr.; Formelov, Z. Cereals and Legumes in Nutrition of People with Celiac Disease. *Int. J. Celiac Dis.* **2014**, *2*, 105–109.

45. Martínez-González, M.A.; Salas-Salvadó, J.; Estruch, R.; Corella, D.; Fitó, M.; Ros, E. Benefits of the Mediterranean Diet: Insights from the PREDIMED Study. *Prog. Cardiovasc. Dis.* **2015**, *58*, 50–60. [CrossRef] [PubMed]

46. Sayón-Orea, C.; Santiago, S.; Cuervo, M.; Martínez-González, M.A.; Garcia, A.; Martínez, J.A. Adherence to Mediterranean dietary pattern and menopausal symptoms in relation to overweight/obesity in Spanish perimenopausal and postmenopausal women. *Menopause* **2014**, *22*, 750–757. [CrossRef] [PubMed]

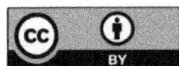

Section 4:
Experts' Guidelines

![nutrients logo] *nutrients*

MDPI

Article

Diagnosis of Non-Celiac Gluten Sensitivity (NCGS): The Salerno Experts' Criteria

Carlo Catassi [1,*], Luca Elli [2], Bruno Bonaz [3], Gerd Bouma [4], Antonio Carroccio [5], Gemma Castillejo [6], Christophe Cellier [7], Fernanda Cristofori [8], Laura de Magistris [9], Jernej Dolinsek [10], Walburga Dieterich [11], Ruggiero Francavilla [8], Marios Hadjivassiliou [12], Wolfgang Holtmeier [13], Ute Körner [14], Dan A. Leffler [15], Knut E. A. Lundin [16], Giuseppe Mazzarella [17], Chris J. Mulder [4], Nicoletta Pellegrini [18], Kamran Rostami [19], David Sanders [20], Gry Irene Skodje [21], Detlef Schuppan [22], Reiner Ullrich [23], Umberto Volta [24], Marianne Williams [25], Victor F. Zevallos [22], Yurdagül Zopf [11] and Alessio Fasano [26]

1   Department of Pediatrics, Università Politecnica delle Marche, 60123 Ancona, Italy
2   Centre for the Prevention and Diagnosis of Celiac Disease/Gastroenterology and Endoscopy Unit, Fondazione IRCCS Cà Granda-Ospedale Maggiore Policlinico, Milan 20122, Italy; lucelli@yahoo.com
3   Clinique Universitaire d'Hépato-Gastroenterologie, CHU de Grenoble, 38043 Grenoble Cedex 09, France; BBonaz@chu-grenoble.fr
4   Department of Gastroenterology, VU University Medical Center, Amsterdam, The Netherlands; g.bouma@vumc.nl (G.B.); cjmulder@vumc.nl (C.J.M.)
5   Department of Internal Medicine, "Giovanni Paolo II" Hospital, Sciacca (AG) and University of Palermo, Sciacca 92019, Italy; acarroccio@hotmail.com
6   Paediatric Gastroenterology Unit, Hospital Sant Joan de Reus, 43201 Reus, Spain; gcastillejo@grupsagessa.com
7   Service d'Hépato-gastro-entérologie et Endoscopie Digestive, Hôpital Européen Georges Pompidou, 75015 Paris, France; christophe.cellier@egp.aphp.fr
8   Interdisciplinary Department of Medicine, University of Bari, Bari 70124, Italy; fernandacristofori@gmail.com (F.C.); rfrancavilla@gmail.com (R.F.)
9   Department of Internal and Experimental Medicine Magrassi-Lanzara, Second University of Naples, 80131 Naples, Italy; laura.demagistris@unina2.it
10 Gastroenterology Unit, Department of Pediatrics, University Medical Centre Maribor, Maribor 2000, Slovenia; jernej.dolinsek@ukc-mb.si
11 Medical Clinic 1, University of Erlangen, 91054 Erlangen, Germany; walburga.dieterich@uk-erlangen.de (W.D.); yurdaguel.zopf@uk-erlangen.de (Y.Z.)
12 Academic Department of Neurosciences and University of Sheffield, Royal Hallamshire Hospital, Sheffield S10 2JF, UK; marios.hadjivassiliou@sth.nhs.uk
13 Division of Gastroenterology and Internal Medicine, Hospital Porz am Rhein, Köln 51149, Germany; w.holtmeier@khporz.de
14 Practice of Nutrition Therapy Allergology and Gastroenterology, Köln 50935, Germany; ute.koerner@t-online.de
15 Division of Gastroenterology, Beth Israel Deaconess Medical Center, Boston, MA 02215, USA; dleffler@bidmc.harvard.edu
16 Seksjon for Gastromedisin, Avdeling for Transplantasjonsmedisin, OUS Rikshospitalet Senter for Immunregulering, Oslo University, 0424 Oslo, Norway; knut.lundin@medisin.uio.no
17 Institute of Food Sciences-CNR, Lab. Immuno-Morphology, 83100 Avellino, Italy; gmazzarella@isa.cnr.it
18 Department of Food Science, University of Parma, IT-43124 Parma, Italy; nicoletta.pellegrini@unipr.it
19 Department of Gastroenterology, Alexandra Hospital, Redditch B98 7UB, UK; krostami@hotmail.com
20 Department of Gastroenterology and Hepatology, Royal Hallamshire Hospital and University of Sheffield Medical School, Sheffield S10 2JF, UK; david.sanders@sth.nhs.uk
21 Division of Clinical Nutrition, Oslo University Hospital, 0424 Oslo, Norway, g.i.skodje@medisin.uio.no
22 University Medical Center of the Johannes Gutenberg University, 55131 Mainz, Germany; detlef.schuppan@unimedizin-mainz.de (D.S.); zevallos@uni-mainz.de (V.F.Z.)
23 Charité—Universitätsmedizin Berlin, Medizinische Klinik für Gastroenterologie, Infektiologie und Rheumatologie, 12203 Berlin, Germany; reiner.ullrich@charite.de
24 Department of Medical and Surgical Sciences University of Bologna, St. Orsola-Malpighi Hospital via Massarenti 9, 40138 Bologna, Italy; umberto.volta@aosp.bo.it

25   Somerset Partnership NHS Foundation Trust, Bridgwater TA6 4RN, UK; marianne@wisediet.co.uk
26   Pediatric Gastroenterology and Nutrition, Mass General Hospital for Children, Boston, MA 02114, USA;
     afasano@mgh.harvard.edu
*   Correspondence: c.catassi@univpm.it; Tel.: +39-071-596-2364; Fax: +39-071-36281

Received: 23 April 2015; Accepted: 15 June 2015; Published: 18 June 2015

Abstract: Non-Celiac Gluten Sensitivity (NCGS) is a syndrome characterized by intestinal and extra-intestinal symptoms related to the ingestion of gluten-containing food, in subjects that are not affected by either celiac disease or wheat allergy. Given the lack of a NCGS biomarker, there is the need for standardizing the procedure leading to the diagnosis confirmation. In this paper we report experts' recommendations on how the diagnostic protocol should be performed for the confirmation of NCGS. A full diagnostic procedure should assess the clinical response to the gluten-free diet (GFD) and measure the effect of a gluten challenge after a period of treatment with the GFD. The clinical evaluation is performed using a self-administered instrument incorporating a modified version of the Gastrointestinal Symptom Rating Scale. The patient identifies one to three main symptoms that are quantitatively assessed using a Numerical Rating Scale with a score ranging from 1 to 10. The double-blind placebo-controlled gluten challenge (8 g/day) includes a one-week challenge followed by a one-week washout of strict GFD and by the crossover to the second one-week challenge. The vehicle should contain cooked, homogeneously distributed gluten. At least a variation of 30% of one to three main symptoms between the gluten and the placebo challenge should be detected to discriminate a positive from a negative result. The guidelines provided in this paper will help the clinician to reach a firm and positive diagnosis of NCGS and facilitate the comparisons of different studies, if adopted internationally.

Keywords: non-celiac gluten sensitivity; diagnosis; double-blind placebo-controlled challenge; gastrointestinal symptom rating scale; irritable bowel syndrome

1. Introduction

Non-Celiac Gluten Sensitivity (NCGS) is a syndrome characterized by intestinal and extra-intestinal symptoms related to the ingestion of gluten-containing food, in subjects that are not affected by either celiac disease (CD) or wheat allergy (WA) [1,2]. The terminology "NCGS" is still a matter of debate. Although NCGS is triggered by gluten-containing cereals, the offending dietary protein has not been identified yet, and could include component/s that are different from gluten itself, e.g., the cereal protein amylase-trypsin inhibitors (ATIs) [3]. Then the terminology "NCGS" could be changed into "Non Celiac Wheat Sensitivity" (NCWS) in the near future, although this would exclude other relevant cereals like barley and rye. The prevalence of NCGS is not clearly defined yet. Indirect evidence suggests that NCGS is more common than CD [4], the latter affecting around 1% of the general population [5]. Treatment of NCGS is based on the celiac-type gluten-free diet (GFD) although it is unknown if long-term, strict avoidance of all gluten-related products is necessary. Since NCGS may be transient, gluten tolerance needs to be re-assessed in patients with NCGS [6].

Clinical presentation of NCGS might be multi-systemic and there have been a range of signs and symptoms reported in association with this condition (Table 1) [7]. The latency between gluten ingestion and the appearance of symptoms is usually short, within hours or days. Common features of NCGS are symptoms usually diagnosed under the umbrella of the irritable bowel syndrome (IBS), e.g., bloating, abdominal pain and irregular bowel movements [4]. Recent clinical studies have opened new insight into the etiology of these symptoms and the current literature suggests that many of the patients previously known under IBS are in fact intolerant to something they eat. Most common food reactions have been reported to gluten, lactose, milk protein and Fermentable Oligo, Di, and Monosaccharides And Polyols (FODMAPs) [8,9]. NCGS patients, however, often report symptoms outside of the intestinal tract, e.g., headache and/or foggy mind [4], which cannot be accounted for by lactose, and/or FODMAPs intolerance.

Table 1. The clinical manifestations of Non-Celiac Gluten Sensitivity (NCGS).

Frequency	Intestinal	Extra-Intestinal
Very Common	Bloating	Lack of wellbeing
	Abdominal pain	Tiredness
Common	Diarrhea	Headache
	Epigastric pain	Anxiety
	Nausea	Foggy mind
	Aerophagia	Numbness
	GER	Joint/muscle pain
	Aphthous stomatitis	Skin rash/dermatitis
	Alternating bowel habits	
	Constipation	
Undetermined	Hematochezia	Weight loss
	Anal fissures	Anemia
		Loss of balance
		Depression
		Rhinitis/asthma
		Weight increase
		Interstitial cystitis
		Ingrown hairs
		Oligo or polymenorrhea
		Sensory symptoms
		Disturbed sleep pattern
		Hallucinations
		Mood swings
		Autism
		Schizophrenia

In recent years, several studies explored the relationship between the ingestion of gluten-containing food and the appearance of neurological and psychiatric disorders/symptoms like ataxia, peripheral neuropathy, schizophrenia, autism, depression, anxiety, and hallucinations [10–14]. One of the hypothesized links between the gut and the brain (*i.e.*, the brain-gut axis) postulates the existence of an increased intestinal permeability, also referred to as the "leaky gut syndrome" [15]. This in turn could allow gluten peptides (or other wheat-derived proteins) to cross the gut barrier, enter the bloodstream, and cross the blood-brain barrier, either causing neuro-inflammation or affecting the endogenous opiate system and neurotransmission within the nervous system. Food-induced modifications could also target the brain through the microbiota-brain-gut axis where the vagus is also a key element [16]. It should however be stressed that the possible relationship between NCGS and certain neuro-psychiatric disorders such as autism and schizophrenia is still far from clear. Furthermore, the cause/effect relationship between gluten ingestion and neuropsychiatric disorders, in terms of time latency, may be particularly difficult to ascertain.

NCGS should not be an exclusion diagnosis only. There is an increasing need for standardizing the procedure leading to the confirmation of suspected NCGS. Ideally we should have a clear diagnosis before starting treatment, however such certainty is not always possible. In clinical medicine this uncertainty can be resolved by using the treatment as the test that confirms the diagnosis. For example, if we are unsure if a patient's airway obstruction has a reversible element, a trial of steroids can test this: a sufficient response is then considered evidence of reversibility [17]. Likewise the strategy of "test of treatment" with the GFD can be used to diagnose NCGS.

On 6–7 October 2014, the 3rd International Expert Meeting on Gluten Related Disorders was held in Salerno, Italy, to reach a consensus on how the diagnosis of NCGS should be confirmed. It was acknowledged that in the absence of sensitive and specific biomarkers, a close and standardized monitoring of the patient during elimination and re-introduction of gluten is the most specific diagnostic approach and hence could be used as the diagnostic hallmark of NCGS. In this paper we report the experts' agreement and recommendations on how the diagnostic protocol should be performed for the confirmation of NCGS.

2. NCGS Diagnostic Protocol

The diagnosis of NCGS should be considered in patients with persistent intestinal and/or extra-intestinal complaints showing a normal result of the CD and WA serological markers on a gluten-containing diet, usually reporting worsening of symptoms after eating gluten-rich food. The aim of the confirmation of the diagnosis of NCGS should be twofold: (1) assessing the clinical response to the GFD; (2) measuring the effect of reintroducing gluten after a period of treatment with the GFD. It follows that a full diagnostic evaluation, including Step 1 and 2 (see below), can only be started in the patient who is on a normal, gluten-containing diet. Unfortunately many of these patients are already on the GFD when first seen at the specialty clinic. A simplified/shortened diagnostic procedure, including only Step 2, may be adopted in these patients.

In both Step 1 and Step 2, the clinical evaluation is performed using a self-administered instrument incorporating a modified version of the Gastrointestinal Symptom Rating Scale (GSRS). The GSRS is a disease-specific instrument, based on reviews of gastrointestinal symptoms and clinical experience, which has been widely used to evaluate common symptoms of gastrointestinal disorders [18]. The instrument presented here includes also items evaluating the extra-intestinal NCGS manifestations. Further items can be included under the box "other" in patients presenting with different symptoms. The patient identifies one to three main symptoms that will be quantitatively assessed using a Numerical Rating Scale (NRS) with a score ranging from 1 (mild) to 10 (severe) (Table 2 and Figure 1).

2.1. Step 1: Definition of a Patient Responsive to the GFD (Patient on a Gluten-Containing Diet)

Patients suspected of suffering from a gluten-related disorder should preliminarily undergo a full clinical and laboratory evaluation to exclude CD and WA while still on a gluten-containing diet, according to a previously outlined diagnostic protocol [19].

The following steps establish responsiveness to the GFD:

1. At baseline the patient has to be on a normal gluten containing diet for at least six weeks. The patient is assessed by the Table 2 diagnostic questionnaire at week-2, -1 and 0 to establish baseline symptoms;
2. At time 0 the GFD is started after detailed explanation (preferably by a dietitian);
3. Timeline: at least six weeks of verified GFD. Although the amelioration of symptoms is expected shortly after starting the GFD, a prolonged observation is needed to properly investigate the causal relationship, particularly for fluctuating symptoms (e.g., headache);
4. Data recording: weekly completion of the Table 2 questionnaire from week 0 to 6. The patient will identify one to three main symptoms. The response parameters are those with an initial score of at least 3 on the numerical rating scale (NRS).

The response is assessed for each parameter separately. A symptomatic response is a decrease of at least 30% of the baseline score. Responders are defined as patients who fulfill the response criteria (>30% reduction of one to three main symptoms or at least 1 symptom with no worsening of others) for at least 50% of the observation time (*i.e.*, at least three of six weekly evaluations).

The diagnosis of NCGS is excluded in subjects failing to show symptomatic improvement after six weeks of GFD. GFD-unresponsive patients should be investigated for other possible causes of IBS-like symptoms, e.g., intolerance to FODMAPs or small bowel bacterial overgrowth.

Table 2. Questionnaire used for Step 1 evaluation (the same items are evaluated during Step 2).

Intestinal Symptoms	Baseline	1 Week	2 Week	3 Week	4 Week	5 Week	6 Week
Abdominal pain or discomfort							
Heartburn							
Acid regurgitation							
Bloating							
Nausea and vomiting							
Borborygmus							
Abdominal distension							
Eructation							
Increased flatus							
Decreased passage of stools							
Increased passage of stools							
Loose stools							
Hard stools							
Urgent need for defecation							
Feeling of incomplete evacuation							
Extra-intestinal symptoms							
Dermatitis							
Headache							
Foggy mind							
Fatigue							
Numbness of the limbs							
Joint/muscle pains							
Fainting							
Oral/tongue lesions							
Other (specify)							

How severe was your symptom in the last week?

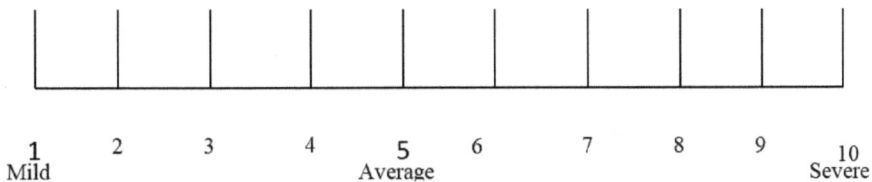

| 1 Mild | 2 | 3 | 4 | 5 Average | 6 | 7 | 8 | 9 | 10 Severe |

Figure 1. The numerical rating scale (NRS) used for rating the intensity of relevant items.

2.2. Step 2: the Gluten Challenge (Patient on the GFD)

Step 2 is required to confirm the diagnosis of NCGS in patients responding to treatment with the GFD. A Double-Blind Placebo-Controlled Challenge with crossover presents a high level of evidence for diagnosing NCGS. Before starting the gluten challenge, the baseline diet needs to be strictly gluten-free to the level of a celiac diet for at least four weeks, *i.e.*, no cross contamination, no gluten traces in the diet. The patient needs to be referred to a dietitian for assessment of the degree of the GFD. Two different types of challenge can be performed depending on the setting: (a) in clinical practice a single blinded procedure could be sufficient; (b) for research purposes, a double blind challenge remains the first choice. Provided there is marked improvement in symptoms with the GFD, the blinded challenges should be undertaken with care. For example, the gluten challenges may need to be repeated to offset the strong *nocebo* effect often seen in these patients.

As far as the daily dose of gluten to be used for the challenge, we suggest an amount of 8 grams, a dose that is both close to the average daily intake of gluten in Western countries (10–15 g) [20] and easy to mix with the vehicle. This dose can be modulated in the research setting. As far as the gluten "vehicle", gelatin capsules are discouraged. The best-suited vehicle is yet to be developed, for instance it could take form of a muesli bar, bread or muffin, possibly different in children and adults. The vehicle should contain cooked, homogeneously distributed gluten, and should be analyzed in order to know exactly the content of the pro-inflammatory factor ATIs. The gluten preparations should be prepared/tested for ATI bioactivity to contain at least 0.3 g of ATIs/8 g of gluten or gluten should be used with defined ATI content. The vehicle should be FODMAPs free.

The placebo vehicle must be completely gluten-free. Gluten and placebo preparations must be undistinguishable in look, texture and taste, and balanced in fibers, carbohydrate, fat and possibly protein content.

The gluten challenge includes a one-week challenge followed by a one-week washout of strict GFD and by the crossover to the second one-week challenge. The duration of the challenge period may occasionally be longer than a week in patients showing fluctuating symptoms, such as headache or neuro-behavioral problems. A questionnaire with the items shown in Table 2 is self-administered and filled in at baseline, and daily during the first seven-day challenge (or less if symptoms prevent completion of seven days), the washout period, and the second seven-day challenge (or less if symptoms prevent completion of seven days). During the challenge, the patient will identify and report one to three main symptoms, without necessarily filling in the full questionnaire. At least a variation of 30% between the gluten and the placebo challenge should be detected to discriminate a positive from a negative result. The threshold of 30% increment in symptoms is somewhat arbitrary and needs scientific validation. Patients showing a negative gluten challenge should be investigated for other possible causes of IBS-like symptoms, e.g., intolerance to FODMAPs or small bowel bacterial overgrowth.

A detailed flow diagram of the diagnostic process is shown in Figure 2.

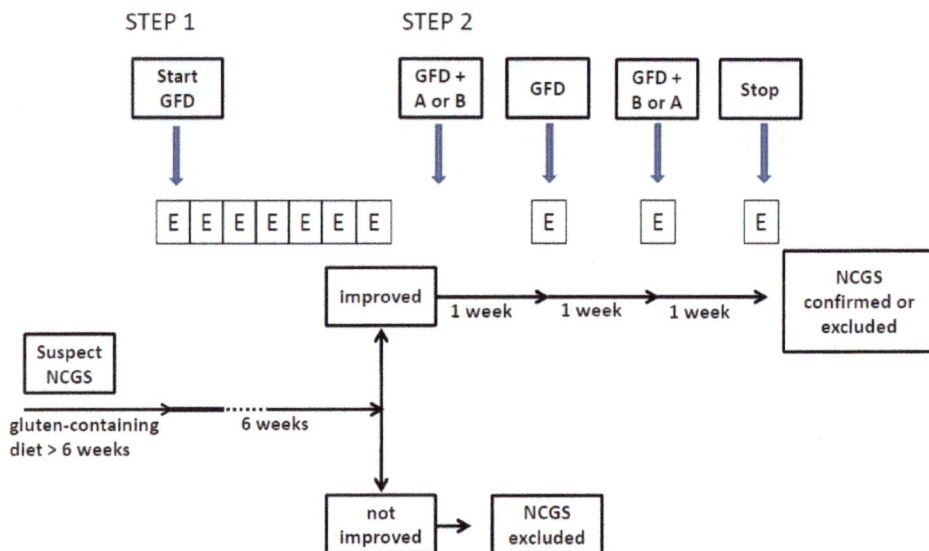

Figure 2. The flow diagram of the NCGS diagnostic process. GFD = gluten-free diet; A = product A (gluten or placebo); B = product B (placebo or gluten); E = evaluation (questionnaire). The evaluation is performed weekly during Step 1 and daily during Step 2.

2.3. Monitoring the Gluten Elimination/Reintroduction Effects by Biomarkers

Ideally the clinical evaluation performed during gluten elimination/reintroduction should include serially repeated specific laboratory tests.

Although the most specific CD serological markers, such as IgA class anti-transglutaminase and anti-endomysial antibodies, are negative in NCGS patients by definition, IgG class antibodies directed against native gliadin (AGA) are found more frequently in these cases (about 50%) than in the general population, when eating a gluten-containing diet. Therefore, the finding of isolated IgG-AGA positivity may be a clue to the diagnosis of NCGS, particularly in subjects with extra-intestinal manifestations. When initially positive, IgG-AGA normalize more quickly in NCGS than CD patients after starting treatment with the GFD [21]. However, it is still unclear whether monitoring the levels of IgG-AGA may be helpful for diagnostic purposes during the rather short period of the gluten elimination/reintroduction challenge.

The hypothesis of a "leaky gut" as a cause of neuropsychiatric disorders found indirect evidence from a study performed by the lactulose/mannitol (L/M) test, a simple clinical investigation exploring the usually divergent trans- and para-cellular permeability of the sugar probes. As a group, autistic children on a regular diet tended to show higher values of the L/M intestinal permeability test when compared with autistic children on a GFD [15]. However, in a subsequent study, a four-week treatment with the GFD did not determine significant changes of the L/M test in a small group of children with autistic spectrum disorder [22]. No L/M test modification has been observed in adult patients affected with typical intestinal manifestations of NCGS [23]. For these reasons, the L/M test cannot be recommended for monitoring the gluten challenge. Recently, Hollon *et al.* investigated the intestinal permeability in human duodenal biopsies mounted in microsnapwells and luminally incubated with either gliadin or media alone. Changes in transepithelial electrical resistance (as an index of intestinal permeability) were monitored over 120 min. Following gliadin exposure, both patients with NCGS and those with active CD demonstrated a greater increase in intestinal permeability than celiacs in disease remission [24]. The clinical significance of these findings remains to be elucidated.

The research on biological marker/s of NCGS is currently very active. Preliminary data observed in intestinal biopsies of NCGS patients showed an increase of intraepithelial lymphocytes (Marsh I) as well as the presence of markers associated with innate, rather than adaptive, immunity [2,23]. Recently, in an intestinal biopsy-based study, NCGS patients showed increased mucosal IFN-γ mRNA after a three-day gluten challenge [25]. Taken together these results suggest the presence of a mucosal immune activation in patients with NCGS. Therefore, the precise mechanisms underlying the induction of the immune response and the identification of reliable biomarkers for the diagnosis of NCGS are relevant issues that should be resolved. A search on www.clinicaltrials.gov performed on 2 January 2015 identified seven studies currently in progress to evaluate serological and mucosal indexes that could eventually find an application for diagnosing NCGS in clinical practice.

3. Conclusions and Future Perspectives

NCGS is a recently "re-discovered" clinical entity distinct from CD for which we have very little certainty and many knowledge "black holes". NCGS was first described in the early 1980s [26], but over the past decade the number of patients diagnosed with NCGS and publications on this topic have increased greatly. However, it is still not clear how to diagnose and manage this condition, and the pathophysiological mechanisms are unclear. Therefore, in terms of knowledge, we are with NCGS now where we were with CD 40 years ago. Since we still do not have validated biomarker(s) for the diagnosis of NCGS, the diagnostic protocol remains cumbersome and not apt for large epidemiological studies aimed at establishing the prevalence of this condition. However specific diagnostic criteria for NCGS are necessary for optimizing clinical care, avoiding self-diagnosis and advancing the science of NCGS. The guidelines provided in this paper will (a) help the clinician to reach a firm and positive diagnosis of NCGS and (b) facilitate the comparisons of different studies, if adopted

Nutrients **2015**, *7*, 4966–4977

internationally. A more practical approach will only be possible with the development of biomarkers or other clinical predictors.

The identification and validation of biomarker(s) will be instrumental to gain insights in NCGS pathogenesis, to establish the trigger(s) of this condition, and ultimately to establish the magnitude of this clinical condition. We will not be able to have a full understanding of NCGS until better diagnostic tools will become available and we have more information on NCGS pathogenesis, following the same path we followed during the last four decades of CD research.

Acknowledgments: The Experts' meeting in Salerno was funded by the Dr. Schär Institute, Merano, Italy. We wish to express our gratitude to Jacqueline Pante and Caroline Mur from the Dr. Schär Institute for taking care of the organization of the meeting.

Author Contributions: All co-authors actively participated in the Salerno meeting discussion that formed the basis for drafting this manuscript, and critically revised the text of this paper. Carlo Catassi coordinated the paper-writing committee including also Alessio Fasano, Luca Elli and Kamran Rostami. All authors approved the final version of the manuscript.

Conflicts of Interest: Carlo Catassi has received consultancy funding from the Dr. Schär Institute and from Menarini Diagnostics. Luca Elli, Gemma Castillejo and Bruno Bonaz are members of the scientific committee of the Dr. Schär Institute. Alessio Fasano owns stock in Alba Therapeutics. Dan Leffler has received funding from Alba Therapeutics, Alvine Pharmaceuticals, Coronado Bioscience, Inova Diagnostics, Ironwood Pharmaceuticals, Sidney Frank Foundation and Glenwood Pharmaceuticals. The other authors declare no conflict of interest.

References

1. Sapone, A.; Lammers, K.M.; Mazzarella, G.; Mikhailenko, I.; Cartenì, M.; Casolaro, V.; Fasano, A. Differential mucosal IL-17 expression in two gliadin-induced disorders: Gluten sensitivity and the autoimmune enteropathy celiac disease. *Int. Arch. Allergy Immunol.* **2010**, *152*, 75–80. [CrossRef] [PubMed]
2. Biesiekierski, J.R.; Newnham, E.D.; Irving, P.M.; Barrett, J.S.; Haines, M.; Doecke, J.D.; Shepherd, S.J.; Muir, J.G.; Gibson, P.R. Gluten causes gastrointestinal symptoms in subjects without celiac disease: a double-blind randomized placebo-controlled trial. *Am. J. Gastroenterol.* **2011**, *106*, 508–514. [CrossRef] [PubMed]
3. Junker, Y.; Zeissig, S.; Kim, S.J.; Barisani, D.; Wieser, H.; Leffler, D.A.; Zevallos, V.; Libermann, T.A.; Dillon, S.; Freitag, T.L.; *et al.* Wheat amylase trypsin inhibitors drive intestinal inflammation via activation of toll-like receptor 4. *J. Exp. Med.* **2012**, *209*, 2395–408. [CrossRef] [PubMed]
4. Volta, U.; Bardella, M.T.; Calabrò, A.; Troncone, R.; Corazza, G.R. Study Group for Non-Celiac Gluten Sensitivity. An Italian prospective multicenter survey on patients suspected of having non-celiac gluten sensitivity. *BMC Med.* **2014**, *12*. [CrossRef] [PubMed]
5. Catassi, C.; Gatti, S.; Fasano, A. The new epidemiology of celiac disease. *J. Pediatr. Gastroenterol. Nutr.* **2014**, *59*, S7–S9. [CrossRef] [PubMed]
6. Fasano, A.; Sapone, A.; Zevallos, V.; Schuppan, D. Non-celiac Gluten Sensitivity. *Gastroenterology* **2015**, *148*, 1195–1204. [CrossRef] [PubMed]
7. Carroccio, A.; Mansueto, P.; Iacono, G.; Soresi, M.; D'Alcamo, A.; Cavataio, F.; Brusca, I.; Florena, A.M.; Ambrosiano, G.; Seidita, A.; *et al.* Non-celiac wheat sensitivity diagnosed by double-blind placebo-controlled challenge: exploring a new clinical entity. *Am. J. Gastroenterol.* **2012**, *107*, 1898–1906. [CrossRef] [PubMed]
8. Biesiekierski, J.R.; Peters, S.L.; Newnham, E.D.; Rosella, O.; Muir, J.G.; Gibson, P.R. No effects of gluten in patients with self-reported non-celiac gluten sensitivity after dietary reduction of fermentable, poorly absorbed, short-chain carbohydrates. *Gastroenterology* **2013**, *145*, 320–328. [CrossRef] [PubMed]
9. Czaja-Bulsa, G. Non coeliac gluten sensitivity—A new disease with gluten intolerance. *Clin. Nutr.* **2014**, *34*, 189–194. [CrossRef] [PubMed]
10. Aziz, I.; Hadjivassiliou, M. Coeliac disease: Noncoeliac gluten sensitivity—Food for thought. *Nat. Rev. Gastroenterol. Hepatol.* **2014**, *11*, 398–399. [CrossRef] [PubMed]
11. Jackson, J.; Eaton, W.; Cascella, N.; Fasano, A.; Santora, D.; Sullivan, K.; Feldman, S.; Raley, H.; McMahon, R.P.; Carpenter, W.T., Jr.; *et al.* Gluten sensitivity and relationship to psychiatric symptoms in people with schizophrenia. *Schizophr. Res.* **2014**, *159*, 539–542. [CrossRef] [PubMed]

12. Catassi, C.; Bai, J.C.; Bonaz, B.; Bouma, G.; Calabrò, A.; Carroccio, A.; Castillejo, G.; Ciacci, C.; Cristofori, F.; Dolinsek, J.; *et al.* Non-Celiac Gluten sensitivity: the new frontier of gluten related disorders. *Nutrients* **2013**, *5*, 3839–3853. [CrossRef] [PubMed]

13. Genuis, S.J.; Lobo, R.A. Gluten sensitivity presenting as a neuropsychiatric disorder. *Gastroenterol. Res. Pract.* **2014**, *2014*, 293206. [CrossRef] [PubMed]

14. Peters, S.L.; Biesiekierski, J.R.; Yelland, G.W.; Muir, J.G.; Gibson, P.R. Randomised clinical trial: Gluten may cause depression in subjects with non-coeliac gluten sensitivity—An exploratory clinical study. *Aliment. Pharmacol. Ther.* **2014**, *39*, 1104–1112. [CrossRef] [PubMed]

15. De Magistris, L.; Familiari, V.; Pascotto, A.; Sapone, A.; Frolli, A.; Iardino, P.; Carteni, M.; de Rosa, M.; Francavilla, R.; Riegler, G.; *et al.* Alterations of the intestinal barrier in patients with autism spectrum disorders and in their first-degree relatives. *J. Pediatr. Gastroenterol. Nutr.* **2010**, *51*, 418–424. [CrossRef] [PubMed]

16. Forsythe, P.; Bienenstock, J.; Kunze, W.A. Vagal pathways for microbiome-brain-gut axis communication. *Adv. Exp. Med. Biol.* **2014**, *817*, 115–133. [PubMed]

17. Glasziou, P.; Rose, P.; Heneghan, C.; Balla, J. Diagnosis using "test of treatment". *BMJ* **2009**, *338*. [CrossRef] [PubMed]

18. Kulich, K.R.; Madisch, A.; Pacini, F.; Piqué, J.M.; Regula, J.; van Rensburg, C.J.; Ujszászy, L.; Carlsson, J.; Halling, K.; Wiklund, I.K. Reliability and validity of the Gastrointestinal Symptom Rating Scale (GSRS) and Quality of Life in Reflux and Dyspepsia (QOLRAD) questionnaire in dyspepsia: A six-country study. *Health Qual. Life Outcomes* **2008**, *6*. [CrossRef] [PubMed]

19. Sapone, A.; Bai, J.C.; Ciacci, C.; Dolinsek, J.; Green, P.H.; Hadjivassiliou, M.; Kaukinen, K.; Rostami, K.; Sanders, D.S.; Schumann, M.; *et al.* Spectrum of gluten-related disorders: consensus on new nomenclature and classification. *BMC Med.* **2012**, *10*. [CrossRef] [PubMed]

20. Van Overbeek, F.M.; Uil-Dieterman, I.G.; Mol, I.W.; Köhler-Brands, L.; Heymans, H.S.; Mulder, C.J. The daily gluten intake in relatives of patients with coeliac disease compared with that of the general Dutch population. *Eur. J. Gastroenterol. Hepatol.* **1997**, *9*, 1097–1099. [CrossRef] [PubMed]

21. Caio, G.; Volta, U.; Tovoli, F.; De Giorgio, R. Effect of gluten free diet on immune response to gliadin in patients with non-celiac gluten sensitivity. *BMC Gastroenterol.* **2014**, *14*. [CrossRef] [PubMed]

22. Navarro, F.; Pearson, D.A.; Fatheree, N.; Mansour, R.; Hashmi, S.S.; Rhoads, J.M. Are "leaky gut" and behavior associated with gluten and dairy containing diet in children with autism spectrum disorders? *Nutr. Neurosci.* **2015**, *18*, 177–185. [CrossRef] [PubMed]

23. Sapone, A.; Lammers, K.M.; Casolaro, V.; Cammarota, M.; Giuliano, M.T.; de Rosa, M.; Stefanile, R.; Mazzarella, G.; Tolone, C.; Russo, M.I.; *et al.* Divergence of gut permeability and mucosal immune gene expression in two gluten-associated conditions: celiac disease and gluten sensitivity. *BMC Med.* **2011**, *9*. [CrossRef] [PubMed]

24. Hollon, J.; Puppa, E.L.; Greenwald, B.; Goldberg, E.; Guerrerio, A.; Fasano, A. Effect of gliadin on permeability of intestinal biopsy explants from celiac disease patients and patients with non-celiac gluten sensitivity. *Nutrients* **2015**, *7*, 1565–1576. [CrossRef] [PubMed]

25. Brottveit, M.; Beitnes, A.C.; Tollefsen, S.; Bratlie, J.E.; Jahnsen, F.L.; Johansen, F.E.; Sollid, L.M.; Lundin, K.E. Mucosal cytokine response after short-term gluten challenge in celiac disease and non-celiac gluten sensitivity. *Am. J. Gastroenterol.* **2013**, *108*, 842–850. [CrossRef] [PubMed]

26. Cooper, B.T.; Holmes, G.K.; Ferguson, R.; Thompson, R.A.; Allan, R.N.; Cooke, W.T. Gluten-sensitive diarrhea without evidence of celiac disease. *Gastroenterology* **1980**, *79*, 801–806. [PubMed]

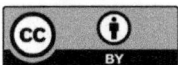

MDPI AG

St. Alban-Anlage 66

4052 Basel, Switzerland

Tel. +41 61 683 77 34

Fax +41 61 302 89 18

http://www.mdpi.com

Nutrients Editorial Office

E-mail: nutrients@mdpi.com

http://www.mdpi.com/journal/nutrients